Introduction to Research in the Health Sciences

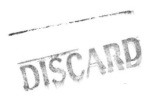

To the memory of Dr George Varnai and Dr George Polgar

To Elizabeth Kearney and June M Thomas

For Churchill Livingstone:

Publishing Manager: Mary Law
Project Development Manager: Dinah Thom
Project Manager: Jane Shanks
Design Direction: George Ajayi

Introduction to Research in the Health Sciences

Stephen Polgar BSc(Hons) MSc

Senior Lecturer, School of Public Health, Faculty of
Health Sciences, La Trobe University, Melbourne, Australia

Shane A. Thomas BA(Hons) DipPubPol PhD

Adjunct Professor, School of Nursing, Deakin University, Melbourne, Australia;
Adjunct Professor, School of Public Health, La Trobe University, Melbourne, Australia;
Visiting Principal Research Fellow, School of Social Work, University of Melbourne,
Melbourne, Australia; Senior Fellow, School of Behavioural Science, University of
Melbourne, Melbourne, Australia

FOURTH EDITION

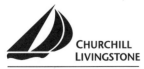
CHURCHILL
LIVINGSTONE

EDINBURGH LONDON NEW YORK PHILADELPHIA ST LOUIS SYDNEY TORONTO 2000

CHURCHILL LIVINGSTONE
An imprint of Harcourt Publishers Limited

First edition 1988
Second edition 1991
Third edition 1995
Fourth edition 2000
  Reprinted 2001, 2003

0 443 06265 X

British Library Cataloguing in Publication Data
A catalogue record for this book is available from the British Library.

Library of Congress Cataloging in Publication Data
A catalog record for this book is available from the Library of Congress.

Note
Medical knowledge is constantly changing. As new information
becomes available, changes in treatment, procedures, equipment and
the use of drugs become necessary. The authors and the publishers
have, as far as it is possible, taken care to ensure that the information
given in this text is accurate and up to date. However, readers are
strongly advised to confirm that the information, especially with
regard to drug usage, complies with the latest legislation and standards
of practice.

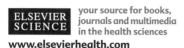
ELSEVIER SCIENCE your source for books,
journals and multimedia
in the health sciences
www.elsevierhealth.com

The
publisher's
policy is to use
**paper manufactured
from sustainable forests**

Printed in China
B/03

Contents

Preface

Consistent with previous versions, the 4th edition of this textbook has two overall aims:

1. To introduce the fundamental principles of research methodology and explain how these principles are systematically applied for conducting research in the health sciences.
2. To demonstrate how these principles and the evidence produced through systematic research are utilized for defining and solving problems in everyday health care.

Both of these aims are consistent with current directions in the education of health professionals. Not only is it taken for granted that health sciences students are formally educated in tertiary institutions but an increasing proportion of students are now enrolling in post-graduate courses which include a research component. It is widely recognized that the advancement of knowledge and practice in an area of health care depends on the education of individuals who are competent in undertaking health research and evaluations.

We recognize that only a relatively small proportion of health sciences professionals have the interest or the opportunity to undertake full blown research. At the same time, *all* contemporary health professionals participate in a 'culture' which privileges knowledge based on the critical review of scientific evidence. In order to participate in discourses concerning health problems and their treatments, practitioners need to understand the methodological principles or 'rules' of evidence as outlined in this book.

It must be emphasized that, in its 4th edition, *Introduction to Research in the Health Sciences* remains an introductory textbook. In order to retain the simplicity and intelligibility of the text we made the following changes for improving and updating the materials in the 4th edition. We have:

- included more revision questions, in particular ones which emphasize the utilization of research for the solution of health problems
- revised and updated clinically relevant research designs such as single case studies and focus groups
- expanded discussion of effect size and clinical significance of quantitative data
- improved the presentation and formatting of the text.

In addition, we have developed Internet-based teaching materials based on *Introduction to Research in the Health Sciences*. Colleagues who are setting this text for their students might be interested in contacting the authors for discussion of relevant teaching programmes and materials on the following E-mail address: s.polgar@latrobe.edu.au.

The scientific method

In this section we will examine some of the basic characteristics of the scientific method. A 'method', in the present context, refers to a systematic method for acquiring knowledge and establishing its truth. Health providers justify their theories and practices on the grounds that they are 'scientific', that is, based on scientific methodology. While not everything we do as health providers is, nor for that matter should be, 'scientific', the scientific method is essential for conducting research and evaluation aimed at improving the effectiveness and cost-effectiveness of health services.

A common view of the scientific method is that it enables us to describe, predict, explain and perhaps to control events in the world. As an example, consider how researchers and practitioners in the health care system responded to the outbreak of the AIDS (acquired immuno-deficiency syndrome) epidemic. One of the first signs of this epidemic was the clinical observation that young men presented with a deadly cancer (Kaposi's sarcoma) which was previously found only in the elderly. This represented the initial *evidence* which indicated that further facts and explanations were required. It was *hypothesized* that the premature failure of the immune system was responsible for the disorder. A hypothesis is a testable prediction about the relationship between observed events. Subsequent clinical evidence supported this hypothesis, leading to a clear definition of the disease as 'AIDS'. As more cases of AIDS were identified it became evident that some groups in the population were most at risk: persons who were involved in multiple homosexual relationships or who were intravenous drug users, or those who required blood products, for example, for haemophilia. An important development was the confirmation of the hypothesis that the disease was caused by a specific virus labelled 'HIV' (human immuno deficiency virus). On the basis of the above clinical, epidemiological and virological evidence it was hypothesized that the HIV was transmitted through body fluids such as blood or semen. In this way it became possible to predict which practices in the population involved a high level of risk for transmitting the virus.

The above findings and hypotheses contributed to constructing *theories* of AIDS, providing systematic and integrated conceptual frameworks for explaining the transmission and integrating the clinical features of the disorder. These theories also inform current practices aimed at controlling the epidemic, such as testing blood products for HIV, or promoting 'safe sex' behaviours in the population. The effectiveness of these practices (at least in some countries) for containing the epidemic is evidence confirming the accuracy of our understanding of the problem. At the same time, we remain sceptical about certain aspects of our theories, recognizing that there are as yet no vaccines or pharmacological cures for AIDS.

You might have recognized that the above brief account of attempting to contain AIDS is deficient in an essential way: it excludes evidence concerning the personal experiences and actions of persons at risk or having HIV. The above account represents a quantitative approach to the scientific method aiming to provide a mechanistic or reductionistic explanation of health and illness. This method is not adequate for researching and theorizing how persons, their families and the community respond to health-related issues and problems. It has been argued that our methods should also include qualitative or interpretive approaches to discover the personal meanings involved in being at risk of or suffering from diseases or disabilities. Qualitative methods are also appropriate for researching the cultural context and social construction of a disorder, for instance, discovering the images of AIDS sufferers communicated by the media in a given community.

The position taken in the present book is that the scientific method, as applied to health care, must include both quantitative and qualitative methods. This more inclusive view of the scientific method may not be supported by all researchers, but in our view the 'biopsychosocial' approach to health care requires both methods for research and theory formation. Regardless of controversies regarding the nature of science and its methodology, there is a broad consensus concerning the conventions and rules for conducting and reporting health sciences research, as outlined in the present book. Our goal is to convey these to our readers.

1

The scientific method and health research

INTRODUCTION

Research is a systematic and principled way of obtaining evidence (data, information) for solving health care problems. Research is *systematic* in that researchers tend to follow a sequential process (see Fig. 1.2) and *principled* in that research is carried out according to explicit rules. These rules or principles constitute the scientific method.

The primary aim of this chapter is to outline the scientific method and to compare it with other methods for conducting enquiry. Special emphasis is placed on the method as a means for conducting applied research and justifying practices in the health sciences.

The general aims of this chapter are to:

1. Define what is meant by a method, and outline some common methods of enquiry.
2. Outline the scientific method.
3. Draw attention to some controversies concerning the nature of the scientific method.
4. Compare qualitative and quantitative approaches to research.
5. Discuss how the scientific method is applied to conducting health sciences research.

METHODS AND KNOWLEDGE

Patient care involves the acquisition of a set of specific skills, the practice of which is justified in terms of a systematic and shared body of professional knowledge. A coherent body of knowledge is based on the use of appropriate methods. The term method refers to a systematic procedure for carrying out an activity, and in the present context implies a set of rules which specify:

1. How knowledge should be acquired.
2. The form in which knowledge should be stated.
3. How the truth or falsity of the knowledge should be evaluated.

Before we begin discussion of the scientific method it is useful, as a means of contrast, to look at some of the other methods of knowing used in the health sciences.

Authority. According to this method, knowledge is considered true because of tradition, or because an experienced and distinguished clinician says that it is true. As a student, you are often asked to accept statements as true because your teachers and clinical supervisors say they are true. To maintain their authority, the 'sources' of knowledge acquire and cultivate various signs of expertise, such as the appellation of 'Professor', or encourage the performance of status rituals. For example, consider the 'Consultant' who sweeps into a hospital ward followed by a retinue of students, registrars and nurses. Who would dare to question the truth of any of the consultant's sacred utterances? However, there are problems with the method of authority: what happens when the statements arising from one authority are contradicted by those made by an equally prestigious authority? For example, say Authority X claims that in their experience psychoanalysis is effective, while Authority Y states that the technique is useless. How can we resolve such conflicting claims? In practice, unless objective and acceptable criteria for resolution can be found, we will have unending disputation, *ad hominem* (personal) attacks, or, in instances of some religious or political disagreements, violence. That is, the controversy is resolved by denigrating or silencing the dissenting authority. In contrast, the scientific method emphasizes the examination of the evidence for establishing the truth of statements.

Rationalism. Reasoning is commonly used to arrive at true knowledge. It is assumed that if the rules of logic are applied correctly, then the

conclusions are guaranteed to be valid. As an example, let us look at the following syllogism:

1. All persons suffering from heart disease are males.
2. Person X has heart disease.
3. Therefore, person X is a male.

Logic guarantees that the conclusion (3) is true, provided that the syllogism is in a valid form and the premises (1) and (2) are true. Clearly, the limitation of formal (that is, 'content independent') reasoning is that it works in practice only if we have means for establishing the factual truth of the premises. In the above example, conclusion (3) might be empirically false, given that the premise (1) is factually false.

Logic and mathematics are very much a part of science but we require evidence to be collected to support logic and mathematical operations.

Intuition. Knowledge is sometimes acquired by sudden insights which arise without conscious reasoning. Truth is judged by the clarity of the experience and its emotional content (the 'Eureka!' experience). For example, after working with a patient without success, you might have a sudden insight about how to change your treatment programme. Unfortunately, even the strongest intuitions are sometimes proven false when put to an empirical test. You might find that your brilliant clinical insights often fail.

New scientific discoveries are sometimes resisted because they seem counterintuitive. Ignaz Semmelweiss, a perceptive and humane 19th century physician, noticed appalling levels of puerperal (child birth-related) fever and maternal death at his hospital. He reasoned that the infection was spread by medical students and staff who went to delivery rooms from the morgue without adequately washing their hands. In 1848, Semmelweiss introduced antiseptic procedures in his wards and demonstrated a substantial reduction in mortality from puerperal fever. However, his colleagues were offended by the notion that physicians were carriers of disease. Semmelweiss was dismissed from his post, ostracized by the medical establishment and died in pitiful circumstances. Clearly, in the light of current evidence we can say that

Semmelweiss' contention was correct, while his colleagues' intuitions were mistaken. Authority, logic and intuition all have their places in health care and research. In a general way, the scientific method can be contrasted with other methods in that it emphasizes the need for empirical evidence. However, as we shall see later in this chapter, what constitutes evidence and what the evidence indicates are complex matters.

THE SCIENTIFIC METHOD AND THE POSITIVIST VIEW

The scientific method crystallized over a period of several centuries, concomitantly with the growth of scientific research. The beginnings of modern western science are generally traced to the 16th century, a time in which Europe experienced profound social changes and a resurgence of great artists, thinkers and philosophers. Gradually, scholars' interests shifted from theology and armchair speculation to systematically describing, explaining and attempting to control natural phenomena. These changed circumstances allowed philosophers such as Descartes and Francis Bacon to challenge tenets of mediaeval thinking, and scientists such as Galileo, Newton and Harvey to propose new models of natural phenomena.

The approaches of such great thinkers had three basic elements, which are the basis of scientific method:

1. *Scepticism*. The notion that any proposition or statement, even those by great authorities, is open to doubt and analysis.
2. *Determinism*. The notion that events in the world occur according to regular laws and causes, not as a result of the caprices of demons or witches.
3. *Empiricism*. The notion that enquiry ought to be conducted through observation and verified through experience.

The scientific method is represented in a simplified form in Figure 1.1. This view is consistent with a view of natural science methodology called 'positivism' by the 19th century philosopher Comte, as well as 'reductionism', a concept introduced in Chapter 8. Both these terms have acquired multiple meanings in the area of philosophy of science. Our interpretations of Figure 1.1 is explained below.

Observation, description and measurement

Considering Figure 1.1 let us start with observations. The description of phenomena involving the precise, unbiased recording of observations of aspects of persons, objects and events forms the empirical basis of all branches of science. Observations can be expressed as either verbal descriptions or sets of measurements (see Section 4). The personal perceptions of the investigator must be transformed into descriptive statements and measurements that can be understood and replicated by other investigators. Some research is based on observation made with instruments (such as recording electrodes, microscopes and standardized clinical tests), while other research calls for observation unaided by instruments. Although advances in instrumentation have contributed enormously to scientific knowledge, the use of complex instrumentation is not a necessary feature of scientific observation. Rather, the key attributes of scientific observation are accuracy and replicability by other scientists. When observations are appropriately summarized and are confirmed by others, they form the factual bases of scientific knowledge.

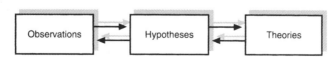

Fig. 1.1   The scientific method.

Generalization and induction

Statements representing observations or measurements are integrated into explanatory systems called hypotheses and theories. The logic underlying scientific generalizations is called induction. Induction involves asserting general propositions about a class of phenomena on the basis of a limited number of observations of select elements. For example, having observed that penicillin is useful for curing pneumonia in a limited set of patients, we make the generalization 'The administration of penicillin cures pneumonia (in all patients)'.

Hypotheses

The statement 'The administration of penicillin cures pneumonia' is called a hypothesis. Scientific hypotheses are statements which specify the nature of the relationship between two or more sets of observations. In this instance, the first set of observations relates to the administration of penicillin and the second set is related to changes in clinical observations or measurements concerning pneumonia. As we shall see in subsequent sections, an important feature of scientific hypotheses is that the terms used must have clear-cut, observable referents. When these hypotheses acquire strong empirical support, they may be called laws.

Theories

Scientific theories are essentially conjectures representing our current state of knowledge about the world. Hypotheses are integrated into more general explanatory systems called theories. A theory will clarify the relationships between diverse classes of observations and hypotheses. For example, a theory to explain why drugs called antibiotics are effective in curing some infectious diseases integrates induction inference evidence from diverse sources, such as micro-biology, pharmacology, cell physiology and clinical medicine. Other examples of theories are the heliocentric theory of the solar system, the DNA theory of genetic inheritance, and the neuronal theory of central nervous system functioning. It is an essential feature of scientific theories that they are statements based on the correct use of language and logic. Some theories entail a model (see Fig. D.1, p. 17), which is a mathematical or physical representation of how the theory works. In this way, theories specify the causes of events and provide conceptual means for predicting and influencing these events. In health care, theories are important for explaining the causes of health and illness and predicting the probable effectiveness of treatment outcomes.

Deduction

A scientific theory should lead to a set of empirically verifiable statements or hypotheses. In addition to being generalizations based on evidence, hypotheses are also deduced logically from the statements and/or mathematical models which specify the causal relationships postulated by the theories. For example, if we hold the theory that the patterns of activity of a set of neurones in the occipital lobe mediates visual sensation in humans, then the hypothesis follows that the activation of these neurones (say, by electrical stimulation) will lead to the report of visual sensations. Such hypotheses have been the bases for subsequent spectacular clinical advances such as artificial vision through cortically implanted electrodes.

Controlled observation

It is desirable that hypotheses are tested under controlled conditions. The aim of control is to discount other competing hypotheses for explaining the predicted phenomenon. For example, if we intend to show that occipital lobe stimulation causes the visual sensations, we must show that we are controlling for any type of brain stimulation causing such changes. Conversely, we would need to show that occipital lobe stimulation does not lead to a host of other types of sensations. Only by discounting alternative explanations through control can we have confidence in the relevance of our observations for our research hypothesis. Of course control must be *ethical* as we shall see in later chapters.

Verification and falsification

After the evidence has been collected, the investigator decides whether or not the findings are consistent with the predictions of the hypothesis. If the hypothesis is supported by the evidence, then the theory from which the hypothesis was deduced is strengthened or verified. However, when the data do not support the hypothesis, the related theory is falsified. If a theory can no longer predict or explain evidence in its empirical domain, it becomes less useful and is usually later discarded in favour of new, more powerful theories. Therefore, scientific theories are not held to be absolute truths, but rather as provisional explanations of available evidence.

The application of the above process has contributed to the spectacular growth of scientific knowledge. Observation and measurement, facilitated by new instrumentation, have resulted in the discovery of an enormous number of accurate and reproducible facts about health and illness. These new facts both challenge existing theories and call for the creation of novel, more powerful theories. The new theories serve as impetus for more research, resulting in new instrumentation and observations. Advances in scientific knowledge have been applied to creating new technologies, which in turn contribute to new discoveries and advances in scientific knowledge. For example, the invention of computers was possible because of advances in electronics, chemistry and mathematics. In turn, the use of computers is now contributing to making and summarizing scientific observations or formulating explanatory models. In addition, the use of computers as information processing systems has generated useful metaphors for theoretical advances, such as explaining the human brain and mental functioning. In this way, the scientific method contributes to furthering our aims by helping us to describe, explain, predict and sometimes control the world in which we live.

CONTROVERSIES CONCERNING THE NATURE OF THE SCIENTIFIC METHOD

The above description is the only interpretation of the scientific method. Rather, there are good reasons why there are controversies concerning the nature of the scientific method as described above.

Firstly, the scientific method is a set of rules devised and applied by philosophers and scientists. They are not eternal truths, but conventions believed to be useful for conducting scientific enquiry. In this way, not only the content but also the methodology of science is open to criticism, debate and change.

Secondly, the interpretation of what constitutes the scientific method is an activity pursued by philosophers of science and epistemologists. In adopting different conceptual frameworks (Realism, Instrumentalism, Anarchism, Idealism, etc.) concerning the nature of reality and knowledge, these philosophers generate unending controversies over the nature of the scientific method.

As scientists or health professionals, we cannot sit around forever waiting for philosophers to decide on the appropriate way of gathering knowledge. However, as the following points exemplify, it would be churlish not to take into account some of the important ideas arising from the history and philosophy of science.

The theory-dependence of observation

Critics such as Chalmers (1976) argued that it is simplistic to believe that observations are made independently of theoretical notions held by the observer. The observer is selective with regard to what is recorded as evidence. Our observations and facts are 'theory-dosed', that is, theories specify what observations are of importance and what aspects of these observations should be recorded or ignored. Schatzman & Strauss (1973) put this point elegantly when they stated that the researcher 'harbours, wittingly or not, many expectations, conjectures and hypotheses which provide him with thought and directives on what to look for and what to ask about'. For instance, in observing the EEG (electro-encephalogram) of an epileptic patient, our perception is guided by theories of the electrical activity of the brain and the nature of brain pathology. We will also hold ideas how the EEG machine works (for example, electrode sensitivity, amplification) and identify artefacts in the evidence. What is observed as evidence of epilepsy by an expert could be perceived as meaningless squiggles by a naive observer. We shall take account of this point in Chapter 12, when we discuss the reliability and validity of measurement.

The validity of induction

Philosophers of science have questioned the logical validity of making general claims on the basis of a limited set of observations. To quote Chalmers (1976): 'any observational evidence will consist of a finite number of observation statements, whereas a universal statement makes claims about an infinite number of possible situations'.

For example, we might have observed that the administration of penicillin cured pneumonia in 100 000 patients. This does not necessarily guarantee the logical truth of the universal statement 'penicillin cures pneumonia', or that patient 100 001 will be cured. We will look at the theories related issue of generalization from samples in Chapter 3. Scientific theories are seen as probabilistic, in the sense that new, inconsistent evidence might emerge in the future, challenging the generality of the theory. Also, it has been argued by some philosophers of science, that hypotheses *need not* be based on induction, but may arise from any source, provided that they have falsifiable empirical consequences.

What constitutes falsification?

It was stated earlier that when novel empirical evidence is inconsistent with the predictions of a theory, the theory is 'falsified' and is eventually modified or discarded. Commentators such as Lakatos (1970) argued that theories are not, in practice, so readily modified or discarded by scientists. Rather, they are structures which have an inner hard core of propositions protected by an outer belt of auxiliary, modifiable hypotheses. Evidence inconsistent with predictions based on the theory results in the modification of auxiliary hypotheses, rather than discarding the 'core'. Consider, for example, the 'germ' theory of infectious disease, on the basis of which one would predict that penicillin (which kills germs) will cure bacterial infections. Suppose that we administer penicillin to a number of patients with an infectious disease and find, contrary to what was predicted, no clinically useful changes. On the basis of this falsification, will we discard the germ theory of disease? No. Rather, we will utilize an auxiliary hypothesis to explain our findings, such as 'the development of penicillin-resistant bacteria'. The methodological issue which remains controversial is the logical basis for discarding one theory and accepting its rival (see Feyerabend 1975). As we shall see in Chapter 22, we judge the outcome of a research programme in the context of an overall pattern of related findings and theories.

SCIENCE AND THE CULTURAL CONTEXT

Science as a human activity

Scientific enquiry is conducted in particular social settings, by individuals with personal aims and values. Some more recent formulations of methodology take into account the social and interpersonal conditions which influence scientists' professional activities (Kuhn 1970, Feyerabend 1975). In this text, we will pay attention to social values, in the context of ethical considerations for designing and conducting research (Ch. 2). Also, we recognize that the formulation of hypotheses and theories are creative acts, rather than the outcomes of the automatic application of induction. In this way, the questions asked by health researchers and the ways in which they explain their findings are influenced in subtle ways by the cultures in which they participate.

The social context of health care research

To understand the nature of scientific research in general, and health research in particular, it is useful to examine how they fit into an overall social context. That is, the way in which persons living in a society view health and illness and the ways in which health workers carry out their professional roles influence the range and scope of health care research (e.g. Taylor 1979).

Until recently, the 'medical model' was by far the most dominant approach to understanding illness in Western society. Briefly, in terms of the medical model, illness is represented by a particular lesion or dysfunction within the human body. The role of the health professional is to identify the location and nature of the lesion or the clinical imbalance and to implement appropriate measures to correct the problem. The patient is assigned a rather passive role in this process, being the 'locus' of the lesion or imbalance and a person complying with the health professionals' recommendations. In the context of the medical model, the most appropriate research is seen as that which improves the technical effectiveness and, therefore, the social power of the health professional.

In Western society the medical model has been, and will continue to be, an influential model for guiding clinical practice and health research. Nevertheless, there have been gradual changes in health care that require the questioning of the generality of the medical model for the following reasons:

1. There have been important changes in the roles and status of health professionals such as nurses, occupational therapists, physiotherapists, speech pathologists and podiatrists. Rather than taking an ancillary, paramedical position, these individuals are becoming directly and independently responsible for a broad range of health care functions, including prevention, assessment, therapy and rehabilitation. However, the perspectives and practices of these health professionals are at times quite different from those involved in the medical model and may require quite different approaches to research and theory. The gradual establishment of university-based education for these professionals has provided an increased opportunity for relevant research, which is not necessarily guided by the medical model.

2. From the 1970s onwards it had become evident that there had been a significant increase in the cost of health care; in part due to the adoption of very expensive diagnostic procedures and the increasing trend for specialization among medical practitioners (Taylor 1979). Attempts to contain health care costs have resulted in several lines of approach including:

(a) increased focus on preventive health care; as shown by anti-smoking campaigns, or drink driving legislation to contain the incidence of road trauma;

(b) increased efforts to enhance the cost effectiveness of current treatment strategies; for example, by improving communications between clinicians and patients or managing patients' fears concerning treatments through the application of psychological techniques;

(c) increased support for self help groups and community managed health centres with a more active involvement of individuals in understanding and managing their own health.

3. Preventative and educational approaches require somewhat different views of the client and the professional to that implicit in the medical model. In turn, research is required which can clarify the relationships between community lifestyles, individual behaviours, health and illness and general economic and social circumstances (e.g. Gardner 1989).

The more holistic approach, which also informs health care research is called the *psychosocial* or *biopsychosocial* model (see Engel 1977), and currently has considerable influence in how we conceptualize health care and how we plan and carry out research. At the same time, the medical model remains influential in research aimed at understanding the workings of the human body and improving the technical aspects of health care, such as clinical assessments and interventions.

QUANTITATIVE AND QUALITATIVE METHODS

The introduction of a biopsychosocial approach has raised questions about the combination of methodologies relevant to health sciences research. We perceive patients or clients in two different but interrelated frameworks: firstly, as broken down or malfunctioning biological systems; and secondly, as persons, like ourselves, living in a society and who are attempting to make sense of, and cope with, their particular health care problems.

As argued earlier, the first view informs a reductionist or *quantitative* approach to research and knowledge. That is, we view our patients objectively, as natural objects, and attempt to identify and measure important variables which represent the causes and expressions of a clinical condition. We develop models and theoretical frameworks which systematically explain how these variables are interrelated and undertake therapeutic actions which serve to diminish the variables representing illness or disability. Our therapeutic actions are the *technical* applications for our scientific theories; their outcomes and effectiveness should be tested under controlled conditions.

The second view informs a *qualitative* or interpretive approach to research and knowledge. We view our patients as persons and attempt to gain insights into their subjective experiences and the reasons for their actions in particular situations. We develop theories for interpreting the nature and development of their personal points of view, and to inform our therapeutic actions so that they seem meaningful and appropriate to our patients. (These concepts are discussed further in Ch. 8).

Take, as an illustration of the above approaches, a patient with cancer. In a quantitative analysis we attempt to quantify the problem by using appropriate instrumentation which measure variables such as the size and location of the tumour and the extent of its spread within the organism. Consistent with current theories of the nature of cancer, various techniques such as surgery, radiology or chemotherapy might be brought into play, the effectiveness of which will be judged in terms of controlling specific variables associated with the condition, such as levels of pain and the weight or time of survival of the patient.

With a qualitative perspective, we would address the meaning of the condition from the patient's personal point of view, within the context of his or her family setting and social circumstances. That is, the patient's value systems must be clarified and understood before actions such as assessments and therapeutic actions are undertaken. Enquiry might uncover conflicting values, for instance, concerning the implementation of a programme of chemotherapy. From the clinician's point of view, a radical programme of chemotherapy might seem appropriate, as probably quantitatively extending the patient's life by several years. However, from the patient's point of view, the quality of life under chemotherapy might seem inadequate, and also they might not wish to be a burden on their families. Clearly, both in clinical practice and in related research, evidence from both quantitative and qualitative enquiries should be integrated to ensure effective health care. This text covers both quantitative and qualitative orientations with an emphasis upon the quantitative orientation. The authors use both approaches in their own research, often in the same project.

THE RESEARCH PROCESS

Although there are differences in how health scientists approach problems, Figure 1.2 shows the sequence of procedures commonly involved in quantitative research. The term 'Data' refers to the complete set of observations or measurements recorded in the course of a research process. You will find that the organization of this book follows the sequential stages of the research process, as outlined below.

1. *Planning.* As we shall show in Section 2,

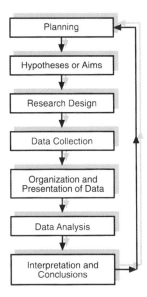

Fig. 1.2 The research process.

research planning involves selecting appropriate strategies and measurements to answer questions or to test hypotheses. It will be argued in Chapter 2 that planning must take into consideration previous research evidence as well as ethical and economic factors before the appropriate research strategy and measurement is selected, and the precise research hypothesis or aim is stated.

2. *Research design*. The usefulness of research depends on plans specifying appropriate sampling methods for ensuring the generalizability of the results. Appropriate designs are selected to ensure controlled observation in order to demonstrate causal relationships. Chapters 3–4 in Section 2 and Chapters 5–8 in Section 3 examine how the uses of appropriate designs and sampling methods ensure the generality and validity of investigations across a variety of research strategies. Chapters 8–11 also outline some basic issues in the collection and interpretation of evidence in the context of qualitative research.

3. *Data collection*. The next step in the research process is collection of data (Section 4). Chapters, 9, 10 and 11 examine data collection methods commonly employed in qualitative

and quantitative health research. Chapter 12 is concerned with appropriate ways of carrying out measurements and different types of measurement scales available for research and clinical assessment.

4. *Organization and presentation of the data*. Section 5 introduces descriptive statistics representing the conventions for summarizing and describing the data. Chapters 13–16 examine basic concepts in this area, outlining how graphs and various descriptive statistics are used to condense and communicate research and clinical findings. The presentation and analysis of qualitative data are discussed in Chapters 8, 9, 10 and 11.

5. *Data analysis*. Data analysis involves applying the principles of probability for calculating confidence intervals and testing hypotheses. The area of inferential statistics, involving decisions concerning whether the data support experimental hypotheses, is outlined in Chapters 17–19 in Section 6.

6. *Interpretation and Utilization of Research*. The final step in any research project involves interpreting one's findings. The findings may support existing theories or practices, suggest that new techniques may be more effective, or, suggest new theoretical notions that are more able to explain phenomena. It is rare that the findings from any single research project are completely definitive, and often the results may suggest the need for further investigation in related subject areas or contexts. This issue will be examined in Sections 6 and 7.

7. *Publication*. For research to be scientifically meaningful, investigators must present their results in professional journals and at conferences. Research findings become part of scientific knowledge only if they stand up to methodological critique and replication. In Chapter 21 we will discuss conventions for preparing publications. In Chapter 22 we will outline steps for critically evaluating published research. It is worth noting that the availability of personal computers and the Internet is changing the ways in which scientific knowledge is disseminated.

The above steps and stages of research represent a logical sequence which is followed in most research projects. An exception, as we mentioned earlier, is in the case of 'qualitative' research (Ch. 8) where a more flexible sequence might be employed. Also, in qualitative research the empirical evidence is not normally summarized and analyzed through statistical methods, but through the use of language and the analysis of narratives.

RESEARCH AND CLINICAL PRACTICE

Research methods cover a wide variety of skills and techniques aimed at the methodologically valid investigation of questions of interest to the researcher. These methods of enquiry are not restricted to research laboratories, nor need they involve expensive equipment or large research teams. Rather, these methods imply an approach to stating and answering questions in any setting.

Applied research in the health sciences focuses on issues such as the prevalence and causes of illness, the usefulness and accuracy of assessment techniques, or the effectiveness of treatments. Applied research which is published aims at producing findings that are of a general interest to groups of professionals working in the health field.

Research methods interact with health practices in multiple and mutually productive ways. An important general aim of this textbook is to discuss the relationships between theories, practices and the ways in which research methods contribute to improving of health care.

Instrumentation and measurement

Individuals working in a modern health care setting are often called upon to use and interpret the results of complex measuring instruments. These instruments include 'high-technology' diagnostic products as well as a variety of standardized clinical tests and measures.

Effective diagnosis involves acquiring skills for using such instruments, understanding the criteria for selecting specific instruments, and being able to interpret the clinical significance of the measurements produced by them.

Therefore, the first aim of this text is to introduce to the student the concepts of validity and reliability, and the procedures involved in interpreting the results of various tests and measures.

Data presentation and analysis

Much of our knowledge of patients, disease processes, or the functioning of health care institutions, is expressed numerically, through the use of descriptive and inferential statistics. The student needs to understand statistical concepts for two reasons:

1. To produce and communicate sets of measurements about patients and treatment outcomes for both clinical and administrative purposes.
2. To be able to interpret research and evaluate data presented in a statistical form.

There is an increasing emphasis on inter-professional interaction in health care. Therefore, it is unfortunate when practising clinicians are unable to present or understand clinically relevant evidence which has been presented in a quantitative form. Much important information is missed this way, often to the detriment of patients.

The second aim of this text is to introduce the student to fundamental procedures in presenting and interpreting quantitative (and to a minimal extent, qualitative) evidence in the health sciences.

Evaluation of treatment procedures

Research and evaluation techniques are typically used by the health professional at two levels:

1. To evaluate the effectiveness of particular treatment techniques in order to improve the quality of therapy available to individuals or groups of clients.
2. To evaluate the relative effectiveness of health care programmes in order to determine the allocation of resources for preventative and therapeutic programmes for a community.

Governments and health care consumers now routinely require evidence demonstrating that their money is well spent. To survive as a health professional in the coming years, it will be necessary to provide hard empirical evidence to justify professional effectiveness. The third aim of the present text is to introduce the student to research strategies appropriate for treatment evaluation.

Conceptual basis for clinical practice

Research methods are based on the application of the scientific method to the conduct of enquiry. As the terms 'health sciences' or 'clinical sciences' imply, there is a close relationship between clinical practice and the scientific approach. Much (although not all) of the systematic knowledge underlying modern health care is based on science. 'Evidence based practice' requires that the evidence is methodologically sound. Therefore, an adequate understanding of the basis for current professional knowledge and practices presupposes some insight into scientific methodology.

The fourth aim of this text is to introduce students to scientific methodology by examining how health related research is planned, conducted and interpreted.

Research contribution

Traditionally, the majority of systematic research contributions to the health sciences emerged from the faculties of Science and Medicine. However, this situation has changed with the emergence of college or university based education for health workers.

In recent years, the allied health professions such as nursing, occupational therapy, physiotherapy and speech pathology have substantially increased the quantity and quality of published research. It should be recognized that, to a considerable extent, the growth, effectiveness and prestige of the allied health professions depend on the production of research of a high standard. We recognize that only some health professionals have the motivation, interest and opportunity to become involved in research. Nevertheless, the emergence of motivated individuals capable of contributing to professional knowledge requires an introduction to research methods during their education.

The fifth major aim of the present book is to introduce students to basic features of the research process, in preparation for further studies in this area of health care. Although not all health practitioners are actively involved in research, it is a necessary condition for professional development that one is able to critique published research.

SUMMARY

There are several common methods used for acquiring, stating and establishing knowledge. The scientific method is one of these and useful in justifying the validity of diagnoses and clinical interventions in the Western health care system. Scientific method is concerned with applying a set of rules or conventions that will allow us to produce scientifically valid knowledge. These rules specify how observations should be made, and theories and hypotheses stated and evaluated.

Theories and hypotheses obtained and verified through scientific enquiry are not held to be absolutely true. An inherent part of the scientific approach is scepticism regarding both the contents of knowledge and the underlying methodology. We have pointed out that there are controversies concerning what constitutes scientific methodology.

It was argued that the scientific method is directly applicable to conducting research in the health sciences. In general, the stages for research include planning, stating aims or hypotheses, and formulating designs; collecting, summarizing and analyzing the data; and drawing conclusions. This process can be applied to ensuring advances in health care and to problem-solving in specific clinical settings. There is a close relationship between professional practices and health sciences research. The rest of the book is organized to follow the stages involved in performing research.

SELF ASSESSMENT

Explain the meaning of the following terms:

authority
deduction
data
determinism
empiricism
falsification
hypothesis
intuition
observation
qualitative
quantitative
rationalism
research programmes
scepticism
theory

TRUE OR FALSE

1. A 'method' specifies how knowledge should be acquired, stated and tested.
2. Very strong intuitions always turn out to be true.
3. The method of authority depends on the status and credibility of the source.
4. When a syllogism is in a valid form, the conclusions should be factually true provided the premises are true.
5. Rationalism calls for correct reasoning for acquiring truth.
6. The case of Ignaz Semmelweiss illustrates that medical decisions are based on the scientific method.
7. Scepticism refers to the notion that all knowledge is false.
8. Empiricism refers to the notion that events in the world occur according to regular laws and causes.
9. Scientific observations are different from ordinary observations because they depend on the use of instruments.
10. Scientific observations must be recorded as numbers.
11. Hypotheses are unproven theories.
12. Hypotheses are statements which specify the nature of the relationship between two or more sets of observations.
13. The logic underlying scientific generalization is called induction.
14. Scientific theories represent notions of natural events and their causes.
15. A good scientific theory is one that cannot be, in principle, falsified.
16. Controlled observation aims to identify the causes of events.
17. Scientific theories should enable the deduction of empirically verifiable hypotheses.
18. When the empirical evidence is found to be consistent with the implications of a hypothesis, we can say that the theory from which the hypothesis was deduced is absolutely true.
19. When we say that a theory was falsified, we mean that hypotheses deduced from it were not supported by empirical evidence.
20. We can question the content but not the methodology of science.

MULTIPLE CHOICE

1. A scientific theory is a set of statements:

   a conforming to the rules of logic
   b explaining the relationships which pertain among apparently diverse phenomena
   c which lead to empirically testable hypotheses
   d all of the above.

2. The statement 'Persons who are highly anxious do not perform well on learning tasks' is:

   a a theory
   b hypothesis
   c false
   d in principle empirically untestable.

3. A scientific hypothesis:

   a should be verified through the use of logic and disputation

   b should be open to empirical verification

   c can not arise through intuition

   d a and c.

4. The results of scientific research:

   a should be made available for critique and replication

   b should not be used to support existing theories

   c must be obtained under controlled laboratory settings

   d must conform to public expectations about the outcome.

5. Descriptive statistics:

   a are based on the principles of probability

   b represent conventions for planning research

   c represent conventions for summarizing and organizing data

   d specify the selection of appropriate measurement scales.

6. The scientific method is a set of rules specifying how:

   a scientific knowledge should be acquired, stated and tested

   b scientists should conduct their life

   c how society should conduct its affairs

   d all of the above a, b, and c.

7. Authority, as a method, is:

   a no longer relevant to the conduct of health care

   b the fundamental source of the scientific method

   c neither a nor b

   d both a and b.

8. A therapist without formal medical qualifications treated cancer patients using an 'alternative' regimen of herbs, massage and medication. Say that there is no scientific evidence available that such a treatment is effective. It follows that:

   a the treatment was ineffective because it lacks scientific evidence

   b the treatment was ineffective because the practitioner was unqualified

   c both a and b

   d neither a nor b.

9. As evidence for the effectiveness of the treatment, the therapist provides 100 signed statements from current or former patients claiming that they were satisfied with the treatment. One reason such evidence lacks scientific validity is that:

   a the opinions of patients can not, in principle, constitute scientific evidence

   b it was not acquired in a manner consistent with the principles of scientific observations

   c we cannot, in principle, generalize from only 100 observations

   d it pertains to an 'alternative', non-scientific treatment regimen.

10. In the context of the scientific method, evidence which would be most indicative of the effectiveness of the treatment would be:

    a the support of medically qualified people

    b the argument that each patient has the right to select their own form of treatment

    c that the survival times of the patients were better than those of equivalent patients being treated with conventional therapies

SELF ASSESSMENT

    d that the patients were willing to pay money to receive the treatment.

11. The statement 'If my theory of schizophrenia is true, then the sun will rise tomorrow morning' is:

    a probably based on the invalid use of deduction

    b untestable

    c based on the method of authority

    d *a* and *b*.

12. According to an astrologer, people who were born under a particular star sign are 'basically kind and very intelligent, although because of their modesty, not sufficiently appreciated by others'. To test the truth of this statement, the astrologer asks a group of individuals if this description fits their personality; 95% of the sample agrees that the description is accurate. One of the problems with this enquiry is that:

    a astrology is inherently false, therefore the evidence must be wrong

    b 'personality' is inherently a misunderstood concept

    c in this case a 100% agreement is required for acceptable evidence

    d it is contrary to the principles of controlled observation.

13. The notion that facts are 'theory-dependent' implies that:

    a what is recorded as evidence is independent of the event being studied

    b theories and hypothesis have no relationship to empirical observations

    c what is recorded as evidence can be influenced by the theoretical notions of the observer

    d only our minds exist, rather than a material world.

14. Lakatos argued that:

    a theories are discarded only when their 'hard core' of propositions are falsified

    b a 'belt' of auxiliary hypotheses protect the fundamental 'hard core' propositions of a theory

    c theories cannot be refuted or falsified on the basis of empirical evidence

    d both *a* and *b*.

15. Which is the least controversial statement concerning the scientific knowledge?

    a There is only one acceptable form of the scientific method independent of the phenomenon being investigated.

    b Scientific theories are derived from the use of induction, rather than creative insights.

    c The principles of the scientific method can be usefully applied to conducting health research.

    d Scientific enquiry is conducted independently of the personal values and social environment of scientists.

16. Which of the following problems might be best approached through the scientific method?

    a The clinical effectiveness of a new instrument needs to be evaluated.

    b The hospital budget is cut by 10%.

    c Personnel refuse to staff an abortion clinic on moral grounds.

    d The nursing staff go on strike.

SECTION 1

Discussion, Questions and Answers

These questions ask you to examine issues concerning the applications of the scientific method to various aspects of health sciences research. Unlike the multiple- choice or true or false questions, these discussion questions do not necessarily have a single correct answer. Rather, they are aimed at promoting a critical, integrative view of conducting research.

Our first discussion question involves theories and examines the relationships between theories, models, hypotheses and empirical observations. Theories are conceptual frameworks (as we discussed in Chapter 1) integrating a range of related observations and explanatory hypotheses. We may deduce empirically testable hypotheses from our theories.

On the basis of observations, in particular when the observations are carried out under controlled conditions, we establish the probable truth of our hypotheses, and thereby support or falsify the theories which were originally the sources for the hypotheses.

Some theories include models which represent specific aspects of a theory. Models are used to explain real situations and predict novel empirical outcomes. Models can be as follows:

1. *Physical models*. These models are constructed from materials, for example a 'pump' model of the heart for showing how the circulatory system works, or a construction of the DNA molecule to show how different nucleotides are organized in order to replicate genetic information.
2. *Mathematical models*. These models contain a series of equations that represent our theoretical interpretations of real-life situations. For example, epidemiologists may employ mathematical models to predict how a given epidemic might spread in a population, or a physiologist may

employ a mathematical model of neuronal membranes to predict the behaviour of action potentials in a neurone. When our theories and related models are sufficiently detailed and well formed, we may use these in simulation research. We now use computers, which are capable of carrying out the complex calculations necessary for the simulation of a real-life situation and predicting numerical outcomes.

3. *'Paper and pencil' models*. Often, our theories are not sufficiently detailed to allow precise numerical predictions. Here the models are 'sketches' of a particular system, defining the key elements of the model and showing how these elements interact to produce various outcomes. Such models enable us to make testable predictions concerning the effects of variables as shown by the following model (Fig. D.1) of the 'Gate Control Theory' of pain (Melzack & Wall 1965). (Note that for teaching purposes this model is an incomplete and modified representation of the original. If you are interested in understanding pain problems, you should consult Melzack & Wall's original work.)

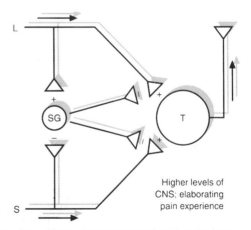

Fig. D.1   Model of spinal gating of nociceptive input (adapted from Melzack & Wall, 1965).

Discussion, Questions and Answers

Elements of the systems

(a) L: 'Large' diameter axons of receptors, which convey information concerning mechanical stimuli, such as pressure and vibration.

(b) S: 'Small' diameter axons of receptors, which convey information concerning noxious (tissue damaging) stimuli.

(c) SG: Neurones within the substantial gelatinosa (SG) of the spinal cord. These receive converging information from L and S axons. The SG neurones control, or gate through pre-synaptic inhibition, the information flowing through to the T neurones.

(d) T: Transmission neurones in the spinal cord, which receive information from both L and S axons. The pattern of activity of T neurones is projected to higher levels of the CNS (central nervous system), where this information is elaborated into the experience of pain.

(e) △: Synapses, which may be either excitatory (+) or inhibitory (–). Excitatory synapses increase, while inhibitory synapses decrease the activity of the post-synaptic neurones.

(f) →: Arrows showing the direction of the information flow; in this case from the periphery towards the spinal cord and, subsequently, to higher levels of the CNS. The activity of large fibres (L) stimulates the gating mechanism (SG) which serves to inhibit nociceptive information conveyed by S axons to the T neurones.

The activity of large fibres (L) stimulates the gating mechanism (SG) which serves to inhibit nociceptive information conveyed by S axons to the T neurones.

The above model is an attempt to produce a representation of the events which take place in the mammalian nervous system when receiving and processing nociceptive input at a spinal cord level. The 'Gate Control' model integrates a broad range of research in the neurosciences and has been applied to explain aspects of pain control in clinical settings.

Questions

After this rather prolonged introduction to the model, we are ready to ask questions about how it may be applied to explaining and predicting observations about pain.

1. Use the above model to describe what happens in the nervous system during noxious (tissue-damaging) stimulation.

2. How would we use controlled observations to demonstrate that small (S), rather than large (L) neurones convey nociceptive information. (Assume that we have instrumentation for measuring the activity of single neurones in response to different kinds of stimuli.)

3. Explain how we would use evidence obtained by recording the activity of single neurones to demonstrate that T neurones are in fact involved in nociception.

4. Describe the effects of large (L) and small (S) axons on the activity of SG neurones.

5. Explain the mechanism by which SG neurones function as a 'pain gating' system.

6. Propose a hypothesis for predicting the effects of selectively damaging T neurones on subsequent pain experience.

7. Propose a hypothesis for predicting the effects of damaging large axons (L) on subsequent pain experience.

8. A virus is identified which damages SG neurones. As a hypothetical case, imagine that people who have this virus report greatly reduced pain sensitivity. What would be the implication of this observation for the validity of the Gate Control theory of pain?

9. Would you discard the Gate Control theory

Discussion, Questions and Answers

on the bases of the hypothetical observations described in question 8? Explain.

10. A clinical technique called Transcutaneous Electrical Nerve Stimulation (TENS) for relieving pain involves the gentle peripheral electrical stimulation of painful areas. Explain in terms of the model how TENS might work to reduce pain. (Hint: TENS does not directly reduce the activity of S axons).

Answers

1. Small diameter S axons convey nociceptive information towards spinal cord neurones, including the SG and the T neurones. The SG neurones are inhibited through nociceptive inputs while the T neurones are excited by the stimulation. Information concerning tissue damage is then conveyed by the axons of the T neurones to higher levels of the Central Nervous System (CNS). There it is elaborated into the experience of pain.

2. By showing that the activity of T neurones was correlated to the levels of peripheral noxious stimulation.

3. Mechanical stimuli—show S axons not responsive while L axons change rate of activity. Noxious stimuli—show S axons change rate of activity while L remain unresponsive.

4. Large axons excite (increase the rate of activity of SG neurones) while small axons inhibit the rate of activity of the SG neurones.

5. The SG neurones inhibit the effect of the S axons on the T cells. As L axons excite the SG neurones, the action of L fibres is to 'close' the pain gate. The S fibres 'open' the

pain gate by inhibiting the SG neurones. In effect, the model is telling us that mechanical stimulation, such as gently scrubbing an injured area will reduce nociceptive input. Conversely, noxious stimulation seems to maintain the effects of subsequent nociceptive inputs.

6. The T cells are crucial for transmitting nociceptive information to higher levels of the CNS. Hypothesis: selectively damaging T neurones will reduce or eliminate pain experience following nociceptive stimulation.

7. Damage to L axons will result in reduced excitatory stimulation of the SG neurones, opening the spinal gate to noxious stimulation. Hypothesis: damaging L axons would increase the pain experienced following nociceptive stimulation.

8. As the model proposes that SG neurones are involved in the gating of noxious stimuli, we would predict that damage to the SG neurones would increase pain sensitivity. Reduced pain sensitivity is evidence which would falsify the Gate Control theory.

9. Probably not; as we discussed in the context of Lakatos' ideas. Theories have a 'protective belt' of assumptions; which means that a single empirical falsification need not result in the rejection of the theory. In this case, we may look for additional effects of the virus; say in destroying CNS tissue involved in elaborating pain experience. However, in the long run, such disconfirmations will lead to discarding the theory.

10. In terms of the model TENS works by stimulating the L axons, and thereby 'closing' the pain gate, as outlined in 4 and 5.

Research planning

The first stage of research involves the detailed planning of the project. The plan for what is to occur in the project is written up in a document called the research protocol. Before the research project may proceed, the protocol is examined by ethics committees and funding bodies to ensure that it conforms with general methodological and ethical principles. The three chapters of Section 2 aim to outline the basic considerations for the successful preparation of a research protocol.

The primary reason for carrying out a research project is to obtain empirical evidence that will advance theory and practice in the health sciences. Before all else, we must be sure that we are asking the right questions, that is, raising issues and problems which are central to progress in contemporary health care. We must convince the critical reader that our aims or the hypotheses which we are attempting to resolve are of central importance. Asking the right research questions depends on being creative, for example, identifying previously ignored patterns in the data, or the construction of novel theories that predict new, as yet unobserved phenomena. Of course, we are not suggesting that researchers are geniuses, or that only brilliant, ground-breaking research is funded. Much important research is carried out by perfectly ordinary men and women, who are interested in their patients and their problems, who have a good knowledge of their professional practices and who understand research methods.

To justify the research proposal it is necessary to write a 'literature review'. The literature review is a summary and critical evaluation of previous research and theory relevant to the problem we are intending to investigate. In this way the literature review both provides a conceptual background for our proposal and justifies the need for further empirical evidence by identifying 'gaps' in our knowledge.

The proposed research may be descriptive, for example, collecting information concerning health needs of a community and/or the impact of illness or injury on a group of patients. In Chapter 3, non-experimental research strategies are described. Non-experimental research which includes both quantitative and qualitative surveys (Section 3) aims to provide a clear picture or description of the health of individuals, groups or whole communities. Experimental research strategies are appropriate when we are testing hypotheses about the causes of illness, and when we attempt to gain control over extraneous variables which may influence treatment outcomes. The notions of causality and control are central for health research and are explored in Chapter 4. Of course, when we write a research protocol, we must be sure that we select the appropriate research strategy.

No research can proceed unless it is judged to be ethical by an appropriate committee. A research proposal is judged ethical if it conforms with our rules and values concerning caregiving. These rules and values are made explicit in documents representing the standards of professional groups and of institutions (e.g. hospitals, universities and research councils). The research protocol must be described in sufficient detail so that a decision can be made as to whether any harm might occur to participants in the research project.

Economic considerations, or the availability of resources also has a strong influence on research planning. For example, you may have designed a qualitative research project which involves 100 'in depth' interviews with persons suffering from a disorder. Say you have only 1 year and a very limited amount of money to complete your project. You would be advised either to reduce your sample size or, if this is not possible, change your topic. Ethics or funding committees will only approve projects which can feasibly be completed with the available resources.

The way in which samples are selected is discussed in Chapter 3. Selection of an appropriate sample is crucial for the generalizability (or external validity) of your findings. Our aim is to select a representative sample of the population but this may not be always possible in health sciences research. We need a sample size which is sufficiently large to identify the phenomena in which we are interested, but not too large or we are simply wasting resources.

Thus, research planning is a process, by which we transform our ideas into well-planned, ethical and economically feasible projects, as described in a research protocol.

2

Research planning

INTRODUCTION

Before the actual data collection begins, researchers invest considerable time and effort in the planning of their investigations. The first step is to select and to justify the selection of the research problem. The second step for quantitative research is to transform the problem into a clear researchable aim or hypothesis. Research planning includes the selection of an appropriate research strategy for providing required empirical evidence. The selection of the appropriate research strategy depends not only on the questions being asked, but also on identifying ethical issues and resource constraints which define the scope and form of the investigation.

The specific aims of this chapter are to:

1. Discuss how research questions are selected and justified.
2. Specify how questions are transformed into empirically testable hypotheses or aims.
3. Broadly outline research strategies available for specific types of investigations.
4. Discuss the ethical and economic constraints on the planning and execution of research.

SOURCES OF RESEARCH QUESTIONS

Advances in health sciences research depend on the identification of questions and problems which promote the development of more powerful theories of health, illness and disability, and then devising more effective ways of assessing, treating and preventing health problems. This advancement depends very much on researchers asking the 'right' questions and identifying solvable problems.

The formulation of research questions depends on the expertise of women and men who have a combination of theoretical knowledge and practical experience for identifying problems and asking the right questions. The professional backgrounds of researchers is an important consideration, to the extent that one's educational background and practices will in part determine what are seen as theoretically and professionally interesting problems.

Whatever the researcher's professional background, it is understood that they are strongly (even passionately) interested in a particular area of the health sciences. The formulation of even apparently simple research questions is often the culmination of intensive preliminary observations, spending long hours in the library reading through and critically analyzing related research, and thinking through the various issues. It is assumed that the researcher already has, or intends to develop, a specialized area of expertise, which is normally a precondition for advancement in health theory or practice.

The health care setting in which the researcher works often has a strong influence on the formulation of research questions. For example, it is an important consideration if the researcher works in a laboratory, a hospital, a community clinic or in private practice. These settings will influence how the patients' problems are perceived, and how researchers define professionally relevant solutions to these problems.

In many areas of health care, such as rehabilitation, community health and neurosciences, researchers sharing similar interests may join together in multidisciplinary research teams. Because of the broad range of expertise and perspectives such teams may be in a position to formulate interesting research questions.

Unfortunately, because of professional rivalries and interpersonal conflicts, such multidisciplinary research groups are sometimes not as productive as they should be. Good research

often requires interpersonal and communication skills.

THE FORMULATION OF RESEARCH QUESTIONS

There is a variety of valid sources for formulating research questions. These include:

1. Hypotheses logically deduced from existing theories, as discussed in Chapter 1.
2. Hypotheses suggested by clinical observations and insights such as that of Semmelweiss, discussed in Chapter 1.
3. Questions raised by previously conducted research which was inconclusive, invalid or incomplete. These questions arise from the critical evaluation of published literature, as outlined in Chapter 22.
4. Questions raised concerning the effectiveness of currently used or new treatment or assessment techniques. These questions arise in the context of evaluating or attempting to improve the outcome of health care.
5. Solutions required to pressing problems faced in professional settings, including problems reported by patients. In effect, much of applied health sciences research may be seen as a process for identifying, clarifying and solving problems.

Whatever the source or sources of the questions or problems, it is understood that they can be answered or resolved by collecting and analyzing relevant empirical evidence.

THE JUSTIFICATION OF RESEARCH QUESTIONS

When researchers call on public funds to conduct their investigations, they must explain in what way their intended investigation will contribute to scientific knowledge or clinical practice. In 'pure' scientific research, a proposed investigation is justified in terms of its potential contribution to existing knowledge. In the context of 'applied' health research, the investigator may be required to demonstrate that the empirical evidence will in some way contribute to the improved practice of health care and benefit patients.

Before embarking on the design and conduct of a research project, the investigator must review previous publications relevant to the aims of the intended project. This process is essential, both for providing the appropriate background and context for the investigation, and for justifying the investigation in contributing to existing knowledge.

Literature searching is carried out at appropriate research centres or libraries where scientific and professional journals are stored. There are now various computerized literature search methods which can simplify the search. Professional library staff can help to locate the relevant literature. However, the critical evaluation of the literature depends on the application of research methods (see Ch. 22) for the identification of controversies or 'gaps' in the available evidence.

FORMULATION OF RESEARCH AIMS OR HYPOTHESES

Hypotheses

A frequent goal in quantitative research is to test a hypothesis. Hypotheses are propositions about relationships between variables or differences between groups that are to be tested. Hypotheses may be concerned with relationships between observations or variables (for example, 'Is there an association between level of exercise and annual health care expenditure for Australians?') or differences between groups (for example, 'Do patients treated under therapy x exhibit greater improvement than those treated under therapy y?'). A *variable* is simply a property that may vary from case to case, for example, the room temperature, the ages of the patients, or their improvement on a measurement scale.

Some research projects do not have a hypothesis to be tested in any formal sense. For example, if you are measuring the health needs of a local community, there need not be any expectation or hypothesis to be tested. This does not mean the research is deficient, it just means it has a different objective from other types of research projects. In

fact, for qualitative research, holding clear cut hypotheses may prejudice the investigation (see Ch. 8). In these cases, we talk about the research having aims or objectives, rather than hypotheses.

An obvious and necessary condition for formulating research aims or hypotheses is that the research questions should have empirical referents. In planning research, the investigator is required to give observable referents to vague and ambiguous concepts. That is, investigators must decide on precisely how the variables are going to be measured. This is called the operational definition of a variable, and will be discussed in Chapter 12 in the context of measurement. Clearly, when formulating research aims or hypotheses we must specify the variables being studied, and how these variables are to be observed or measured.

Let us look at an example for illustrating how concepts should be specified in terms of empirical (observable) referents. Consider the concept 'coronary disease'. What are its observable referents (or symptoms)? They include:

- severe periodic pain in the chest and upper left arm
- occlusion (blockings) of coronary arteries, reducing blood flow
- sudden death.

Now suppose a new drug, x, is introduced to help people with coronary disease. The researchers hypothesize that 'The new drug x is effective for helping patients with coronary disease'. Using the observable symptoms as referents, the research hypothesis is then restated:

- Patients diagnosed with coronary disease taking drug x will report fewer incidents of pain in the chest and upper left arm than patients taking traditionally used drug y or
- Patients diagnosed with coronary disease taking drug x will have greater volume of blood flow through their coronary arteries than patients taking traditionally used drug y or
- Fewer patients diagnosed with coronary disease taking drug x will die during a 5-year period than those taking traditionally used drug y.

A published example of formulating hypotheses

Let us look at a published example for illustrating how concepts can be defined in operational terms. This paper is titled: *Effects of preoperative teaching on postoperative pain: a replication and extension*, by Mogan et al (1985).

Firstly, the proposed intervention 'preoperative teaching' is a rather vague concept. What do the authors mean by this? In effect, this involved 'brief relaxation training', which is more precise. However, there are a variety of possible brief relaxation techniques. Therefore, quite appropriately, the authors explained that: 'The present study was designed to replicate, at least conceptually, and extend a method ... described by Flaherty & Fitzpatrick (1978)' (Mogan et al 1985).

Now, by reading through the reference and noting the modifications of the authors described in the paper, we are in a position to understand the precise nature of the intervention.

Secondly, we may ask how the outcome (post-operative pain) was defined and measured. After all, as the authors pointed out, pain is a subjective experience and its quality and meaning may be different for patients. Having reviewed the relevant literature, Mogan et al (1985) decided to operationally define pain in terms of:

1. The amount of analgesic required by individual patients following surgery: in general, the less pain the smaller the quantity of analgesic required.
2. The self-reports of patients on a 10-point pain rating scale, reporting the 'sensory' and 'distressing' aspects of pain.

Although we may argue about the validity of these means for measuring pain, the authors provided operational definitions for the variables studied in their clinical experiment. The following hypotheses guided their research:

1. Patients taught a relaxation technique will have lower vital signs (blood pressure, pulse and respiration) than those not taught a relaxation technique.
2. Patients taught a relaxation technique will

experience less pain than those not taught a relaxation technique as indicated by:
   (a) consuming fewer analgesics
   (b) less self-reported pain sensation
   (c) less distress from these sensations.
3. Patients taught a relaxation technique will be discharged from the hospital earlier than those not taught a relaxation technique (Mogan et al 1985, pp 269–270).

The formulation of an adequately formed research hypothesis or aim is a process during which the researcher gradually refines a broadly based issue into specific operationally defined statements. This process must take into account the logical requirements of designs for the data collection and ethical standards for conducting health sciences research. In addition, the aims or hypotheses must inform a realistic data collection procedure which can be supported by the resources available for researchers. We will examine these issues in the rest of this chapter.

RESEARCH STRATEGIES

Research planning also involves the selection or formulation of research strategies. Research strategies are established procedures for designing and executing research. Research strategies outlined in this book include experimental and quasi-experimental strategies, single case research, surveys, and qualitative field research. Before detailed discussion of the differences between these strategies is undertaken in following sections, it is instructive to compare the basic structures of non- experimental (surveys) and experimental research. As we shall see in subsequent sections, these are fundamentally different ways of conducting research.

Non-experimental strategies

The three essential steps involved in non-experimental strategies are shown in Figure 2.1. You will note in the Figure that the researcher defines the population of interest, selects the cases to be studied (this process is described in

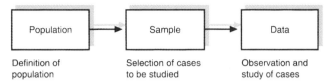

Fig. 2.1 Structure of a non-experimental study.

some detail in Ch. 3) and then observes or studies them, generating the data. There is no active intervention in the situation by the researcher. Indeed, intervention that would change the phenomenon being studied is discouraged and avoided. In this type of research strategy there is a constant tension between the requirements for close and detailed observation and the possibility that the behaviour of the cases may change because they are being studied. There are techniques for dealing with this problem, such as the use of unobtrusive measures and participant observation, which will be discussed in subsequent chapters. An important class of non- experimental research strategies are called 'qualitative' or 'interpretive' (Ch. 8).

Experimental strategies

Experimental research strategies involve more steps, as illustrated in Figure 2.2. As with the non-experimental strategy, cases are selected for study from a defined population. However, these cases are then assigned (generally by chance or random method) to a treatment or non-treatment group, and then treated. (The term 'treatment' is used here in the sense that the subject or event is being systematically influenced or manipulated by the investigator; that is, in a broader sense than as medical or physical treatment.) The two groups are then observed and compared. If everything went according to plan, any differences in the data of the treatment and non-treatment groups should be a result of the effects of the treatment. Unfortunately, there are often other factors (sources of error) that are responsible for the differences. Good experimental technique attempts to eliminate these errors through control (Ch. 4).

Thus, there is quite a difference in the structure of experimental and non- experimental research strategies. Cook and Campbell (1979) have proposed a third class of *'quasi-experimental'* strategies (which are really just tightly structured non-experimental strategies) that we will also cover later (see Ch. 6).

The decision of the investigator to adopt experimental or non-experimental strategies depends on the phenomenon being studied and the specific question type of research (causal or descriptive) being investigated.

RESEARCH PLANNING: ETHICAL CONSIDERATIONS

In health research, where the health and lives of people participating in the study may be at stake, ethical considerations play a decisive role in research planning and execution. For instance, consider the question of the effects of cigarette smoking on health. A convincing way of investigating this question would be through experimental strategies, which (as we will see) are best suited for establishing causal relationships. However, it would be ethically unacceptable to have a number of people randomly assigned to a group involved in long-term, heavy cigarette smoking. Clearly, evidence must come from quasi- or non-experimental strategies, where investigators observe the effects of smoking in persons who have chosen to smoke.

A research process is judged to be *ethical* by the extent to which it conforms to or complies with the set of standards or conventions in the context in which the research is to be carried out and community standards. Most health settings and higher education institutions now have ethics committees to oversee health research involving humans and/or animals. Ethics committees,

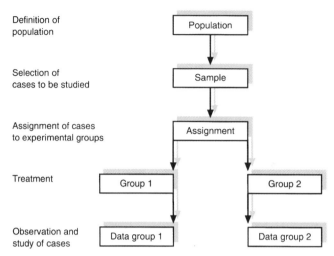

Fig. 2.2 Experimental research strategies.

along with the researcher, are responsible for interpreting and enforcing ethical standards. It should be noted, however, that even when a given research proposal is judged to be ethical, it may not be seen as *moral* by specific individuals or groups in a community. A good example is animal experimentation when the research involves painful or stressful procedures such as surgery. According to the value systems of some persons and groups, such work is considered to be intrinsically immoral. From this viewpoint, there may be no justification for inflicting suffering on animals, even when the results may be beneficial for humans. Others argue that such procedures are morally justified, given that they are necessary for the advancement of the biological and medical sciences and provided that reasonable steps are taken to limit the suffering of the animals. There are no absolute solutions for such controversies but, often, discussing these issues in public helps to establish a degree of consensus in the community and guidance for the ethical decisions of researchers.

It is beyond the scope of this subsection to examine in full the ethics of health research, but the following issues are central to making decisions in these areas:

1. *Benefits*. Who is to benefit from the research? One likes to think that 'humanity', 'the

subjects', or 'health science' are going to be the beneficiaries. A slightly more cynical analysis points to the investigators as having the most to gain, at least in the short term. After all, given a successful outcome for the research project, they stand to satisfy their curiosity, improve their career prospects, or to raise their esteem before colleagues. In practice, benefits accruing to the investigator, the participants and health science have to be carefully weighed in relation to the conduct of any project. The protection of the rights and welfare of the participants is the primary consideration of scientific ethics.

2. *Informed consent*. Informed consent by human participants is a necessary condition for ethically acceptable research. This means that all the risks involved in the investigation must be explained, as well as the possible benefits. Honest explanation of the procedures to the participant takes considerable skill, if disclosing the design of the study (say with placebo treatments) influences the expectations and performances of the participants. Special care needs to be taken when the participants are in some way limited in understanding the risks; for example, people who are intellectually disabled, or confused under the influence of drugs. Informed consent implies a freedom of

choice: the participant must feel confident that refusal to participate will not prejudice their subsequent clinical treatment.

3. *Protection of participants.* It is the investigator's responsibility to minimize the chances of long-term deleterious effects to subjects. Dangers can arise from administering new interventions or treatments with unknown side-effects, denying treatments of known effectiveness, or using invasive assessment techniques. The welfare of laboratory animals must not be ignored. There are now enforceable constraints on the conditions for using non-human subjects in research.

4. *Minimizing discomfort.* The investigator must also minimize even short-term pain, anxiety, discomfort or embarrassment involved in an investigation, especially if it is not part of routine therapeutic practice. This is an important issue, as some therapists and researchers take a mistakenly 'proprietary' view of their patients, imagining that they should put up with some discomfort for the good of medical science. In the past, patients in public wards of hospitals and long-term prisoners have been most vulnerable to questionable ethical practices.

5. *Privacy.* Health care research may involve collecting information which can lead to the embarrassment or stigmatization of the participants. The identity of participants must be protected (for example, by 'coding' their real names).

6. *Community values.* Some research, such as that involving the assessment of sexual functioning or the investigation of human fetuses, calls for very sensitive planning. Anatomical research involving the use of human cadaver material must be planned to ensure respectful handling and disposal. Even if the investigator does not agree, the values and taboos of groups in the community must be taken into consideration when planning the investigation.

7. *Conservation of resources.* A fundamental value is that the time and effort of researchers and subjects and the resources of the community should not be wasted on a badly planned investigation. There is never a guarantee that an investigation will produce clinically useful results, but some poorly designed projects are doomed to failure even before the data collection begins and lead to confusion and controversy in the professional literature. Therefore, the correct use of research methods is not only useful for solving problems, but constitutes an ethical necessity. Many ethics committees also vet projects for scientific merit before the project is approved.

A responsible investigator is required to take into consideration ethical principles and to plan research projects accordingly, so that no harm is caused. Therefore, the health researcher must use considerable ingenuity in designing valid investigations, while maintaining ethical values. One of the roles of ethics committees is to guide investigators on complex issues and to ensure that research is conducted in accordance with accepted community principles.

SELECTION OR RESEARCH STRATEGIES: ECONOMIC CONSIDERATIONS

Selection of appropriate research strategies is also influenced by the resources of investigators. Some projects involving the evaluation of the safety and effectiveness of new drugs, or the identification of risk factors in cardiac disease, have taken tens of millions of dollars to finance. Research planning takes into account economic issues, such as:

1. *Availability of participants.* Here the investigator has to consider if enough people can participate in the project under the required conditions. Attention has to be paid to issues such as the frequency of the disorder in the community, problems in identifying participants, and their level of voluntary participation. As will be shown in Chapter 3, selection of participants is crucial for the validity of a study.

2. *Availability of equipment.* Some equipment is costly to acquire or to operate (for example, CT scanners, biochemical assays,

experimental drugs). Research planning should take these expenses into account.

3. *Availability of expertise*. Specialized assessment techniques and the administration of clinical treatments require professional expertise. If these are beyond the investigator's competence or if the experimental design requires an unbiased, 'blind' therapist or assessor (see Ch. 5), there must be means for securing them.

4. *Availability of time*. Research projects have a tendency to take considerably longer than an inexperienced researcher might expect, owing to the erratic and at times disastrous workings of Murphy's Law: 'If anything can go wrong, it will'. Equipment breaks down and needs to be repaired, subjects 'disappear', collaborators might not deliver services promised. Research planning should take into account possible problems and how these might affect the time scale of investigations. This is a particularly important issue for post-graduate students.

The availability of resources strongly influences the scope of the research programme and also the research strategy selected by the investigator. A research project must be shown to be economically feasible before it is initiated. It is only after the ethical constraints and economic resources have been evaluated that the researchers' questions can be transformed into clearly defined hypotheses or aims.

STEPS IN RESEARCH PLANNING

The following steps should be considered in quantitative research before actual data collection begins. The term 'data' refers to the set of observations recorded during an investigation.

1. Identification of the research problem
2. Retrieval and critical evaluation of relevant

literature for justifying and giving the context of the research problem.

3. Formulation of precise research aims or hypotheses in the light of:
   (a) the relevant variables selected for study
   (b) the appropriate research strategies
   (c) the ethical restraints necessary to protect subjects
   (d) the projected cost of the project.
4. In addition, as to be discussed in this book, research planning takes into account:
   (a) how the sample is to be selected (Ch. 3)
   (b) the design of the investigation (Chs 4–8)
   (c) how the data is to be collected (Chs 9–12)
   (d) how the data is to be analyzed (Chs 13–20).

The above points are written up in the form of a *research protocol*. This is submitted to supervisors, colleagues or ethical committees, for scrutiny of methodological and ethical problems. It is only when the protocol is acceptable that the actual data collection begins. It is often desirable to carry out a small-scale preliminary study, called a 'pilot'. This is an economical way of identifying and eliminating potential problems in the large-scale investigation.

SUMMARY

The planning of a research project requires the transformation of a vague question or problem into clearly stated aims or hypotheses. To achieve this, the researcher should review the relevant literature and evaluate ethical considerations and economic constraints in conducting the investigation. Next, an appropriate research strategy needs to be selected. On the basis of the above, the researcher is in a position to state precisely the aims or hypotheses being investigated.

Before data collection begins, a protocol for the complete investigation is scrutinized by colleagues to correct methodological problems, or to prevent unethical research.

SELF ASSESSMENT

Explain the meaning of the following terms:

> ethics
> informed consent
> literature review
> Murphy's law
> non-experimental study
> pilot study
> research strategy
> variable

TRUE OR FALSE

1. Scientific research always involves the testing of hypotheses.
2. A sample is a subset of the data.
3. The population being studied is defined after the sample has been selected.
4. A research protocol is a summary of the data obtained in an investigation.
5. A pilot is a small-scale research program to demonstrate the feasibility of an investigation.
6. Human cadavers are not sentient beings, therefore their treatment falls outside the scope of medical ethics.
7. Planning quantitative research includes specifying the variables to be studied and how these are to be measured.
8. Abstract constructs, such as 'intelligence' or 'motivation' cannot have empirical referents.
9. A literature review is necessary for providing the appropriate background and rationale for an investigation.
10. Well-established data collection techniques are called research findings.
11. A non-experimental design involves the random assignment of subjects to treatment groups.
12. Both experimental and non-experimental designs involve the drawing of an appropriate sample from the population being studied.
13. An anthropologist studying how ethnic groups relate to illness would tend to adopt an experimental research strategy.
14. The clear explanation of the risks involved in a research project is a necessary condition for obtaining informed consent from a subject.
15. The use of correct research methods does not constitute an ethical necessity.
16. A hypothesis is a proposition about the relationship existing between variables or prediction of differences between groups.
17. Some scientific research projects do not involve the testing of hypotheses.
18. Existing theories are the only appropriate sources for experimental hypotheses.
19. In a non-experimental study there is no need to pay attention to sampling.
20. Experimental designs involve the random assignment of the sampled subjects into treatment groups.
21. Experimental designs are more appropriate than non-experimental designs for demonstrating causal relationships.
22. The subjects participating in medical research are generally the most likely beneficiaries of the project.
23. Informed consent of human subjects is necessary even when the investigation is not apparently embarrassing or dangerous.
24. It is unethical to study human sexual behaviour because people find it embarrassing to serve as subjects in such research.
25. Medical researchers should expect that patients who receive free hospital treatment should participate in medical experiments.
26. The correct use of research methods in conducting an investigation is useful, but not an ethical necessity.
27. A well-designed, relevant research project will be always financed, regardless of the expense.
28. A variable is a property or attribute which varies from subject to subject.

SELF ASSESSMENT

MULTIPLE CHOICE

1. The aim of research planning is to:

   a generate appropriate aims or clear-cut research hypotheses
   b select an appropriate research strategy
   c identify possible ethical or economic limitations in conducting the investigation
   d a and b
   e all of the above.

2. A literature review:

   a is a list of research publications relevant to an investigation
   b should discredit research findings which are inconsistent with the hypothesis
   c should include only findings which directly support the hypothesis being investigated
   d should be a critical review of findings relevant to an investigation.

3. Which of the following is common to both experimental and non- experimental research strategies?

   a assignment
   b selection of cases to be studied
   c experimental hypothesis
   d participant observation
   e field research.

4. Which of the following is unique to the experimental research strategy?

   a assignment
   b selection of cases to be studied
   c definition of population
   d participant observation
   e field research.

5. The availability of resources to conduct an investigation:

   a is not the concern of a scientific researcher

   b has an influence on the scope and design of the investigation
   c is determined by Murphy's Law
   d none of the above.

6. 32° Centigrade is an example of:

   a a variable
   b the value of a variable
   c a ratio
   d a null hypothesis.

7. A variable is:

   a a property which can take different values across different individuals
   b a property which can take different values within an individual
   c both a and b
   d neither a nor b.

8. Which of the following represents the most explicitly formulated research aim?

   a The aim of the present project was to investigate if health care workers were satisfied with their current rates of pay
   b The aim of the present project was to identify the number of persons living in the Newcastle metropolitan area
   c The aim of the present project is to examine pay rates.

9. Which of the following represents the most explicitly formulated research aim?

   a The aim of the present project was to investigate if health care workers in Gotham City were satisfied with their pay and career prospects
   b The aim of the present project was to investigate if emotionally disturbed persons living in Gotham City received adequate medical care
   c The aim of the present project was to

identify the reasons why health professionals in Gotham City leave their professions, and turn to other types of employment

d The aim of the present project was to identify the proportion of teenagers in Gotham City smoking more than 10 cigarettes a day.

10. A research protocol should make explicit:

a the justification for undertaking the research project

b the way in which the data is to be collected

c the empirical evidence provided by the investigation

d *a* and *b*.

11. Which of the following represents a non-researchable problem (in the context of the scientific method)?

a Is aspirin preferable to steroids in reducing the symptoms of arthritis?

b Does the use of alcohol result in greater levels of brain damage than the use of marijuana?

c Are painful experiments involving animals justified if they lead to benefits to patients?

d Do people coming from a low socioeconomic class receive poorer health care than people from a higher class?

3

Sampling methods and external validity

INTRODUCTION

Research in the health sciences usually involves the collection of data on a sample of cases, rather than on the entire population of cases in which the investigator is interested. A sample is studied because it is usually impossible or extremely costly to study complete populations. For example, when individuals suffering from conditions such as diabetes, cerebral palsy or emphysema are being investigated, it is not possible to study everyone because of the large size of such populations, and because many people do not seek treatment or may be wrongly diagnosed. Therefore, in both experimental and non-experimental investigations, the researcher routinely studies a subset or sample of the population and then attempts to generalize the findings to the population from which the participants were drawn.

The aim of this chapter is to examine ways samples should be drawn so as to ensure that they permit the investigator to make valid generalizations from the sample to the population.

We will also consider the question of generalizing the findings of an investigation to other samples and situations. This is referred to as 'external validity', a concept related to induction, as discussed in Chapter 1.

The specific aims of this chapter are to:

1. Define what is meant by sampling and representative samples.
2. Outline the relative advantages and disadvantages of commonly used sampling methods.

3. Discuss the relationship between sampling error and sample size.
4. Examine the concept of external validity for generalizing research findings to other settings.

WHAT IS SAMPLED IN A STUDY?

This chapter will focus on the selection of the research participants or subjects in a study. However, in most studies, many other things are also selected or sampled. These include:

- the information to be collected
- the procedures for the collection of the information
- where the research is conducted
- the clinicians and researchers involved.

Many researchers focus on the selection of the research participants and do not pay enough attention to the other factors they are sampling. It is not unusual to see studies that employ large and sophisticated participant samples with only one or two clinicians involved in the research in one health setting. Although not always the case, many quantitative studies are very weak in their consideration (and sampling) of research context but strong in participant sampling. Many qualitative studies, again unnecessarily, have strong consideration of context but are weak in their sampling of research participants.

BASIC ISSUES IN SAMPLING

Often, because of the number of cases involved, it is not within the resources of the researcher to study the whole population. In any event, in most situations it would be wasteful to study all the population. If a sample is representative, one can generalize validly from the sample's results to the population.

The population is the group of individuals in which the researcher is interested. For example, all English women under 25, all children with diagnosed spina bifida in the state of Alberta or all the students at a particular Australian college. The researcher defines the population to which they wish to generalize. Note that a population

Table 3.1 Examples of populations and samples

Population	Possible sample selection
All working podiatrists in a state	50 podiatrists selected for a study of job satisfaction
All working pathologists in a state	25 pathologists selected for detailed tax evaluation by an inspector
The temperature of a patient during a 24 h period	Hourly measurements of patient's temperature recorded by staff
Stuttering in a child's speech	Number of stutters made during 5 min of reading a standard piece of material
All patients in a state with frontal lobe damage	30 patients with frontal lobe damage selected for evaluating a rehabilitation programme
All surgical gauzes held by a given hospital	10 gauzes selected by a bacteriologist to test for sterility

need not consist of human or animal subjects. Objects or events can also sampled, as shown in Table 3.1.

As shown in Table 3.1, a *population* is an entire set of persons, objects or events which the researcher intends to study. A *sample* is a subset of the population. *Sampling* involves the selection of the sample from the population.

REPRESENTATIVE SAMPLES

There is a variety of different ways by which one can select the sample from the population. These are called sampling methods.

The aim of all sampling methods is to draw a representative sample from the population. The advantage of a representative sample is clear: one can confidently generalize from a representative sample to the rest of the population without having to take the trouble of measuring the rest of the population. If the sample is biased (not representative) one can generalize less validly from the sample to the population. In addition, this might lead to quite incorrect conclusions or inferences about the population. This would mean that the results obtained in the study would not necessarily generalize to other experiments or studies using the same population. Figure 3.1 illustrates the concept of a representative sample.

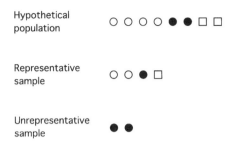

Hypothetical population

Representative sample

Unrepresentative sample

Fig. 3.1 A simple representative sample.

Figure 3.1 illustrates a hypothetical population composed of three different types of elements. A representative sample is a precise miniaturized representation of the proportion of elements of the population. An unrepresentative or biased sample does not represent the elements in correct proportions, leading to mistaken conclusions about the state of the population.

The selection of the appropriate sampling method depends upon the aims and resources of the researchers. For instance, if someone is designing a very expensive social welfare programme on the basis of a survey of clients' needs, it is imperative that the researcher uses a good sampling method and obtains a representative sample, so that appropriate inferences may be made about the population. Good sampling methods are more expensive and more difficult to implement than poor methods. The main sampling methods used in scientific and clinical research are incidental and random sampling.

Incidental samples

Incidental sampling. This is the cheapest and easiest sampling method to use. It involves the selection of the most easily accessible members of the target population. For example, a political scientist who stands in the middle of a city street and quizzes people about their voting intentions is practising incidental sampling. However, it is likely that this sample would not be representative of the general voting population. There would probably be an over-representation of businessmen and white-collar workers, and an under-representation of factory workers and housewives. Thus, the political scientist's predictions of any election results might not represent the actual results because of these sampling anomalies. The sample is likely to be unrepresentative and biased.

A further example of incidental sampling might involve a researcher surveying the needs of a group of spina bifida children at a local community health centre. Their measured needs may be representative of those of other spina bifida children but then again they may not.

Thus, incidental sampling is cheap and easy to implement but may give a biased sample that is not representative of the population.

Quota sampling. Sometimes it is known in advance that there are important subgroups within the population that need to be included in the sample because they may affect the results of the study. Two important groups within the human population are males and females. Further, it is known that they occur in the ratio of approximately 49:51 in the general population. Our intrepid researcher might decide that it is very important that the sexes are proportionally represented in the sample. Thus, the researcher would set two quotas (of 49 male and 51 female respondents in a sample of 100 and sample accordingly in a city street. This is still a form of incidental sampling but has some advantages over simple incidental sampling. Even more complicated examples involving more than two groups can be accommodated as shown in Table 3.2.

We can see from Table 3.2 that if we were to be representative regarding both sex and occupational status, in a sample of 100 people we would need 19 blue collar males, 15 blue collar females, and so on.

Table 3.2 Distribution of percentages of gender and occupational variables in the general population

	Blue collar	White collar 'no collar'	Not employed	Total
Male	19	21	9	49
Female	15	15	21	51
Total	34	36	30	100

Quota sampling still has a number of short-comings: before it can be used, one has to know which population groups are likely to be important to a particular question and the exact proportions of the various groups in the population. Also, the members of the sample are still incidentally chosen. The blue collar males, for example, selected in a city centre on a week-day may still be quite different from those working elsewhere.

Random and systematic samples

Random sampling. This is one of the best but most difficult sampling methods to implement. A random sample is one in which all members of the population have an equal chance of selection. Thus a random sample is more likely to be representative of the relevant population than an incidental sample.

The procedure for drawing a random sample involves:

1. The construction of a list of all members of the population.
2. Using a method such as dice, coins or random number tables to select randomly from the list the number of members required for the sample.

A simple example of a random sample is provided by a common raffle, where names on equal size papers are put in a hat, shaken and selected 'blind'. Many lotteries use numbered balls that are drawn randomly from a barrel. Another way to draw a random sample is to construct a list of all the members of the population and assign a number to each element. A table of random numbers, generated by a computer, could then be used to select a random sample. Computers can do this efficiently, even when large populations are involved.

The cases selected from the list constitute a random sample. Sometimes, because of refusal to participate in the study, mortality, etc., it is necessary to select replacements for some cases. This can introduce bias into the sample, as the refusers may differ consistently from those who accept. An example of this would be seen in a survey of sexual behaviours: persons who would refuse to participate might have different sexual behaviours from those who consent to participate.

However, random sampling methods have important advantages over incidental or non-random methods:

- because the exact sizes of the sample and population are known, it is possible to estimate exactly how representative the sample is, that is, the size of the sampling error. This cannot usually be done with non-random sampling methods.
- Because random samples are usually more representative than non-random samples, the sample size needed for good representation of the population is smaller.

The major disadvantages of random sampling methods are:

- The researcher needs to be able to list every member of the population. Often this is impossible because the full extent of the population is not known. For example, it would be very difficult to sample randomly from the population of Australians with coronary disease, because no such list exists.
- Cost. It is much easier to use conveniently available groups. Random sampling usually involves considerable planning and expense, especially with large populations.

Stratified random sampling. This is the same as quota sampling, except that each quota is filled by randomly sampling from each subgroup, rather than sampling incidentally. For example, if one was drawing a sample stratified with respect to sex, one would have to prepare a list of all females and all males in the population and then sample randomly from these lists with the numbers of each group in the sample corresponding to the population proportions.

The advantages of stratified random sampling are:

- all the important groups are proportionally represented. This is particularly important when key subgroups in the population occur in low proportions.

- the exact representativeness of the sample is known. This has important statistical ramifications.

The disadvantages are:

- a list of all members of the population, their characteristics and the proportions of the important groups within the population need to be known
- cost
- the gain in accuracy is usually very small in comparison to simple random sampling.

Area sampling. In area sampling, one samples on the basis of location of cases. For example, on the basis of census data, the investigator may select several areas in a city or county with known characteristics, such as high or low unemployment rates. The areas could then be further divided into specific streets and the occupants of, say, every third house contacted for participation in the study. In other words, the locations are randomly selected and then one interviews the occupants of those locations. This can be a very effective, cheap method of sampling in social surveys. It does not require a list of the individual members of the population, merely the location where they live.

Systematic sampling. This involves working through a list of the population and choosing, say, every 10th or 20th case for inclusion in the sample. It is not a truly random technique but will usually give a representative sample. It is based on the (usually justified) supposition that cases are not added to the list in a systematic way which coincides with the sampling system. Provided that a list of cases is available, systematic sampling is an easy and convenient sampling method. In clinical practice we are using systematic sampling when, for instance, we measure temperature and blood pressure every hour.

SAMPLE SIZE

One of the most poorly understood aspects of sampling is the optimal number of cases that should be included in a sample.

It is obvious that in one sense the more cases selected the better, but the costs associated with the data collection must be balanced against the greater accuracy of making inferences with larger samples. Also, some health related studies involve discomfort, pain, or even danger to patients or laboratory animals. Therefore, it is ethically necessary (see Ch. 2) to ensure that no more than the bare minimum of subjects is used. The fact is that clinical researchers 'walk a tightrope' in deciding the optimum sample sizes for these kinds of studies. However, there are some principles available to guide the researcher.

First of all, let us say quite definitely that there is no magic number that we can point to as an optimum sample size. We cannot say what percentage of the population should be sampled. Rather, the optimum number in the sample depends on the characteristics of an investigation, in the context of which the sample is drawn. In general, the optimum sample size is one which is adequate for making correct inferences from a sample to a population. Let us try to illuminate this in relation to the concept of sampling error.

Sampling error

Sampling error is reflected in the discrepancy between the true population parameter and the sample statistic. For example, if I happen to know from census data that the average age of males in a district is 35 years and the average age of a sample of males I have surveyed from the district is 30 years, then I have a sampling error of 5 years. However, if we do not know the actual population parameters, we can only estimate the probable sampling error.

Sampling error is related to sample size by the following relationship:

$$\text{Sampling error} \propto \frac{1}{\sqrt{n}}$$

What the above equation claims is that the greater the sample size n, the smaller the probability of sampling error. In fact, the sampling error is inversely proportional to the square root of the sample size. For the calculation of probable sampling error, see Chapter 17.

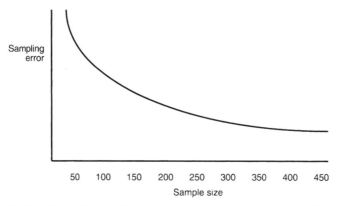

Fig. 3.2 The relationship between sample size and sampling error. The scaling but not the form of the curve will alter with the variability of the data.

From this relationship it can be seen that doubling the sample size would only result in a reduction of the error by a factor of the square root of 2 (1.414). Similarly, a ninefold increase in sample size would result in only a threefold reduction in the sampling error. Figure 3.2 illustrates this point by showing the graphical relationship between probable sampling error and sample size.

It can be seen from this graph that not much is gained from a sample size of over, say, n_1. Yet the cost of the sampling and data collection can be very high with large numbers, (such as n_2) for relatively little gain in reducing sampling error. In some research situations, even large probable sampling errors have relatively little potential influence on our decisions. In such situations, we can live with a relatively small sample size. In other situations, we need large samples to justify our confidence in the truth of our decisions.

As an illustration, suppose that we are attempting to predict the outcome of an election fought between two political parties, A and B. A representative sample of 100 respondents is polled before the election. Say the outcome is as follows:

Intends to vote for A	Intends to vote for B	Estimate sampling error
25%	75%	10%

In this instance, the estimated sampling error is very small in relation to the size of the *effect*

(that is, the difference between the percentage of intended votes for the two parties). We can predict confidently, assuming that the respondents were truthful and do not change their minds before the elections, that political party B will romp into government. Increasing sample size, say to 10 000 would enormously increase the cost of the survey. The corresponding reduction in sampling error would not justify this cost, as we would still come to the same conclusion. However, say the following sample statistics were obtained in the pre-election poll of n = 100 respondents:

Intends to vote for A	Intends to vote for B	Estimate sampling error
48%	52%	10%

Now, the same level of estimated sampling error is too large, in relation to the apparent size of the effect, to make a decision concerning which party is likely to win the election. The poll would have to be repeated using a substantially increased sample size to reduce the sampling error.

The example illustrates the notion that the adequacy of the sample size is affected by the specific investigation in which we are making inferences. A sample size which is adequate in one situation might be inadequate in another. One benefit of a pilot study is that it allows the investigator to estimate the size of the effect, and thereby make an educated guess of the sample size required to demonstrate it. In addition, a pilot study indicates the adequacy of the sampling model being employed by the investigator.

EXTERNAL VALIDITY AND SAMPLING

The term *external validity* refers to the extent to which the results of an investigation can be generalized to other samples or situations. External validity can be classified into two types: *population* and *ecological* (Huck et al 1974).

Population validity. This refers to generalizing the findings from the sample to the population from which it was drawn. We have already examined the importance of having a representative sample in the generalizing of results from a sample to a population. However, an investigator in the health sciences might face another problem: the accessible population from which the sample was taken might not be the same as the target population, that is, the one of general interest. Let us illustrate this point with an example: a physiotherapist working in a large private maternity hospital intends to examine the effectiveness of a new antenatal exercise procedure for pregnant women for controlling levels of pain during delivery. A random sample of 50 pregnant women is chosen for the investigation from the population attending the hospital. The sample is then randomly assigned into two groups: one receiving the new antenatal exercise procedure, the other receiving the traditional programme. The researcher finds a statistically and clinically significant difference between the two procedures, such that the new programme is shown to be effective.

Strictly speaking, these findings can be generalized only to the population of women who attend the hospital. However, if the target population is *all* women having babies, then the generalization lacks external validity because women attending different hospitals or having children at home had no chance of being included in the sample. They might have different characteristics in relation to the variable measured and these different characteristics may interact with the treatment in different ways to that of the sample. For instance, women who chose to deliver at home might respond better to the traditional intervention.

Ecological validity. There is also another limitation to external validity: the situation in which an investigation is carried out might not be generalizable to other situations. This is called ecological validity. Consider the following examples:

1. It has been shown that for clinical pain (due to disease or injury), morphine is an excellent analgesic. However, in laboratory studies of pain induced by electric shocks, morphine had little effect on subjects' reports of pain threshold. Clearly, generalizing from laboratory to clinical settings, or vice versa, has to be done with extreme caution (Beecher 1959).

2. Coronary arteriography involves the insertion of a small-gauge catheter into the coronary arteries, and injecting a dye for X-ray visualization. It was initially reported that the mortality rates for this rather dangerous-sounding practice were only 0.1% (1 per 1000) in a first-class medical institution. However, later reports from various other institutions showed mortality rates as high as 8% (80 per 1000) (Taylor 1979). Clearly, the effectiveness of treatments or the usefulness of clinical evaluations can well depend on in whose hands they are carried out.

The above examples illustrate the caution necessary in generalizing findings.

SUMMARY

Appropriate sampling strategies ensure the external validity of both experimental and non-experimental investigations. The aim of sampling strategies is to ensure the selection of a sample which is *representative* of the population of objects, persons or events the investigator aims to study. Incidental and quota samples are chosen for convenience, but these sampling strategies do not guarantee a representative sample. Random and stratified random sampling methods ensure that all elements of the population have a chance to be selected. Random sampling strategies are the most desirable to obtain a representative sample, although unfortunately random sampling is not always possible in health sciences research. Area sampling and systematic sampling are also strategies which can be used to obtain representative samples.

An adequate sample size reduces the probability of random sampling error. More precisely, the probable sampling error is inversely proportional to the square root of the sample size. It was argued that optimum sample size is not the maximum number of subjects obtainable or a constant number or proportion. Rather, it has to be estimated for a specific investigation on the basis of the parameters of the phenomenon being studied. Two types of external validity were discussed: population and ecological. External validity is related to inference, which involves using evidence from a limited set of elements to formulate general propositions.

SELF ASSESSMENT

Explain the meanings of the following terms:

area sample
biased sample
ecological validity
external validity
incidental sample
population
population validity
random sample
random sampling
representative sample
sample
sampling error (probable)

TRUE OR FALSE

1. The basic idea underlying sampling is to select a representative sample from which the investigator can make inferences to the population.
2. A sample is said to be random when it is not representative of the population.
3. If a population contains 50% males and 50% females, and our sample has 10% males and 90% females, then our sample is said to be biased.
4. When you take a patient's blood pressure daily, you are in fact sampling from a population of potential blood pressure readings.
5. If the patient's blood pressure fluctuates considerably during the day, then a single reading will be an inadequate sample.
6. Stratified random sampling involves the selection of the most accessible elements of the population.
7. Assume that important subgroups of the population are known and subjects are sampled incidentally in proportion to these subgroups. This sampling method is known as area sampling.
8. A random sample is one in which 50% of the elements of a population have equal chances of being sampled.
9. Random sampling in health sciences is the least expensive and time-consuming strategy for selecting a sample.
10. When you take blood pressures hourly, you are in fact using a random sampling method.
11. The larger the sample size, the larger the sampling error.
12. The problem of internal validity might emerge when we generalize results obtained in one research setting to another.
13. An incidental sample can not be, in principle, representative of the population.
14. If a sample is representative, it yields valid data for making generalizations about the population from which it was drawn.
15. The main difference between random and quota sampling is that in quota sampling particular subgroups of the population are represented proportionately.

16. Incidental sampling generates less bias than systematic sampling.
17. Area sampling involves selecting an area at random and assessing the inhabitants of that area.
18. A sample that is unbiased is a representative sample of the population from which it is drawn.
19. Sample error decreases as the sample size increases.
20. If the sample size is halved, the sampling error will be doubled.
21. If a sample is large (say $n > 500$) then the sample must be representative.
22. Generalizing findings from laboratory to clinical settings raises questions of ecological validity.
23. The problem of population validity refers to a population which contains invalid elements.

MULTIPLE CHOICE

1. As sample size increases:

   a the sampling error decreases
   b the ecological validity of the investigation increases
   c the population becomes more accessible
   d the sample becomes more biased.

2. A representative sample:

   a consists of at least 500 cases
   b must be a random sample
   c is defined as the inverse of the square root of the sample size
   d reflects precisely the crucial dimensions of a population.

3. An incidental sample is:

   a not necessarily biased
   b generally obtained through costly and difficult sampling procedures

   c used only in non-experimental investigations
   d none of the above.

An investigator wishes to study individuals suffering from agoraphobia (fear of open spaces). The investigator places an advertisement in the newspaper asking for subjects. A total of 100 replies are received, of which the investigator randomly selects 30. However, only 15 subjects actually turn up for their appointment.

Questions 4–6 refer to the above information.

4. Which of the following statements is true?

   a The final 15 subjects are likely to be a representative sample of the subjects selected by the investigator
   b The final 15 subjects are likely to be a representative sample of the population of agoraphobics
   c The randomly selected 30 subjects are likely to be a representative sample of those agoraphobics who replied to the newspaper advertisement
   d None of the above is true.

5. The problem with drawing a representative sample of subjects with clinical conditions such as agoraphobia is that:

   a The subjects who consent to participate may be unrepresentative of the target population
   b no sampling strategies are appropriate
   c no complete lists of sufferers' names are usually available
   d a and c.

6. The basic problem confronted by the investigator is that:

   a the accessible population might be different from the target population

SELF ASSESSMENT

b the sample has been chosen using an unethical method

c the sample size was too small

d agoraphobics are impossible to study in a scientific way.

7. Say that it is known that coronary disease occurs twice as frequently among males as females and three times more commonly among over 50-year-olds than those under 50. Given a sample of 120 obtained by quota sampling, how many subjects would you expect to be female and under 50?

a 60
b 40
c 30
d 10

8. Referring to the population in Question 7, and given a sample obtained by stratified random sampling, how many females over 50 would you expect in the sample?

a 40
b 30
c 10
d 5

9. If a study is externally valid then:

a its results can be generalized to other equivalent settings

b it must have been an experiment

c quota sampling must have been used

d all the subjects in the sample must have been equivalent.

10. A random sample is one in which:

a all the elements had an equal chance of selection

b a chance method was used to select the elements included in the sample

c both *a* and *b*

d neither *a* nor *b*.

11. When we say that a study lacks ecological validity we are implying that:

a the study was carried out in a laboratory

b the results cannot be generalized to other settings

c the target population is the same as the accessible population

d all of the above.

12. Pilot studies are useful for establishing:

a the approximate sample size necessary for the investigation

b the appropriateness of the sampling model being employed

c both *a* and *b*

d neither *a* nor *b*.

13. If a pilot study indicates that the effect is likely to be small in relation to the sampling error then the investigator should:

a abandon the research project

b use a relatively small sample

c use a relatively large sample

d use an incidental method of sampling.

4

Causal research and internal validity

INTRODUCTION

Some types of research are purely descriptive: the aim of the investigator is to gather descriptions and measurements about phenomena. For example, we may gather statistics on the incidence of schizophrenia or neonate deaths. However, in the health sciences much research is aimed at identifying the causes of illness and disabilities. It is by understanding these causes that we can formulate and justify our assessments and treatments. Furthermore, we can justify the treatments we use in that we can point to empirical evidence that demonstrates that the treatments are causing the beneficial changes in patients' symptoms. In scientific research, the concept of internal validity is related to the design of research projects.

The specific aims of this chapter are to:

1. Examine the concept of causality.
2. Examine how threats to internal validity generate plausible alternative explanations.
3. Discuss how control arising from correct designs increases internal validity.
4. Discuss some limitations of control in clinical research.

CAUSALITY

In scientific research, we look for the following important criteria for the demonstration of causality:

1. Antecedent occurrence of cause to effect (C occurs before E).

2. Covariation of cause and effect (if C occurs then so does E).
3. Elimination of rival causal explanations of the effect (If C does not occur, then E does not occur).

The first criterion is quite obvious. For example, if we say that injury to the person's arm is the cause of their reported pain, we assume that the injury was sustained prior to the onset of the pain. Clearly, if the pain had been already present, the injury would not be seen as the cause of the pain. Second, we assume that there will be concomitant variation between the injury and the pain. The worse the injury, the more severe the pain. As the injury clears up, a decrease in the level of pain can be expected. In general, we are establishing a lawful functional relationship between the cause and the effect.

However, observing a relationship between two events is not enough to demonstrate causality. Night follows day in a predictable, lawful fashion. But we do not say that day causes the night. In scientific research, we look for *control* over phenomena, so that we can reproduce or change them at will. Of course, such control is not always possible, for instance, in the fields of astronomy, geology and cultural anthropology. One cannot invoke an earthquake or a supernova at will, or return to times past. All we can do is to describe, point out patterns or covariations and then formulate hypotheses and theories which offer a causal explanation for the findings. In particular, we must attempt to eliminate plausible alternative explanations or hypotheses which offer rival causal explanations for the findings. What constitutes plausible alternative explanations changes from situation to situation. However, we will examine some of these in the next subsection, in the context of threats to internal validity.

THREATS TO INTERNAL VALIDITY

Cook and Campbell (1979) defined a number of threats to the internal validity of experiments and quasi-experiments. These threats to internal validity compromise the ability of the researcher to conclude that the different treatments administered to groups of subjects are in fact responsible for the differences or lack of differences observed. Threats to internal validity are in fact sources of alternative explanations for the outcome of an investigation.

These threats to internal validity include:

1. *History*. This refers to events that intervene between the pre-test and post-test (see Ch. 5) that do not form part of the treatment being investigated by the researcher. For example, in a study of the effects of an exercise programme on hypertension, some of the patients might take up additional exercise, such as playing tennis.

2. *Maturation*. In a study over time, the patients may naturally mature. This is a particular problem with paediatric and geriatric populations and studies that are conducted over an extended time period (so called longitudinal studies). In a more general sense, maturation refers to any time-dependent internal changes in patients (for example, an infection clearing up by 'itself').

3. *Testing*. The patient may, as a result of familiarity with the testing procedures, appear to improve spontaneously. These are sometimes called practice effects. For instance, the re-administration of an IQ test might lead to better performance without an actual improvement in the subjects' intellects. Alternatively, a test may be so boring that upon second administration, the patients apparent performance may decline owing to boredom and fatigue.

4. *Instrumentation*. During the time between measurements, the measuring instrument might change, for example, start reading heavier or lighter, leading to apparent improvement or deterioration when no such change has occurred.

5. *Regression to the mean*. This is a special effect that originates from the unreliability of test measures. Often, clinical research involves the selection for study of patients who have achieved particularly low or high scores on one or more measures, for example, the most depressed patients or those with the highest measured cholesterol levels. It is often found that such patient groups, when retested, will show apparent spontaneous improvement or regression towards the mean. This happens because, on the

second measurement, the measurement error tends to be less than on the first measurement. If patients are chosen on the basis of very good or very poor performance on an initial assessment, they are likely to include a number of cases in which measurement error is quite high, and proportionately few with small measurement error. In such cases the regression to the mean phenomenon is a possibility, as on the second measurement there is likely to be, on average, less extreme measurement error.

6. *Selection or assignment errors*. The groups being compared may be different at the outset because of inadequate assignment or selection procedures, rather than as a result of any treatment effects. This might well happen if the subjects were not randomly assigned into treatment groups. If the groups differ before treatment, it is very difficult to attribute differences after treatment to the treatments alone.

7. *Mortality*. You do not have to have anyone die in a study to have mortality. Mortality in a study refers to when a participant withdraws from the study before its completion. There may be more dropouts in one group than in others, making the groups different. For example, subjects in a placebo group might reject an ineffectual treatment and refuse to participate to the conclusion of the study. Since the subjects who drop out might be different from those who stay, the experimental and the control group no longer remain equivalent. Once again, if the groups are different, it is difficult to ascribe these differences to their different treatments.

The following investigation illustrates the effects of some of the above threats to validity. A recent study attempted to demonstrate the effects of an exercise programme in patients with occlusions (blockage) of some of the major arteries in the leg. The *dependent variables* measured included the distance walked by the patient to 'limit of pain tolerance'. The *independent variable* was the exercise programme, which included daily walking, with encouragement to increase the distance daily. Patients were also strongly advised to stop smoking and were given a diet low in animal fats and carbohydrates.

More than half the patients were smokers and reported that their smoking declined markedly by the end of the programme. The method of the experiment involved pre-tests on the dependent variables (including walking), the administration of the treatment, and then a re-test 6 weeks after the programme commenced. The results were not evaluated statistically, but the results (Fig. 4.1) appeared to indicate an increase in the walking distance. The study was done under the guidance of a vascular surgeon, who also selected the patients.

Figure 4.1 shows that there was an increase in the patients' average walking distance. The question here is: 'Was this change in the dependent variable caused by the independent

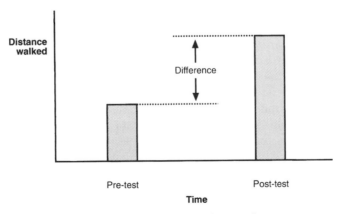

Fig. 4.1   Walking tolerance: before and after exercise programme.

variable or by other uncontrolled extraneous variables?' To answer this question, let us examine some of the possible threats to the internal validity of the study.

1. *History*. The threat here is from simultaneous changes in walking, smoking pattern, and diet; any of which might have been responsible for some or all of the changes in the dependent variable reported in the study.
2. *Maturation*. The degree of this threat depends on the natural history of the illness. Natural improvement in the condition might account for at least some of the difference in walking.
3. *Testing*. Both the pre-test and the exercise programme included walking. It is possible that the difference between pre-test and post-test is simply due to practice effects, the patients becoming more confident in walking to real tolerance limits.
4. *Instrumentation*. This threat is not relevant in this instance, in that no sophisticated or potentially inaccurate measuring devices were used to measure the dependent variable.
5. *Regression to the mean*. Possibly, the vascular surgeon selected extreme cases for the study: those most in need of treatment. Their performances might have drifted back towards the mean on the post-test.
6–7. *Selection errors and mortality*. These threats are not relevant, as no control group was included in the study.

We have not shown that the extraneous variables described above necessarily caused the reported difference. Rather, the point is that, because of the lack of control, the investigator cannot claim that the differences found in the dependent variable *necessarily* reflect changes due to the independent variable, i.e. that the change observed in the outcome measure was *caused* by the treatment.

THE NEED FOR CONTROL

We have seen how uncontrolled extraneous variables can result in plausible alternative explanations for the outcomes of an investigation. In causal research, the adoption of an appropriate design enables us to remove the confounding influences of extraneous variables. If we can do this—correctly attribute any effects we observe and eliminate the effects of other factors—we can say that the experiment is internally valid or has *internal validity*.

In the context of laboratory research, an investigator can use several types of strategy to achieve control over extraneous variables. For example, a physicist studying electrical phenomena will make sure that the apparatus is insulated against extraneous electrical disturbances; a researcher studying bio-feedback would make sure that the subjects were in a noise-insulated, temperature-controlled room. In 'field' research, in applied clinical settings, such tight control is not feasible. Other methods, such as the inclusion of control groups in the design are used to ensure internal validity.

A control group consists of subjects that undergo exactly the same conditions as the group receiving the treatment, the causal effect of which is being investigated. For example, in drug trials control groups will often receive an injection of saline solution if the experimental treatment is administered via injection, in order to control for the effects of actual injection. If the medication were administrated orally, similar-looking inert tablets would be used for control subjects. It has been found that if people receive any form of 'therapy', improvement may occur even when the 'treatment' is physiologically and biochemically inert. The effect is called a *placebo effect*. The control group allows the experimenter to measure the size of this and other effects, and to control for these effects.

If we are to include a control group in our experiments, it is essential that at the outset the experimental and control groups are as similar as possible. We have to take the group of subjects participating in the study and split them up into the experimental and control groups as equally as possible.

The methods we use to decide to which groups the subjects are to be assigned are termed *assignment procedures*. As we have seen in Chapter 2, the assignment of subjects to their groups by the investigator is an essential feature of an experiment. The two main assignment methods used will be discussed in more detail in Chapter 5.

In later chapters, we will see that control is possible for non-experimental designs as well as experimental designs. Control is a matter of degree, rather than an absolute. Even some tightly designed investigations allow for plausible alternative explanations arising from unexpected extraneous variables. Furthermore, a trade-off exists between internal and external validity. In order to maximize internal validity of an experiment, the researcher ought to eliminate as many external influences as possible. In a hypothetical study of resident psychiatric patients, this could include suspension of visits, removal of furniture, cessation of all other medication, elimination of contact with other patients and so on. How representative would this be of everyday life? Could these results be usefully generalized to any other context? Therefore, to ensure the ecological validity of the investigation, we may sacrifice control and, to some extent, internal validity. The inclusion and appropriate use of control groups improves the internal validity of an investigation.

THE USE OF CONTROL GROUPS IN CLINICAL RESEARCH

Let us re-examine the investigation outlined on page 47 and see how it stands up to threats of internal validity, with the use of a control group included in the study.

1. Select the sample of subjects with arterial occlusions to participate in the study. To ensure external validity we would need a better sampling strategy than some surgeon's say-so. However, for ethical reasons the subjects might need to be checked out, to minimize possible adverse side effects of the treatment.
2. Assess the walking distances of the patients in a pretreatment test.
3. Assign subjects into experimental or control groups by matching on basis of pre-test performance, and random assignment within pairs. We will examine such research designs in Chapter 5.
4. Administer:
   (a) experimental treatment (total package of exercise plan, walking, diet and smoking reduction) and
   (b) control treatment (an alternative activity, walking, diet and smoking reduction). The *only* difference between the two groups is that one group receives the exercise programme, and the other some alternative activity.
5. Test both groups on walking distance, following the treatment.

The results of this fictional study are presented in Figure 4.2.

Let us examine how this new design stands up to threats of internal validity in contrast to the original investigation outlined on page 47.

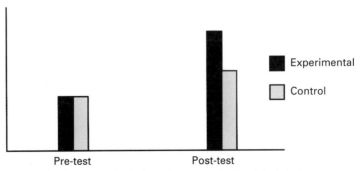

Fig. 4.2 Hypothetical results of a pre-test/post-test study.

1. *History*. Both groups had walking, smoking decrement and diet; it is unlikely that the difference between post-test results shown in Figure 4.2 is due to these variables.
2. *Maturation*. Both control and experimental groups had the same time to recover or deteriorate; it is unlikely that this factor explains the difference.
3. *Testing*. Both groups had the pre-test and the walking; unlikely that this factor explains difference.
4. *Instrumentation*. Not relevant, as discussed on page 48.
5. *Regression to mean*. Both groups were similar on pre-test performance, given that they were matched.
6. *Selection error*. Random or matched assignment would have controlled for this, so initial differences between the two groups is minimized.
7. *Mortality*. This depends on the actual data; internal validity is preserved if drop-out rates are equivalent in the two groups.

We can see that using a design with a control group resulted in an improvement of the internal validity of the investigation. Note that the use of a control group has not removed the effects of history and other extraneous variables in this study. It is still possible, but much less likely, that the differences in the outcomes for the two groups were *not* a result of the different treatments they received. Now the investigator has a much sounder basis for deciding whether or not the exercise programme was effective.

It should be noted that there are ways, other than control groups, to minimize the effects of uncontrolled extraneous variables. For example, if 'noise' is a possible extraneous variable in administering a test, we may 'insulate' from it by using a quiet setting. However, if noisy settings are the norm in real life, then the search for higher internal validity may be at the cost of external validity.

SUMMARY

The demonstration of causality involves the discounting of plausible alternative explanations for the outcome of an investigation. When uncontrolled extraneous variables generate alternative explanations to the research hypothesis then the investigation lacks internal validity. The aim of designing an investigation is to reduce the threats to internal validity. It was shown that when the design includes an appropriate control group, the causal effects of the treatment on the outcome becomes more convincing.

However, in field research involving human subjects, complete control over the phenomena is not possible. To some extent, control might have to be sacrificed in order to ensure the external validity of the results. In the next chapter, we examine a variety of research strategies and the designs used within these strategies aimed at maximizing internal and external validity.

SELF ASSESSMENT

Explain the meaning of the following terms:

    assignment errors
    causality
    causal explanations
    control
    history
    instrumentation
    internal validity

    maturation
    mortality
    regression to the mean
    testing

TRUE OR FALSE

1. It is possible to have an effect occur prior to its cause.

2. If a group of children were found to have improved their reading skills in a long-term treatment programme, it would be easy to eliminate maturation as a rival explanation to treatment for their improvement.
3. If two groups in a study start off on an unequal basis, this would probably be an example of assignment errors.
4. In a test of skill that is easily learned, testing effects are unlikely to be a problem.
5. Control groups will eliminate assignment errors.
6. If the researcher can attribute the outcomes in a study to the treatment programmes employed and not other factors, then the study is internally valid.
7. If a study is internally valid then it must be externally valid.
8. Mortality refers to the difficulty of patients dying while undergoing the treatment programme.
9. Regression to the mean occurs mainly in studies where groups have been selected to participate on the basis of some form of extreme score in a pre-test.
10. Control refers to the need to eliminate alternative conflicting explanations for the outcomes observed in a study.

MULTIPLE CHOICE

1. If a group of participants in a study are selected on the basis of a particularly poor pre-assessment, it is likely that they will appear to 'improve' when reassessed soon after, without any treatment. This phenomenon is known as:

   a regression to the mean
   b maturation
   c history
   d assignment error.

2. If, after a 12-month programme, a group of children with reading problems had improved their reading ages by an average of 9 months, a viable alternative explanation for the results, other than the effectiveness of the programme, would be:

   a regression to the mean
   b maturation
   c history
   d assignment error.

3. If, after the evaluation of the effectiveness of two different rehabilitation programmes, it was found that the participants in the 'better' programme had all attended a disability workshop together, a viable alternative explanation for the results other than the programme would be:

   a regression to the mean
   b maturation
   c history
   d assignment error.

4. If, after the evaluation of the effectiveness of two different rehabilitation programmes, it was found that the participants in the 'better' programme were selected from a less-impaired group, then a viable alternative explanation for the results other than the programme would be:

   a regression to the mean
   b maturation
   c history
   d assignment error.

5. The advantage of including a control or comparison group in a study of treatment effectiveness is that:

   a effects such as maturation can be eliminated
   b effects such as maturation can be reduced
   c effects such as maturation can be measured

SELF ASSESSMENT

d effects such as maturation can be ignored.

6. If a well-designed study demonstrates a convincing advantage of one therapeutic technique over another, but is based on a sample of five people in the two groups, then the study is likely to have:

   a high internal and low external validity
   b high external and low internal validity
   c low internal and external validity
   d high external and internal validity.

7. Those patients that receive inert treatment in a control comparison group yet respond as if they had received real treatment are demonstrating:

   a the placebo effect
   b external validity
   c internal validity
   d regression to the mean.

8. In a long-term treatment study with a single group with no comparison or control group, it is possible to attribute any improvements observed to:

   a the treatment
   b history effects
   c maturation
   d all of the above.

SECTION 2

Discussion, Questions and Answers

Our next discussion question takes us back over 50 years in time, to the setting of the closed psychiatric institutions where persons with serious mental illnesses were often confined under dismal and overcrowded conditions. Psychiatric researchers were desperately seeking new and effective treatments which could enable the residents to return to the community and thus to relieve the pressure on the institutions. A team of Italian researchers, led by the psychiatrist Cerletti, were working on a new technique which they hoped would provide a quick and effective treatment for schizophrenia.

Unfortunately, their research programme was guided by what was later shown to be a false hypothesis: that persons who suffered from epilepsy did not develop schizophrenia. On the basis of this false hypothesis it was predicted that inducing epileptic convulsions would help to reduce the signs and symptoms of schizophrenia. Thus, in the late 1930s thousands of mentally ill persons were administered convulsants, such as the drugs cardiazol and metrazol. The drugs induced convulsions that were difficult to control and proved to be very dangerous. Cerletti argued that the use of electrical shocks to induce epileptic convulsions would be a safer approach than the drugs.

In an article which outlines the historical development of electroshock, Krzyzowski (1989) reported what happened when Cerletti and his assistant Bini first presented these ideas to their colleagues.

Bini, at a conference in Munich in 1936, and Cerletti in the same year in Milan, mention the possible application of electric current to cause therapeutically desired epileptic attacks. The idea was almost unanimously rejected on the grounds of its barbarity and associated hazard. It should be noted that the electric chair had just been introduced in America.

(*Krzyzowski 1989*), *p. 51*.

Despite this hostile reaction, Cerletti and his team continued research into electric shock, experimenting with animals in Rome's slaughterhouses. According to Krzyzwoski (1989, pp. 51–52) the team was ready for their first human subject by 1938.

On April 15 1938, a patient manifesting distinct symptoms of mental illness was admitted into the clinic in Rome after having been arrested by the police for travelling on a train without a ticket. The condition of the patient was then as follows: fully normal orientation, expressed distinct introversion, and persecution delusions often using neologisms. He considered himself to be under telepathic influence directing his behaviour. At the same time he exhibited hallucinations thematically related to the delusions. He was depressed and altered neurological conditions were found. Schizophrenia was diagnosed.

Having selected their first subject, the team administered the first ECT (electroconvulsive therapy) procedure.

Two electrodes were attached symmetrically in the vicinity of the crown and forehead and then a relatively low 80 V current was passed for 1.5 s. On switching the current on, the patient sat upright on the bed, his muscles contracted and he fell back onto the bed, not losing consciousness, however. He cried out for a while and then became quiet.

It appeared that the voltage applied was too low to induce the convulsion required for the therapeutic effectiveness of the ECT procedure. What happened next is discussed by Krzyzowski:

Continuation of the treatment was postponed until the next day. The patient, on hearing of such suggestions, roused himself and shouted normally: 'No more. It could kill me'. The words were spoken aloud normally, while previously he used only a specific and hardly understandable jargon, self-devised and full of neologisms. This normal utterance confirmed and assured Cerletti of the effectiveness of the method and, in spite of the strong reservations

Discussion, Questions and Answers

of his assistants, he decided to repeat the ECT without delay. This time a 110 V current with a pulse duration of 1.5 s was used. Once again a short lived, general contraction of all muscles was observed followed by a full classic epileptic type attack of convulsions. All those present uneasily watched the pallidness and cyanosis accompanying the attack, relaxing as the patient gradually recovered.

The story, you will be pleased to hear, had a happy ending.

After prolonged treatment consisting of 11 full and 3 incomplete shocks, the patient was discharged from the clinic in good health. At follow-up a year later, the mental state of the patient was seen to be good and stable. Subsequent years evidenced a widening application of ECT.

(Krzyzwoski 1989, p. 52)

As a matter of interest, ECT is still used by contemporary psychiatrists, but in a greatly modified fashion:

- it is used with anesthetized patients, with electrodes placed only on one side of the head
- it is not used with persons with schizophrenia (for whom it was found to be ineffective) but rather with persons who are profoundly depressed.
- It is used as a 'last resort' when current pharmaceutical treatments are ineffective.

Questions

The following questions concerning research planning are related to the above narrative:

1. On the basis of the information given propose aims and/or hypotheses which might have guided the above study.
2. Given the state of psychiatric knowledge and practice of the late 1930s; do you think the above study was justified?
3. Give 3 or 4 reasons why a contemporary ethics committee might reject such a research project.
4. By present ethical standards, what should have been done after the patient shouted

'No more, it could kill me'?
5. Cerletti proceeded with a more severe shock on the grounds that the previous shock 'improved' the patient's condition. Comment on this logic, in the context of scientific methodology?
6. Do you think such dangerous experiments are ever justified in the context of health care? If yes, under what conditions?
7. Discuss 2 or 3 problems with the 'internal validity' (Ch. 4) of this study. Suggest simple changes in 'control' which may help to improve internal validity.
8. Comment on the 'external validity' of this study in the light of the fact that subsequent studies ECT was shown to be ineffectual as a treatment for schizophrenia.
9. Do you think Cerletti and his colleagues were guided by a rather simplistic paradigm of schizophrenia? Explain, by comparing the biomedical and biopsychosocial approaches discussed in Section 1.

Answers

1. The research seems to have been guided by several interrelated aims and/or hypotheses.
   (a) The first aim was to find the electrical shock intensity that was sufficient to induce an epileptic seizure in a human.
   (b) The second aim was to demonstrate that the seizure did not result in death or disability; that is, that the treatment was 'safe'.
   (c) The hypothesis implicit in the research might be stated as: 'A course of ECT is effective for reducing the signs and symptoms of schizophrenia'.
   You may be able to suggest other aims and hypotheses. None of the outcomes was stated precisely in the paper quoted.
2. As you may have judged from this brief

Discussion, Questions and Answers

excerpt, the state of knowledge concerning the biological causes of mental illness was confused and had a weak empirical basis. Biological treatments, such as drug-induced epileptic seizures were poorly theorized, dangerous and generally ineffective. In this context, in the late 1930s, it could be argued that experimenting with new and safer treatments was justified.

3. We outlined some relevant ethical guidelines in Chapter 2 in terms of which the present study would be judged as problematic, e.g. questionable benefits for patients, lack of informed consent, dangerous and painful intervention, lack of consultation with the relatives/guardians of a mentally ill person.

4. Obviously, discontinue the research. Even though the person was confused when admitted to the hospital, his request was rational and reasonable. There was no doubt whatsoever concerning the patient's desires, and by present ethical standards researchers must comply with such requests.

5. The first electrical shock did not induce the epileptic convulsion which was postulated as the factor 'causing' the therapeutic change. As the first shock simply hurt the man, there was no theoretical or empirical justification for his apparent improvement being due to this shock.

6. One could argue that risking people's health and lives in the context of 'heroic' medicine is never justified. Rather, we should look to prevention or gentler, more natural treatments.
The other point of view is that aggressive medical treatment is justified if there are incapacitating and chronic problems, such as schizophrenia. According to this approach, painful and potentially harmful experimental treatments are justified provided that the study is well designed

and the participants are well informed and have consented.

7. The issue is whether or not the apparent improvement in the patient's condition was due to the ECT or to other 'extraneous' factors or variables. There are several possibilities which provide plausible alternative explanations, such as:
   (a) *History.* The patient may have been frightened by the treatment and 'pretended' to be better to escape the situation
   (b) *Maturation.* The patient may have recovered anyway, their condition may be cyclical
   (c) *Testing or instrumentation.* There may have been inaccuracies and bias in the way in which the patient's condition was assessed.
   Control may be introduced by using groups of persons who have (a) no treatment and/or (b) another treatment for schizophrenia. The appropriate designs for showing causal effects are outlined in Section 3. However because of the poorly designed research in the area, there were almost 2 decades of useless treatments before it became evident that ECT was not an effective treatment for schizophrenia.

8. Clearly, there was no evidence that the improvement claimed in this study was caused by ECT. In addition, it is tricky to make inferences from unrepresentative samples to populations. In this study, the patient may have shown symptoms of depression, which perhaps responded to the treatment. But this may not be generalizable to persons who show other patterns of schizophrenia. External validity is ensured by appropriate sampling procedures (Ch. 3) and clear operational definition and assessment of the condition, as outlined in Chapter 12. Without

Discussion, Questions and Answers

appropriate sampling and assessment procedures, we may use inappropriate treatments, unsuitable for the specific needs of our patients.

9. The researchers were working in the context of a 'biomedical' model, assuming that schizophrenia was simply a biological disorder which could be suddenly cured by an heroic treatment such as ECT. A biopsychosocial approach takes a more complex view of chronic disorders, and research programmes include identifying and treating both psychological disabilities and social handicaps entailed in schizophrenia. Biopsychosocial research may involve both quantitative and qualitative methods.

Research designs

In the previous section, we identified broad categories of descriptive (non-experimental) and causal (experimental) strategies for conducting research. The aim of Section 3 is to discuss these issues in more detail, by examining various research designs and outlining their applications for conducting health sciences research. As in other areas of creative human activity such as architecture or the fashion industry, *designs* refer to explicit plans for completing an object or an activity.

The conceptual basis for experiments is the need for control, as outlined in Chapter 4. In experimental research (see Ch. 5) we manipulate one or more variables (independent variables), while controlling the extraneous variables, by using appropriate controls such as control groups. If the experiment is well designed and properly conducted we are in a position to demonstrate the causal effects of the independent variables on the outcome or dependent variables. The random assignment of subjects to experimental groups is a common way to achieve control. However, health and illness outcomes often have multiple and interacting causes requiring multivariate experimental designs.

Another issue we need to address is reactivity of human beings to social situations, such as being involved in research. Well-designed experiments attempt to control for the biases of both the subjects and the experimenters involved in a research project.

There are situations where for practical or ethical reasons we cannot randomly assign subjects to control or treatment groups. Here we use quasi-experimental methods which involve comparing pre-existing groups undergoing different treatments (see Ch. 5). There are other research designs discussed in Chapter 6, including naturalistic comparisons, correlational designs and surveys. Naturalistic comparisons and correlational designs enable us to describe and predict relationships among variables, but should be used only with extreme caution in attempting to understand causal effects. Surveys that include the use of questionnaires and interviews to study a person's knowledge, attitudes and beliefs concerning aspects of health and illness are essentially a tool for descriptive research. The accuracy of the information collected within the framework of non-experimental designs depends to a large extent on the use of appropriate sampling strategies for selecting the subjects.

An interesting and commonly used design in clinical settings is the $n = 1$ or 'single case' design. The advantage is that using $n = 1$ designs we may be able to demonstrate causal effects using only one or two subjects, without the need for separate control groups. The major limitation of $n = 1$ (and other types of clinical case studies) is that the findings may not be generalizable to other cases or situations.

Chapter 8 describes some of the elementary characteristics of qualitative 'field research' designs. This chapter aims to compare and contrast quantitative and qualitative research, and describes the importance of qualitative research for understanding the personal experiences of our clients and/or patients. Specific qualitative designs (such as indepth interviewing and participant observation) and strategies for interpretive data analysis are outlined in Section 4.

5

Experimental designs

INTRODUCTION

Experimental research involves the active manipulation of variables under the control of the researcher. These are termed *independent variables*. The experimental approach attempts to study how subjects or phenomena will react to the manipulated conditions through monitoring one or more outcome measures. The outcome variables are termed *dependent variables*. If an experiment is well designed, the experimenter may, in principle, detect causal relationships between the independent and the dependent variables. However, there are many threats to the satisfactory detection of such relationships.

The experimental approach has been used extensively in the 'hard' sciences and therefore is worthy of close study.

The specific aims of this chapter are to:

1. Examine the basic structure of experimental research designs.
2. Consider threats to the validity of the results obtained from experiments.
3. Discuss how researchers and participant may react to experimental situations.

EXPERIMENTAL RESEARCH

Experimental studies involve the following steps:

1. *Definition of the population.* Researchers define the population to which they wish to generalize. For example, this might be males over 55 years with coronary heart disease or the

local community or a certain type of health care organization.

2. *Selection of the sample.* Using an appropriate sampling method, the sample is selected from the population. It is important that the sample is representative of the population. (It is important to note that steps 1 and 2 are common to most research designs and have been previously discussed in detail.)

3. *Assignment procedures.* Using an assignment procedure, the participants are allocated to groups. For example, in an experimental study of the effectiveness of different types of weight-loss programme, one group might receive an instructional manual, another might receive supervised dietary training, and others may receive no treatment. The purpose of the assignment procedure is to ensure that the groups are as similar as possible or equivalent to begin with. If they are substantially different, it will be very difficult to attribute any differences in final outcome to the 'treatments' administered. That is, internal validity will be under threat.

4. *Administration of intervention (treatment).* The researcher then administers the intervention(s) to the various groups participating in the experiment. This is called the independent variable(s). It is important that the intervention is administered in an unbiased way, in order that a fair test of any differences in outcomes may be provided. As will be discussed later, awareness of the expected outcomes on the part of participants often leads to a spurious promotion of the phenomena under study. Therefore, the true aims and expectations of the researcher are sometimes concealed from the participants.

5. *Measurement of outcomes.* The researcher assesses the outcome of the experiment through measurement of the dependent variable. Sometimes, the dependent variable is measured both before and after the experimental intervention (pre-test, post-test) and other times only afterwards (post-test only).

Thus, in an experimental study the researcher actively manipulates the independent variable(s) and monitors outcomes through measurement of the dependent variable(s).

Assignment of subjects into groups

The most straightforward approach is to assign the subjects randomly to *independent* groups. Say, for instance, we were interested in the effects of a specific drug (we will call this Drug A) in helping to relieve the symptoms of depression. We also decide to have a placebo control group, which involves giving patients a capsule identical to A, but without the active ingredient.

Given a sample size of say 20, we would assign each subject randomly to either the experimental (Drug A) or the control group (placebo control). In this case, we would end up with the two treatment groups:

Levels of the independent variables

	Control group (Placebo)	Experimental group (Drug A)
Number of subjects	$n_c = 10$	$n_e = 10$

Here n_c and n_E of course refer to the number in each of the groups, given that the total sample size (n) was 20.

Matched groups

Random assignment *does not guarantee* that the two groups will be equivalent, rather the argument is that there is no reason that the groups should be different. While this is true in the long run, with rather small sample sizes even chance differences among the groups may have an impact on the results of an experiment. Matched assignment of the subjects into groups minimizes group differences caused by chance variation.

For example, following the hypothetical example discussed previously, say that the experimenter required that the two groups should be equivalent for the measure of depression being used in the experiment. Here the subjects would be assessed for level of depression before the treatment and paired for scores from highest to lowest. Subsequently, the two subjects in each pair would be randomly assigned to either the experimental groups or the placebo. In this way, the two groups would be the same for the average pre-test scores on depression.

DIFFERENT EXPERIMENTAL DESIGNS

Three types of experimental design will be discussed. These are the pre-test/post- test, post-test only and factorial designs.

Pre-test/post-test design

In this design, measurements of the outcome or dependent variables are taken both before and after intervention. This allows the measurement of actual changes for individual cases. However, the measurement process itself may produce change, thereby introducing difficulties in the clear attribution of change to the intervention on its own. For example, in an experimental study of weight loss, simply administering a questionnaire concerning dietary habits may lead to changes in those habits by encouraging people to scrutinize their own behaviour and hence modify it. Alternatively, in measures of skill, there may be a practice effect such that, without any intervention, the performance on a second test will improve. In order to overcome these difficulties, many researchers turn to the post-test only design.

Post-test only design

At first it may appear that this would make measurement of change impossible. At an individual level this is certainly true. However, if we assume that the control and experimental groups were initially identical and that no change had occurred in the controls, direct comparison of the post-test scores will indicate the extent of the change.

This type of design is fraught with danger in clinical research and should only be used in special circumstances, such as when pre-test measures are impossible or unethical to carry out. The assumptions of initial equivalence and of no change in the control group often may not be supported and, in such cases, interpretation of group differences is difficult and ambiguous.

Table 5.1 Example of a factorial design

	Drug A	No drug
Rogerian therapy	1	2
No psychological treatment	3	4

Factorial designs

A researcher will often not be content with the manipulation of one variable in isolation. For example, a clinical psychologist may wish to manipulate both the type of psychological therapy and the use of drug therapy for a group of patients. Let us assume that they were interested in the effects of therapy versus no psychological treatment, and of drug A versus no treatment. These two variables lead to four possible combinations of treatment (see Table 5.1).

This design enables us to investigate the separate and combined effects of both independent variables upon the dependent measure(s). If all possible combinations of the values or levels of the independent variables are included in the study, the design is said to be *fully crossed*. If one or more is left out, it is said to be *incomplete*. With an incomplete factorial design, there are some difficulties in determining the complete joint and seperate effects of the independent variables.

In order that the terminology in experimental designs is clear, it is instructive to consider the way in which research methodologists would describe the example design in Table 5.1 This is a study with two independent variables (sometimes called factors), namely, type of psychological therapy and drug treatment. Each independent variable or factor has two levels or values. In the case of psychological therapy, the two levels are Rogerian therapy and no psychological therapy. This would commonly be described as a 2 by 2 design (each factor having two levels). There are four groups (2 × 2) in the design.

If a third level, drug B, was added to the drug factor, then it would become a 2 by 3 design with six groups required. Two groups, drug B with Rogerian therapy and drug B with no psychological therapy, would be added. It is possible to overdo the number of factors and levels in experimental studies. A $4 \times 4 \times 4$ design would require 64 groups: that is a lot of subjects to find for a study.

Repeated measures and independent groups

In order to economize with the number of subjects required in an experimental design, the researchers will sometimes re-use subjects in the design. Thus, at different times the subjects may receive, say, drug A or drug B. If it were the case that every subject encountered more than one level of the drug variable or factor, then 'drug' would be termed a repeated measures factor. An important consideration is using a 'counter-balanced' design to avoid series effects. For example, half the subjects should receive drug A first, and half drug B. If *all* the subjects received drug A first and then drug B, the study would *not* be counterbalanced and we would not be able to determine whether the order of administration of the drugs was important. Time is a common repeated measures factor in many studies. A pre-test post-test design involves the measurement of the same subjects twice. If 'time' is included in the analysis of the study, then this is a repeated measures factor. In statistical analysis, repeated measures factors are treated differently from factors where each level is represented by a separate, independent group (see Ch. 19). This is true *both* for matched groups discussed earlier as well as for repeated measures discussed above.

Multiple dependent variables

Just as it is possible to have multiple independent variables in an experimental study, it is also permissible to have multiple outcome or dependent measures. For example, in order to assess the effectiveness of an intervention such as icing of an injury, factors such as extent of oedema and area of bruising might both be important outcome measures. In this instance, there would be two dependent measures.

It is nevertheless true that the statistical treatment of studies with two or more outcome measures (multivariate designs) can be somewhat

problematic, and hence researchers are often more disposed towards multiple independent variables than multiple dependent variables.

EXTERNAL VALIDITY OF EXPERIMENTS

We have already discussed external validity in Chapter 3. There are further criteria for ensuring the generalizability of an investigation, depending on the procedures used, and the interaction between the patients and the therapist.

The Rosenthal effect

A series of classic experiments by Rosenthál (1976) and other researchers have shown the importance of expectancy effects, where the expectations of the experimenter are conveyed to the experimental subject. This type of expectancy effect has been termed the *Rosenthal effect* and is best explained by consideration of some of the original literature in this area.

Rosenthal and his colleagues performed an experiment involving the training of two groups of rats in a maze learning task. A bright strain and a dull strain of rats, specially bred for the purpose, were trained by undergraduate student experimenters to negotiate the maze. After a suitable training interval, the relative performances of the two groups were compared. Not surprisingly, the bright strain significantly outperformed the dull strain.

However, what is surprising is that, the two strains were not different. The two groups of rats were genetically identical. The researchers had deceived the student experimenters for the purposes of the study. The students' expectations of the rats had resulted in different methods of treatment which had affected the rats' learning ability. These results have been confirmed time and time again in a variety of experimental settings, and with a variety of subjects.

If the Rosenthal effect is so pervasive how can we control for its effects? One method of control is to ensure that the subjects do not know the true purpose of the study, that is, the experimental hypothesis. This can be done by withholding information—just not telling people what you are doing—or by deception.

Deception is riskier and less ethical. Most organizations engaged in research activity have ethics committees which take a dim view of this sort of approach. Whatever the mechanism, if the subjects are unaware of the hypothesis being tested we say that they were *blind* to the hypothesis.

Often, however, blinding of the subjects is not enough. In many studies it is critical that the person taking the measurements, administering the treatments, etc., is also blinded. Thus, if both the experimenter (not the researcher) and the subjects do not know the researcher's hypothesis, we say that *double blinding* has been employed. Both subject expectations and experimenter expectations are Rosenthal effects.

Hawthorne effect

Quite apart from the issue of the expectations of participants in experimental studies, there is the issue of whether the attention paid to subjects in the experimental setting alters behaviour.

In the late 1920s, a group of researchers at the Western Electric Hawthorne Works in Chicago were investigating the effects of lighting, heating and other physical conditions upon the productivity of production workers. Much to the surprise of the researchers, the productivity of the workers kept improving independently of the actual physical conditions. Even with dim lighting, productivity reached new highs. It was obvious that the improvements observed were not due to the manipulations of the independent variables themselves, but some other aspect of the experimental situation. The researchers concluded that there was a facilitation effect caused by the presence of the researchers; perhaps the workers were afraid they would lose their jobs. This type of effect has been labelled the Hawthorne effect and is prevalent in many settings.

Of particular interest to us is the manifestation of the Hawthorne effect in clinical research settings. It must be taken into account that even 'inert' treatments might result in significant improvements in the patient's condition. The existence of the placebo effect reinforces the importance of having adequate controls in applied clinical research. Although we cannot eliminate it, we can at least measure the size of it through observation of the control group, and evaluate the experimental results accordingly.

WHEN SHOULD EXPERIMENTAL STUDIES BE USED?

Some philosophers and methodologists would say 'never'. This position is adopted by those who argue that by intervening in the situation under study, the experimenter irrevocably changes it. This is an extreme position and not a terribly popular one in the health sciences since intervention in natural situations in an attempt to ameliorate conditions may be considered to be the primary activity of health scientists.

There are many situations in which the experimental approach is the best available. The study of the effectiveness of interventions is an area of particular suitability, often allowing definitive conclusions about the relative effectiveness of different treatment approaches to be reached. The control of extraneous factors provided in a well-designed and executed experiment strengthens the conclusions reached.

There are many situations in which other approaches are better suited. For example, if it is wished to estimate the health needs and wants of a community, experimental methods would be less suitable than, say, survey or observational approaches.

It is a matter of matching the research aims with an appropriate investigation method. If these aims include the study of the effects of interventions, especially in clinical populations, then experimental methods are a prime candidate. However, in many studies, experimental designs are implemented with an emphasis upon the maximization of internal rather than external validity. That is, the results are methodologically pure but of doubtful validity in the field. This is not an inherent feature of the experimental approach, but a common failing.

SUMMARY

The experimental approach involves the active manipulation of the independent variable(s) and the measurement of outcome through the dependent variable(s). Good experimental design requires careful sampling, assignment and measurement procedures to maximize both internal and external validity.

The Hawthorne and Rosenthal effects are important factors affecting the validity of experimental studies, and we attempt to control for these by 'blinding', when ethically possible.

Common experimental designs include the pre-test/post-test, post-test only and factorial approaches. These designs ensure that investigations can show causal effects.

SELF ASSESSMENT

Explain the meaning of the following terms:

> control group
> factorial design
> Hawthorne effect
> history
> independent variable
> internal validity
> instrumentation
> matching
> mathematical model
> maturation
> mortality
> physical model
> pre-test/post-test design
> post-test only design
> random assignment
> Rosenthal effect
> selection error

TRUE OR FALSE

1. The dependent variable is the variable measured by the investigator.
2. Selection or assignment error arise when, after the assignment of the subjects, the groups are not equivalent.
3. If in a clinical investigation more people die in the control group than the experimental group, the investigation lacks internal validity.
4. Ideally, the control group and the experimental group should receive exactly the same treatments.
5. Given that a placebo is an inert substance, its administration has no effects on the subjects' behaviours.
6. The random assignment of subjects is always preferable to assignment by matching.
7. Persons can serve as their own controls.
8. We reduce the effects of subject and experimenter expectancies by blindfolding.

MULTIPLE CHOICE

1. The aim of controlled observation is to:

   a remove the effects of confounding influences
   b identify the effects of the independent variable on the dependent variable
   c establish causal relationships
   d all of the above.

2. To say that an investigation lacks internal validity means that:

   a the independent variable had no effect
   b the dependent variable was not measured
   c uncontrolled variables may have affected the outcome
   d there were several dependent variables.

3. Which of the following is most representative of a placebo effect?

   a Headache is reduced when an anti-depressant is administered
   b Headache is reduced one second after

swallowing an analgesic, well before it is absorbed by the body

c Headache is increased after a fierce argument with a 'significant other'

d Headache is decreased after the use of biofeedback.

A researcher is studying the effect of a new drug on healing of ulcers. Patients are assigned randomly, by the physician who treats them, to receive either the standard treatment or the new drug. Patients are informed that they are being studied, but they do not know which treatment they are getting. The measure of rate of healing is the number of days until the ulcer is completely healed.

4. The independent variable in the above study was:

   a ulcers
   b the new drug
   c type of treatment
   d rate of healing.

5. The dependent variable in the above study was:

   a ulcers
   b the new drug
   c type of treatment
   d rate of healing.

6. This study is:

   a double blind because the patients do not know what treatment they are getting or which is expected to be more effective
   b double blind because neither the researcher nor the patients know what treatment each person is getting
   c single blind because the patients do not know what treatment they are getting but the physician who treats them does
   d not blind at all as the patients know they are being studied.

7. Which of the following threats to internal validity is not controlled for in this study?

   a maturation
   b regression to the mean
   c repeated testing
   d history
   e none of the above.

8. This investigation is an example of:

   a an experiment, because patients are assigned randomly
   b a study, because the treating doctor did the assigning
   c an experiment, because two treatments are compared
   d a study, because there is no control group.

9. If an experiment is internally valid, this means that:

   a the study's results cannot be generalized to other equivalent settings
   b the sampling method is appropriate
   c the study is not really an experiment
   d the independent variable is responsible for any trends observed
   e the dependent variable has face validity.

A researcher wishes to study the effectiveness of a new drug for treating arthritis. Subjects are selected randomly from patients attending a clinic and are assigned randomly to treatment with the new drug (A) or with the current standard treatment (B). A pre-test/post-test design is used. A number of arthritic symptoms is assessed using a checklist of seven items.

10. The dependent variable in this study is:

   a the number of arthritic symptoms
   b the new drug
   c the method of assignment
   d the type of treatment.

SELF ASSESSMENT

11. The independent variable in this study is:

    a the number of arthritic symptoms
    b the new drug
    c the method of assessment
    d the type of treatment.

12. The actual outcome of the study is illustrated by the following graph. Even though the subjects were assigned randomly, the graph indicates possible threat(s) to internal validity due to:

    a maturation
    b regression to the mean
    c assignment
    d b and c
    e all of the above.

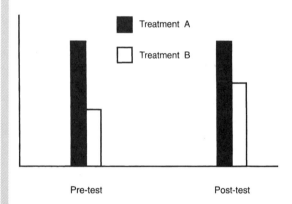

Pre-test   Post-test

13. A factorial design involves:

    a more than one independent variable
    b more than one dependent variable
    c only one independent variable, but with more than one level
    d no control group
    e none of the above.

14. Simulation research means:

    a using computers to analyze data
    b studying differences between different artificial limbs

    c studying a model of a situation to reach conclusions about a situation
    d pretending to research one behaviour while actually studying another.

15. An appropriate design for an investigation will be one which:

    a minimizes all possible sources of error
    b is experimental
    c gives you the answer you expect
    d none of the above.

16. If a study is externally valid, then:

    a it must have been an experiment
    b the dependent variable has face validity
    c it cannot be internally valid
    d its results can be generalized to other equivalent settings.

17. The placebo effect:

    a happens only in drug studies
    b occurs in experimental as well as control groups
    c is another name for relaxing subjects
    d occurs only if you do not have double blinding.

18. Random selection of subjects in a study is typically employed to:

    a maximize generality of the results
    b minimize random measurement error
    c control assignment errors
    d minimize Rosenthal effect
    e minimize Hawthorne effect.

19. Random assignment of subjects in an experiment is typically employed to:

    a minimize random measurement error
    b minimize Rosenthal effect
    c minimize Hawthorne effect

d ensure that the experimental and control groups are similar at the outset

e maximize generality of the results.

20. The principal advantage of a factorial design is that:

a all important factors are taken into account

b only one factor is considered

c the dependent variable is more reliable

d the joint effects of two or more independent variables may be assessed

e the independent variable has more levels.

6

Surveys and quasi-experimental designs

INTRODUCTION

In the previous chapter, the basic features of the experiment were presented. Experiments, when properly designed and implemented, allow the study of causal relationships between variables. However, the detection of causal relationships may not be the goal of the researcher and, even if it is, experimental procedures may not be feasible. Most health sciences research does not use the experimental design. Bloch (1987) reported that of the 757 articles on back pain published in 1985, only eight employed a randomized control (experimental) design. In this chapter we will examine a variety of 'naturalistic' approaches used for investigation of phenomena which do not lend themselves to true experimental designs.

The specific aims of this chapter are to:

1. Examine the uses of naturalistic designs.
2. Discuss the use of surveys in health sciences research.
3. Outline the characteristics of designs involving naturalistic comparisons, correlations and quasi-experiments
4. Identify some of the limitations of naturalistic designs.

NATURALISTIC DESIGNS

If experimental designs provide the tightest possible control, why should we resort to alternative methods? There are a number of reasons why non-experimental research designs may be employed instead of experimental designs.

1. Many variables are not amenable to experimental manipulation. For example, if the research question is concerned with sex differences in responses to heart surgery, then sex cannot be manipulated by the researcher. Similarly, if the researcher is interested in age differences, the ages of the participants cannot be altered by her or him. Many such variables cannot be manipulated and hence cannot be incorporated in this way in an experimental study.
2. Often, it is ethically inappropriate to investigate research questions using an experimental design. For example, if a researcher wished to perform a study on the effects of smoking upon health, to do this in an experimental design would require the experimenter to randomly allocate participants to the smoking or non- smoking group, i.e. force some to smoke and others to not smoke. In experimental designs using a non-treatment control group, valuable and effective treatment might be withheld from participants. Would you agree to be harmed for the sake of science?
3. Experiments are best used to study simple causal relationships between variables. Yet, many human diseases and illnesses are not determined by a single cause but rather by a number of causes interacting in a complex fashion. For example, heart disease may be caused by factors such as smoking, excessive stress, inappropriate diet or genetic factors. To identify such possible causal (or risk) factors, we need to study systems as they function in nature. That is, we should investigate patients in their natural setting, even with the difficulties this entails.

Therefore, we use naturalistic designs when experimental methods are inappropriate, as a result of the nature of the characteristics of the variables or individuals being investigated.

SURVEYS

Surveys are investigations aimed at describing accurately the characteristics of populations for specific variables (see Fig. 2.1). Surveys are commonly used in health care research for the following purposes:

1. To establish the attitudes, opinions or beliefs of persons concerning health related issues. The data collection techniques often include questionnaires or interviews (see Chs 9 and 10).
2. To study characteristics of populations on health related variables, such as utilization of health care, blood pressure, emotional problems or drug use patterns.
3. To collect information about the demographic characteristics (age, sex, income, etc.) of populations. A government census can be an important source of knowledge concerning population characteristics.

The statistics obtained from the above types of surveys present us with an overview of the state of health, illness and treatment patterns in a given community. In this way, we can gain insights into issues such as the prevalent causes of death or the health related requirements of the population. The above statistics might present us with patterns in the data, that is, significant differences or interrelationships. Such patterns can be the bases for hypotheses and theories concerning the causes of illness in a community. The area of health science concerned with such matters is called *epidemiology*.

NATURALISTIC COMPARISONS AND CORRELATIONAL STUDIES

We can use surveys to study differences or interrelationships between health related variables in select populations.

Naturalistic comparison

Essentially, this type of survey or study involves the comparison of two or more naturally occurring groups or populations, in relation to one or more measures. For example, a researcher may be interested in the relative performances of males and females on a test of spatial abilities. The researcher might take a sample of each sex studying at a university and then compare the relative performances of the males and females on the test. Alternatively, a researcher might be interested in whether people growing up in different cultures have different pain reactions. Here, the researcher would select a sample of volunteers from the cultural groups of interest and compare their pain responses to standard noxious stimuli.

There are extraneous variables which can be controlled in this type of investigation. In both studies, the researcher could (and should) control variables such as the ages or educational backgrounds of the subjects. Note, however, that the researchers have not manipulated the variables being studied. All that has been done is to measure differences between naturally occurring groups, whereas in a true experiment, the independent variable is actively manipulated by the researcher. One could not seriously claim that the researcher had manipulated the sexes or the cultures of the participants. It is important to maintain this distinction between experimental and natural comparison studies. Although there is a similarity in that groups are compared, in the experiment the researcher actively controls who receives what treatment. In a natural comparison study, there is no such control and groups may differ in many uncontrolled variables other than the one chosen by the researcher.

To relate this to our first example, if our researcher determines that there is indeed a statistically significant difference in the performance of males and females on the measure(s) chosen, well and good. If our researcher then claims that biological factors are solely responsible for the differences, this is another matter altogether. This inference is only one of a number of alternative explanations that could be advanced to account for the differences observed. It is possible, for instance, that males and female in a sample have been exposed to different types of toys and games during their development, so that males might perform better or worse on some tasks. In the second example, any significant results in the pain responses might not be due to 'culture', but rather to systematic biological differences among the

groups or a complicated interaction between these factors.

The simple fact of the matter is that it is impossible to unequivocally determine causation in natural comparison studies. However, with logically interrelated studies, investigators may gain crucial information about the differences between groups on clinically relevant measures. Natural comparison studies are vital components of the researcher's methodological tools.

Correlational studies

The aim of correlational studies in the health sciences is to identify *interrelationships* among clinically significant variables. The term 'correlation' will be examined in detail in Chapter 16. At this point, let us just say that correlation expresses numerically the strength of association that might exist between two or more variables.

Let us look at a simple illustration of correlational studies. Say that clinical observations indicate that people who suffer from coronary heart disease tend to be overweight. Such observations might generate the hypothesis: 'there is a significant positive correlation between being overweight and the probability of coronary heart disease.'

Here, the investigator will need to draw a representative sample of the population of interest (500 men and 500 women randomly selected from a population of healthy men and women aged 40 living in a specified district). The next step would be to determine the values of the first variable, that is, the subjects' weights and heights. These measures might be monitored over a period of time to check for drastic changes in weight. The second variable would be measured by the criterion of whether or not the subject suffered from heart disease during a specified period (e.g. 10 years) representing the length of the study. The incidence of coronary disease can then be converted into a probability for a particular category of weight (see Table 6.1.)

It can be seen from Table 6.1 that the higher an individual scores on one variable (percentage overweight) the higher the scores on the other

Table 6.1 Fictional data representing the relationship between variables 'percentage overweight' and 'probability of coronary heart disease' (for a 10-year period)

Percentage overweight	Number of subjects	Number suffering coronary heart disease	Probability of coronary heart disease
Underweight or normal	600	30	30/600 = 0.05
10–19% overweight	200	20	20/200 = 0.10
20–29% overweight	100	15	15/100 = 0.15
30–39% overweight	75	20	20/75 = 0.27
40% or more overweight	25	10	10/25 = 0.40

variable (probability of coronary heart disease). In this way, the fictional data presented in Table 6.1 are consistent with the predictions of the hypothesis stated above.

Two points should be considered at this stage. First, no evidence has been presented that one variable is *causally* related to another. This sort of investigation does not, by itself, allow us to conclude that, for instance, 'being overweight causes coronary heart disease'. There are several alternative hypotheses, such as 'stress causes both being overweight and heart disease', which can also account for the findings. Second, it is clear that, at least for the period of the investigation, the variable 'percentage overweight' does not account for all of the other variable 'probability of coronary heart disease'. That is, according to the data presented in Table 6.1, there are normal or underweight individuals who suffer from coronary heart disease and very overweight people who do not. Clearly, there must be other variables which are also related to the incidence of coronary heart disease. In fact, we find that there are many other variables, such as smoking, blood cholesterol level, personality type, stress and family history of heart disease, which also correlate with the probability of coronary heart disease.

Some human diseases, for example, lung cancer and chronic back pain, have complex, interacting causes. Natural comparisons and correlational designs can help us to identify risk factors, that is, variables which *might* be causally related to the onset or progress of these illnesses.

QUASI-EXPERIMENTAL DESIGNS

If clinical interventions are to be undertaken to reduce the risk factors associated with a disease, then clinicians require reasonable evidence that these factors are, in fact, causally related to the disease. Quasi-experimental designs are often used for this purpose.

Quasi-experimental designs can resemble experiments, with the important difference that there is no random assignment into treatment groups. However, the investigator can control the time at which a treatment is introduced or withdrawn. One such method is time-series design.

Time-series designs

Time-series designs involve repeated observations before and after a given treatment. In this way, changes in the sequence of observations following the introduction of a treatment may represent the effects of the treatment on the observed variable. Let us look at an example illustrating the use of time series designs in health sciences research.

Returning to the risk factor of 'being overweight' we discussed previously, the following investigation using a time-series design could provide evidence for a causal relationship between this variable and cardiac disease.

1. Select an appropriate population to study.
2. Specify the dependent variable, that is, some clear-cut measure of 'coronary heart disease'. A commonly used measure may be the incidence of the disease. By 'incidence' we mean the number of new cases of the disease reported in relation to the population within a specified period of time (for example, 50 per 100 000; 1 year).
3. Introduce an appropriate treatment which

reduces the magnitude of the risk factor. In our example, a health promotion package could be introduced, emphasizing exercise and good eating habits. Let us assume that this intervention is adequately financed and a significant proportion of the population adheres to the programme. It could then be hypothesized that: introduction of the health promotion package will result in a decrease in the incidence of coronary heart disease in the community.

4. Monitor the dependent variable over a period of time. It is essential to have readings of the variable both before and after the introduction of treatment. In this instance, the incidence of coronary illness would be determined from the medical records of hospitals, clinics and physicians. Public health authorities often gather and make available such statistics.

Figure 6.1A and B represent two of the many possible empirical outcomes using time-series designs. We will assume that the incidence of the illness was monitored for 6 years before and after the introduction of the treatment.

There are, of course, other possible outcomes. However, in this case, Figure 6.1A would be consistent with the predictions of our hypothesis, while the outcome shown on Figure 6.1B would be inconsistent with our hypothesis. Discussion of the way in which data generated by time-series designs are analyzed is beyond the scope of the present text. Briefly, it involves the analysis of trends (increase or decrease) found in the dependent variable.

Time-series designs suffer from various problems of internal validity. What assurance have we, after all, that the decrease in the incidence of coronary heart disease, shown in Figure 6.1A, was caused by the introduction of the health promotion programme? Perhaps there was another cause, such as the introduction of drugs to control high blood pressure.

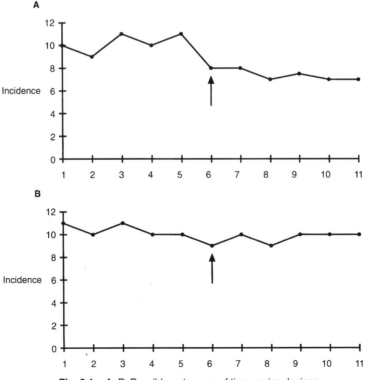

Fig. 6.1 A, B. Possible outcomes of time-series designs.

Multiple-group time-series designs

The introduction of multiple-group time-series designs involves the comparison of two or more naturally occurring groups. Let us examine a simple illustration of such designs by a fictional further investigation of the coronary heart disease problem.

Using a multiple-group time-series design, the investigator would select a community which is as similar as possible on demographic variables (socioeconomic classes, age, size of the community, etc.) to the community being studied. In this way we would have:

- *Community A*. Control. Do not introduce health promotion programme
- *Community B*. Introduce health promotion programme.

Figure 6.2 shows two of the several possible outcomes for such an investigation.

Where the two communities show different trends, the outcome shown on Figure 6.2A is consistent with our previously stated hypothesis. However, in Figure 6.2B there is a trend for decrease in both A and B, therefore, the evidence is not consistent with the prediction of the hypothesis.

Even with multiple-group time-series designs, some threats to internal validity remain. There are no guarantees that the communities A and B were equivalent on all relevant factors, or that there were no important changes during the study in the communities which might have influenced the incidence of coronary heart disease. The best that researchers can do is to identify and try to estimate the effect of such extraneous factors on the dependent variable. There are problems such as insulating the two groups: when people in Community B learn about the programme being carried out in Community A they, by themselves, might initiate aspects of the programme.

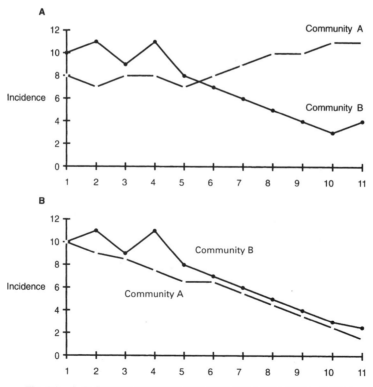

Fig. 6.2 A, B. Possible outcomes of multiple-group time-series designs.

THE INTERNAL AND EXTERNAL VALIDITY OF NATURALISTIC DESIGNS

We have noted several types of problems concerning the internal validity of investigations using natural comparison, correlational and time-series designs. These are similar to the problems of internal validity found in experimental investigations. However, because researchers have generally less control over the phenomena being investigated, the use of natural comparison designs makes it more difficult to evaluate causal hypotheses. That is, given uncontrolled extraneous variables, a variety of plausible alternative hypotheses might be offered to account for the findings (Ch. 4). Therefore, in areas such as epidemiology, researchers use evidence arising from a variety of investigations using different types of designs to evaluate their theories and models of the causes of human diseases.

When evaluating evidence from natural comparison designs, the external validity of the findings must be considered. In Chapters 3 and 5, we stated that external validity refers to the generalizability of the results of an investigation. Strictly speaking, the results of an investigation should be generalized only to the population from which the sample was selected. For instance, consider the example discussed previously, where a sample of male and female students were compared on a test of spatial ability. Any differences between these two groups can be generalized validly *only* to the population of students from which the samples were drawn. Investigators sometimes forget this obvious point, and try to make inferences about males and females in general. Such sweeping generalizations are invalid. For instance, other cultures with alternative child-rearing practices might well have males and females with completely different relative spatial abilities. Just because a variable is found to be a risk factor in one community, does not guarantee that it will have the same influence on diseases in another community. Clearly, the finding that cigarette smoking is a serious risk factor for coronary heart disease in Western societies does not *necessarily* mean that cigarette smoking is a risk factor for coronary heart disease among Zulus. Given the complex, inter-acting causes of coronary heart disease, there may be different risk factors in communities which follow different lifestyles or have different physical constitutions.

It is not surprising, therefore, that advances in knowledge concerning systematic differences between culturally, racially, or sexually different groups have been slow and controversial.

SUMMARY

Descriptive surveys were shown to be important for establishing the attitudes, behaviours and health problems of a community. These statistics might be used to propose theories or test hypotheses of the nature and causes of illness. We examined several types of non-experimental research designs, including naturalistic comparisons, correlational designs and time-series designs. It was argued that these designs are appropriate when experimental designs cannot be used, having the advantage that we can study systems as they are in nature.

Just as with true experimental designs, investigations using natural comparison designs must confront problems of internal and external validity. Unlike experimental designs, quasi-experiments do not involve random subject assignment into treatment groups. However, we can control the nature of the treatments and the times at which they are introduced. Because control over subject selection and the administration of treatments is more difficult, evaluation of causal hypotheses using naturalistic designs tends to be more controversial than with experimental designs. This does not mean, however, that their use is invalid. Rather, researchers and clinicians working in areas such as epidemiology need to integrate evidence arising from investigations using a range of research designs.

SELF ASSESSMENT

Explain the meanings of the following terms:

> correlational studies
> epidemiology
> multiple-group time-series
> naturalistic comparisons
> risk factors
> surveys
> time-series
> quasi-experimental designs

TRUE OR FALSE

1. If it is impracticable to manipulate an independent variable, the investigator might adopt a non-experimental design.
2. The finding that the incidence of birth abnormality has increased in a community since the fluoridation of the water supply is sufficient evidence that fluoridation caused the birth defects.
3. If there is a high correlation between levels of stress and heart disease, we can say that stress is a risk factor in heart disease.
4. Time-series designs involve the repeated observation of subjects before and after treatment.
5. An important difference between experimental and quasi-experimental designs is that in a quasi-experimental study the subjects are not assigned into treatment groups by the investigator.
6. A quasi-experimental design affords greater control over extraneous variables than an experiment.
7. It might be invalid to infer that there are general differences between males and females on the basis of findings involving a sample.
8. An investigator compares the IQs of two ethnic groups, but does not control for systematic differences in socioeconomic status. Therefore, the study lacks internal validity.
9. When we speak of the 'insulation' of one group from another, we mean attempting to prevent subjects in a control group learning about and adopting the treatment given to an experimental group.
10. If a risk factor is, in fact, a cause for a disorder, we can predict that reducing the risk factor should lead to a reduction in the incidence of the disorder.
11. Surveys are utilized in the social, but not in the medical sciences.
12. 'Naturalistic' designs are useful when it is physically or ethically impossible to manipulate the independent variable.
13. The advantage of naturalistic designs over experimental designs is that they enable the investigator to exercise more control over the independent variable.
14. Naturalistic designs should not be employed to investigate conditions which have complex, interacting causes.
15. Naturalistic comparisons yield data which unequivocally establish the causal effects of the independent variable.
16. A risk factor is a possible cause of a disease.
17. Quasi-experimental designs can involve the production of 'time-series'.
18. Time-series designs involve the calculation of correlation between time and space.
19. A multiple-group time-series design involves the comparison of two or more naturally occurring groups over a period of time.
20. A multiple-group time-series design can be employed only if the subjects can be randomly assigned into treatment groups.
21. For a factor to be recognized as a 'risk factor' it must be shown that it correlates with aspects of a disorder across cultures.
22. Epidemiologists are interested in the frequency and causes of diseases.

MULTIPLE CHOICE

1. Naturalistic designs are appropriate when:

   a It is ethically inappropriate to manipulate the independent variable

  b when only a small sample of subjects is available
  c when the independent variable is extremely difficult or impossible to manipulate
  d *a* and *c*
  e all of above.

2. Naturalistic comparisons differ from experimental designs in that:

  a random selection of subjects is not possible with naturalistic comparisons
  b random assignment of subjects is not necessary with naturalistic comparisons
  c naturalistic comparisons lack external validity
  d all of the above.

3. A risk factor is:

  a a sufficient cause for a complex disorder
  b a necessary cause for a complex disorder
  c both *a* and *b*
  d neither *a* nor *b*.

We compare a representative sample of Kamchatkans and Patagonians currently resident in Australia on a test of visual acuity. Questions 4 and 5 refer to the above.

4. The design employed in the above investigation is:

  a a naturalistic comparison
  b a true experiment
  c a factorial design
  d a time-series design.

5. Given that the sample of Kamchatkans are found to have higher visual acuity than the sample of Patagonians, we can conclude that:

  a Patagonians have poor eyesight
  b Kamchatkans have higher visual acuity than Patagonians

  c living in Kamchatka improves one's visual acuity
  d Kamchatkans living in Australia probably have higher visual acuity than Patagonians living in Australia
  e both *a* and *d*.

6. We employ correlational designs in order to:

  a establish the magnitude and direction of association between variables
  b to establish unequivocally causal effects
  c to identify the possible causes of disease entities
  d both a and c.

7. We intend to investigate if the use of ice is more effective than an exercise program in treating a particular type of physical injury. The design most appropriate for investigating this problem is:

  a an experimental design
  b a correlational design
  c a model
  d a time-series design.

8. An investigator intends to establish if there is a relationship between levels of atmospheric lead and learning deficits in children. The design most appropriate for investigating this problem is:

  a an experimental design
  b a correlational design
  c a model
  d a time-series design.

The graph below summarizes changes in infant mortality rates over a period of years in two communities, A and B. In community A, a programme of intensive fetal monitoring was introduced at the time indicated by the arrow. No such programme was introduced in community B.

SELF ASSESSMENT

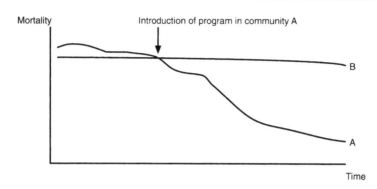

Questions 9–10 refer to the above information.

9. The investigation should be described as:

   a a correlational study
   b an experiment
   c a time-series design
   d a multiple-group time-series design.

10. The findings summarized in the above graph appear to be consistent with the conclusion that:

    a the introduction of fetal monitoring had no effect on infant mortality rate
    b the introduction of fetal monitoring decreased mortality rate
    c the introduction of fetal monitoring increased infant mortality rate
    d none of the above conclusions is consistent with the data.

11. Risk factors of diseases:

    a can be identified by correlational designs
    b are not necessarily the sole causes of diseases
    c are not necessarily the same across cultures
    d all of the above.

A multiple-group time-series design is introduced to study the effects of an insecticide on the number of spontaneous abortions. The insecticide was introduced (not by the investigator) in community A, but not in a similar community B. The graph below represents the hypothetical data.

12. On the basis of the graph below, one can conclude that:

    a there is evidence that the introduction of

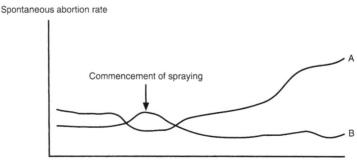

the insecticide increased spontaneous abortions in community A

b there is no evidence that the introduction of the insecticide increased spontaneous abortions in community A

c there appears to be a contamination of community B by the insecticide

d a and c.

13. An investigator distributes a questionnaire to a sample of ex-nurses in an attempt to discover their reasons for leaving the profession. This is best described as:

a a quasi-experiment

b an experiment

c a survey

d a social model.

14. In an attempt to demonstrate the causal relationship between intake of animal fat and heart disease, an investigator studies the eating habits and heart disease rates of demographically defined groups. Which of the following (hypothetical) findings, is most inconsistent with the hypothesis that 'The intake of high levels of animal fats causes heart disease'.

a Vegetarians have a lower rate of heart disease than meat eaters

b Canadian males have a lower rate of heart disease than Canadian females

c The increase of protein and fat intake in China has correlated with an increased incidence of heart disease

d Eskimos, whose diet consists mainly of animal fats, have lower incidence of heart disease than Egyptians who eat mainly grains.

7

Single subject ($n = 1$) designs

INTRODUCTION

We have discussed designs involving the comparison of groups of subjects selected from a population. These designs can provide evidence concerning the general causes of diseases, or the overall effectiveness of treatment. However, health professionals most often work with individual patients and need to understand the specific causes of their problems and the effectiveness of treatments as applied to them as individuals. $N = 1$ designs are useful for demonstrating the close relationship between the principles for conducting research and every day clinical practice.

The aim of the present chapter is to examine single subject ($n = 1$) designs, as applied by a variety of health professionals in natural settings. You will be able to recognize close similarities between these designs, and the quasi-experimental designs discussed in Chapter 6.

The specific aims of the present chapter are to:

1. Identify methodological similarities between clinical problem solving and designing $n = 1$ studies.
2. Examine the use and comparative advantages of AB, ABAB, and multiple-baseline designs
3. Comment on the validity of $n = 1$ designs.
4. Demonstrate how the interpretation of single case studies is related to generally applied methodological principles.

AB DESIGNS

Let us look at a simple example to illustrate the

basic procedures involved in using $n = 1$ designs. Say that a patient is admitted to your ward suffering from a condition which involves having a high temperature. Before an appropriate treatment is devised, the patient's temperature is recorded every 15 min, for 2 h. Following this time interval, the patient is given medication to reduce their temperature. The question here is: 'How do we show that the medication was effective for reducing the patient's temperature?' Obviously, we need to show that the patient's temperature had fallen following the administration of the medication. Figure 7.1 illustrates a possible outcome.

Let us assume that the drug is known to act quickly, say in 20 min. The evidence shown in Figure 7.1 would be clearly consistent with the hypothesis that the medication caused a decrease in the patient's temperature. Let us generalize this example to $n = 1$ designs used in various settings. Figure 7.2 illustrates the general conventions used in $n = 1$ designs.

1. We can see that the y-axis (y) represents the *dependent variable* (DV); observations made of specific physical characteristics of behaviours.
2. The x-axis represents the time over which the observations were carried out.
3. The period A represents the sessions during which no treatment was administered. This is the 'control' level of the *independent variable* (IV). The observations recorded during A form the *baseline*.
4. Period B represents the sessions during which treatment was administered, that is, the active stage.
5. The observations taken during A are compared with those taken during B. Systematic changes in the DV between A and B phases (increases or decreases) are assumed to reflect the influence of the treatment.

Therefore, an AB design involves the taking of observations during phase A, introducing

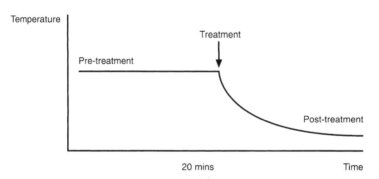

Fig. 7.1 Possible outcome of an AB design.

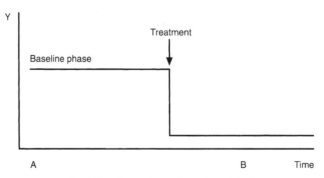

Fig. 7.2 General structure of $n = 1$ designs.

an appropriate treatment (B), and then taking observations during B.

It might have occurred to you that several of the threats to validity (outlined in Chapter 4) can be identified in AB designs. An obvious one is maturation, that is, recovery or deterioration occurring in the patient which might influence the readings on the dependent variable. Another possible threat is history, that is, influences on the patient other than the actual treatment. In the example we just looked at, one could also argue that perhaps the patient's temperature would have gone down, even without the drug, because of the condition improving by itself, or the environment of the ward (maturation) or perhaps the ward was air-conditioned and the patient would have cooled down anyway, drugs or not (history). Next, we shall look at ABAB designs, which provide stronger control for extraneous variables than AB designs.

ABAB DESIGNS

The basic feature of ABAB designs is the introduction of a reversal condition. That is, the researcher attempts to reintroduce the conditions under A. In this way, the design allows the examination of the observations as they occur when the treatment variable is withdrawn again and, therefore, control for threats to validity discussed above.

Developing the above example, an ABAB design would involve the withdrawal of the drug and its subsequent reintroduction. Figure 7.3 illustrates this procedure.

Figure 7.3 illustrates the outcome that when the drug is withdrawn (second A) the patient's temperature returns to previous levels. When the drug is reintroduced (second B), the patient's temperature declines. Clearly, such an outcome is consistent with a causal relationship between the independent variable (treatment) and the dependent variable (observations of temperature). Figure 7.4 demonstrates the graph expected using ABAB designs.

Although the above design is useful for demonstrating causal effects in a single individual, there are situations where it is inappropriate. ABAB designs are not particularly useful when there is a good reason to expect that the variable underlying the observations is *irreversible* following the treatment. For example, if the medication used in the previous example involved antibiotics, then the discontinuation of such drugs after a period might not result in the re-emergence of the symptoms since the antibiotics might well cure the underlying problem. Even when reversal is possible, it might not be ethical. Clearly, if we have succeeded in establishing desirable effects in our client during the first B period, we might well be reluctant to reverse this for the sake of demonstrating causal relationships.

MULTIPLE BASELINE DESIGNS

Multiple baseline designs involve the use of

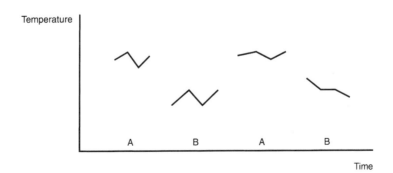

Fig. 7.3 Graph of patient's temperature under different treatment conditions.

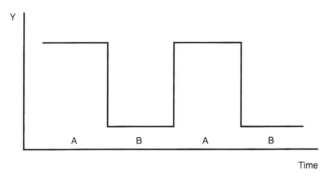

Fig. 7.4 General structure of ABAB designs.

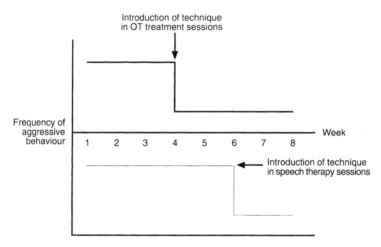

Fig. 7.5 Aggressive behaviour of a brain-damaged patient in two situations.

concurrent observations to generate two or more baselines. Given two or more baselines, the investigator has the opportunity to introduce treatment affecting only one set of observations, while using the other(s) as a control. We will examine a hypothetical clinical problem to illustrate these designs.

Say that we have a brain-damaged client showing aggressive behaviours which disrupt therapy. Therapy is offered in two situations, say occupational therapy (Situation 1) and speech therapy (Situation 2). A behavioural programme is devised, aimed at reducing the frequency of the aggressive outbursts. A multiple baseline design involves the observation of the frequency of the target behaviour in both Situations 1 and 2. After establishing a baseline, the treatment is

introduced first in one of the situations and then in the other. Evidence demonstrating the effectiveness of the behavioural treatment is shown in Figure 7.5.

The fictional data presented in Figure 7.5 indicates that the frequency of the target behaviour (aggression) declined in Situation 1 when the treatment was introduced, while it remained stable in Situation 2. The subsequent introduction of the treatment in Situation 2 resulted in a decrease of the behaviour.

Multiple baseline designs can be introduced also by generating baselines for two or more behaviours, or for two or more individuals. Just as in the example involving the different situations, the treatments would be introduced first for one of the behaviours or individuals and,

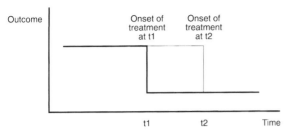

Fig. 7.6 General structure of multiple baseline designs.

subsequently, for the others. Figure 7.6 illustrates a general example for multiple baseline designs.

Clearly, by introducing the treatment at different times, we are controlling for the effects of extraneous variables that might have influenced our dependent variable. Both ABAB and multiple baseline designs are appropriate for demonstrating the benefits of therapeutic procedures in individual patients.

THE INTERPRETATION OF THE RESULTS FOR *n* = 1 DESIGNS

The principles for conducting and interpreting health research are also relevant for evaluating the effectiveness of every day health practices. The need for control and accurate measurement arises when we intend to demonstrate that particular treatments or preventative interventions are causally related to beneficial outcomes.

As we have seen previously we can exercise control by systematically introducing and withdrawing treatments and measuring concomitant changes in the signs and symptoms of a disorder.

HYPOTHETICAL EXAMPLE

Let us look at a hypothetical example for illustrating four different methodological principles relevant to the interpretation of *n* = 1 studies. Imagine that you are caring for a young man called John who had suffered a severe fracture of the femur following a motorbike accident. He is gradually recovering with intensive rehabilitation but he is still in severe pain when narcotic analgesics are not provided.

Previous research has shown that trans-cutaneous electrical stimulation (TENS) was a safe and effective modality for managing acute pain (see Section 1, Discussion Question). However the treatment is not equally effective for *all* patients so that there are no absolute guarantees that TENS will control pain in this specific patient. Also, even biologically inert pain control techniques can reduce pain through placebo effects. In this case you decide to investigate two clinically relevant research questions:

1. TENS is effective in reducing John's pain.
2. The pain reduction is causally related to the action of TENS.

Having obtained your patients informed consent you decide to conduct an ABAB, *n* = 1 design for obtaining evidence to answer the above research questions. The variables here can be defined as follows:

1. *I.V.* The independent variable is the pain control strategy using the TENS machine. The electrical stimulation produced by the TENS machine can be regulated such that you are in a position to vary the output of the machine. Two settings are selected:
   (a) A represents TENS output which is known to be physiologically *ineffective* for activating the 'pain gating' mechanisms (see Section 1). A represents the 'placebo control' level of the I.V.
   (b) B represents TENS output which is known to be physiologically effective in activating 'gating' mechanisms. B represents the 'treatment' level of the I.V.
2. *D.V.* The dependent variable is an explicit measure of aspects of the signs and symptoms of the patent's condition. In this case we can select 'pain intensity' as a relevant dependent variable, measured on a 10 point scale (on this scale 0 represents 'no pain at all' and 10 excruciating pain). We will discuss specific issues in measurement in Chapter 12, however, for the time being let us assume that this scale constitutes an appropriate measure of pain.
3. *E.V.* Extraneous variables are variables other

Table 7.1   Data collection procedure for hypothetical example

Time period	I.V. level	D.V.
Week 1	A phase (placebo)	Daily assessment of pain
Week 2	B phase (treatment)	intensity (at 0800 hours)
Week 2	A phase (placebo)	
Week 3	B phase (treatment)	

than the IV which can influence the D.V. and may 'confound' the demonstration of causal effects (Chapter 4).

In the present $n = 1$ study we are controlling for extraneous variables by:

(a) Using a placebo control condition

(b) Introducing and withdrawing the active treatment over time (ABAB).

The therapeutic effectiveness of the TENS for pain control will be represented by the changes in the pain intensity or the *differences* between the A and B phases of the intervention. Table 7.1 provides the procedure for conducting the data collection.

The 'A' phase gives us the baseline against which we can compare the effectiveness of the active TENS treatment for reducing pain intensity. The outcome indicates a large and consistent difference between the A and B levels of the independent variable and the large difference between A and B indicates a clinically useful reduction in the pain intensity experienced by John, your patient. You are now justified in continuing the treatment until he is sufficiently recovered to be pain free.

We hope you will agree that this was an inspiring little story, the problem with it being that things just do not normally happen this way in the real world. The data we hypothesized above clearly illustrates an ideal, easily interpreted outcome appropriate for educational purposes. But what happens with 'real' results?

1. *Variability*. The above results are idealized, as opposed to 'variable'; that is to say appearing to be all over the place. We will look at the concept of variability in Chapters 14 and 15. At this stage it suffices to say that the more

variable the findings the more difficult it is to identify the trends and differences in results of $n = 1$ studies.

2. *Effect Size*. The effect size is indicated by the difference between the Baseline (A) and the Treatment (B) phases. If the effect size is large in relation to the variability of the data, changes in pain intensity will be easy to see. However, if the effect size is small in relation to the variability of the data, then changes in pain intensity will be hard to see. Thus, the ability to detect the effects of interventions is affected by natural variability in the measured variable. We will look at these issues further under the interpretation of the evidence in Chapters 18, 19 and 20.

THE VALIDITY OF *N* = 1 DESIGNS

We examined three (AB, ABAB, multiple baseline) designs in the previous subsections. However, more complicated, 'mixed' designs are available for $n = 1$ investigations. The mixed designs include elements of both reversal and multiple baseline strategies. We will not discuss these in detail in this text; interested readers are referred to Hersen and Barlow (1976).

A basic requirement for the valid interpretation of all $n = 1$ designs is the production of a stable baseline. Unless this requirement is met, the interpretation of the results is extremely difficult. In some clinical situations, the production of a stable baseline might be unethical as it could involve withholding treatment. The treatment phase must also be long enough for the effectiveness of the treatment to emerge. Some treatments, such as those involving physical rehabilitation or psychotherapy, might need to be administered for months before their effectiveness, or lack of it, becomes apparent. Clearly, we can not (and need not) assume that the baseline and treatment phases are of equal duration.

It is essential that the observations should be valid and reliable. Some observations are straight-forward, such as those based on taking temperatures. However, given a more complex variable such as 'aggression' we need to establish with clarity that different observers agree on the type of behaviours we are going to observe; behaviours which might seem 'aggressive' to one observer might not be classified as such by another. This issue is discussed further in Chapters 9 and 12.

We have already discussed how $n = 1$ designs attempt to control for the influence of extraneous variables. Although the $n = 1$ designs can be conceptually adequate to demonstrate causality, the patients, being in their natural setting, can be influenced by all sorts of uncontrolled events. After all, it is not possible (or desirable) to insulate individuals from their environment. Therefore, sources of invalidity must be evaluated with respect to each $n = 1$ investigation. It must also be remembered that no matter how sophisticated the $n = 1$ design, the observed outcomes for any given case may not generalize to other cases. Using techniques known as meta-analysis it is possible to combine the data from a number of such single case studies to investigate overall trends. Thus, $n = 1$ designs do not side-step sampling or generalizability issues.

SUMMARY

In this chapter, we examined three (AB, ABAB and multiple baseline) of the designs available for studying single individuals in their natural settings. It was argued that ABAB and multiple baseline studies provide a valid means for evaluating the causal effects of variables on therapeutic outcomes. These $n = 1$ designs are particularly useful for establishing the usefulness of treatment procedures for individual patients. Although some limitations and ethical constraints might emerge in conducting $n = 1$ studies, they provide a useful tool for the practising clinician interested in evaluating the effectiveness of treatments.

Although the statistical analysis of $n = 1$ studies is beyond the scope of this introductory text, it should be noted that graphing our observations, as discussed in this chapter, provides evidence for possible causal relationships. A precondition for interpreting the results of $n = 1$ studies is, of course, having a sufficient number of stable observations across the various conditions.

The $n = 1$ designs are quite similar to quasi-experimental designs, in that the investigator has control over the type and timing of the treatments.

SELF ASSESSMENT

Explain the meaning of the following terms:

    AB design
    ABAB design
    baseline
    multiple baseline
    designs reversal

TRUE OR FALSE

1. $n = 1$ designs are most appropriate for conducting epidemiological investigations.
2. The graphing of $n = 1$ findings involves graphing the magnitude of the dependent variable along the y-axis and time or sessions along the x-axis.
3. With an AB design, the time period A represents the time period during which the treatment is introduced.
4. A baseline is a series of observations recorded during a period when the treatment is administered.
5. With an AB design, a treatment is introduced, withdrawn and then reintroduced.
6. A limitation in using ABAB designs in clinical investigations is that it might be possible, but unethical, to withdraw a treatment.
7. Using multiple baselines across two situations involves establishing baselines,

SELF ASSESSMENT

then administering treatments simultaneously in both situations.

8. An advantage of using multiple baseline designs over AB designs is the increased control over threats to internal validity.
9. AB designs involve a period of initial treatment followed by the withdrawal of the treatment.
10. For $n = 1$ designs, the 'B' period is when the treatment is administered.
11. $n = 1$ designs cannot, in principle, indicate causal effects.
12. The major advantage of $n = 1$ designs is that no ethical issues need to be taken into account in planning such research.
13. An ABAB design involves introducing the treatment twice.
14. An ABAB design provides a more powerful control over possible extraneous variables than an AB design.
15. ABAB designs are particularly useful when changes in the symptoms following treatment are irreversible.
16. The production of a stable baseline might be unethical in some clinical situations.

MULTIPLE CHOICE

1. Quasi-experimental and $n = 1$ designs are similar in that:

   a they can both involve time dependent sets of observations
   b both can involve control over the time at which a treatment is introduced
   c both a and b
   d neither a nor b.

2. An ABAB design:

   a involves the use of two individuals, A and B
   b has two baseline periods
   c depends on manipulating A and measuring B
   d involves correlating AA with BBC.

Consider the following outcome for an $n = 1$ type investigation.

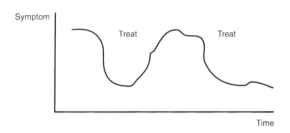

Questions 3 and 4 refer to the graph above.

3. This is a(n):

   a AB design
   b ABA design
   c ABAB design
   d 'mixed' design.

4. The above graph indicates that:

   a the treatment appears effective in reducing the symptom
   b the treatment appears to exacerbate the symptom
   c the treatment appears to have no effect on the symptom
   d no conclusion can be reached on the basis of the obtained data.

A child with a serious behavioural problem at home is institutionalized. After a 1-week period of observation, a behavioural treatment is introduced. The graph below represents the fictitious results.

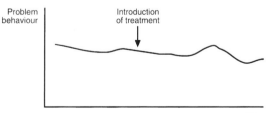

SELF ASSESSMENT

Questions 5–6 refer to the above data.

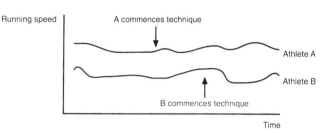

5. This is a(n):

   a AB design
   b ABA design
   c ABAB design
   d multiple baseline design.

6. The above graph indicates that:

   a the treatment appears to have improved the child's problem behaviour
   b the treatment appears to have exacerbated the child's problem behaviour
   c the treatment appears to have had no effect on the child's behaviour
   d a factorial design should have been used.

7. Treatment is undertaken to attempt to reduce anxiety in an individual. An ABAB design is used to evaluate treatment effectiveness. Because of different shifts at a hospital, six different observers are used to record the anxiety related behaviours. Problem(s) with this investigation is (are) that:

   a the observers might not record exactly the same behaviours as reflecting 'anxiety'
   b the presence of the different observers might influence the behaviours in different ways
   c both *a* and *b*
   d neither *a* nor *b*.

A new technique to improve running speed in athletes is evaluated. The graph below represents fictional results for two athletes.

Questions 8 and 9 refer to the above data.

8. This design is a(n):

   a AB
   b ABAB
   c multiple baseline
   d factorial.

9. The above graph indicates that:

   a the new technique appears to improve running speed
   b the new technique appears to reduce running speed
   c the new technique appears to have no effect on running speed
   d further investigations on the effects of the technique are necessary.

10. The use of an ABAB design is most useful for reducing threats due to:

   a placebo effects
   b experimenter expectancy
   c maturation
   d assignment.

8

Qualitative field research

INTRODUCTION

The research strategies discussed in previous chapters can be called 'quantitative' in that the data obtained consists of measurements which can be statistically treated. It has been argued by some researchers that such quantitative statistical portrayals miss the essence of what constitutes health and illness in humans. Qualitative or interpretive field research involves the investigation of specific individuals in their social settings. The investigator seeks to understand the thoughts, feelings and experiences of individuals, focusing on direct, face-to-face knowledge of patients or clients as human beings coping with their conditions and treatments in a given social setting. The use of evidence from qualitative studies has traditionally been a fundamental source of knowledge in the clinical and social sciences.

The specific aims of this chapter are to:

1. Outline different conceptual approaches to qualitative research.
2. Compare and contrast specific dimensions of qualitative and quantitative approaches to research.
3. Examine the scope and limitations of qualitative research in health sciences.

WHAT IS QUALITATIVE FIELD RESEARCH?

Qualitative field research is disciplined enquiry examining the personal meanings of individuals' experiences and actions in the context of their social environments.

'Qualitative' refers to the nature of the data or evidence collected. Qualitative data consists of detailed descriptions, based on language or pictures recorded by the investigator. 'Field' research indicates that the investigation is preferably carried out in the natural environment in which the phenomenon occurs, rather than in controlled laboratory settings. By 'disciplined' we mean that the enquiry is guided by explicit methodological principles for defining problems, collecting and analyzing the evidence, and formulating and evaluating theories.

'Personal meaning' refers to the way in which individuals subjectively perceive and explain their experiences, actions and social environments. Qualitative field research provides systematic evidence for gaining insights into other person's views of the world, 'putting ourselves into someone else's shoes', as it were.

There are a variety of approaches to qualitative field research and these take somewhat different positions concerning how data should be collected and analyzed. There are also, several diverse schools of thought which have contributed to the historical development of qualitative field research. The most noteworthy contributions were made in the following areas (for brief reviews, see Taylor and Bogdan 1984, Cohen and Manion 1985):

1. *Phenomenology*. Phenomenology, which is both a system of philosophy and an approach to psychology, emphasizes the direct study of personal experience and the understanding of the nature of human consciousness. Research in this area involves 'bracketing' or putting aside the usual preconceptions and prejudices that influence everyday perception so that we can uncover the pure constituents of conscious experience. Conscious experience is in turn seen as the basis for personal meaning as we reflect on our experiences in the context of our goals and purposes. An important concept adopted from phenomenology is the notion of 'multiple realities', that is, different people may consciously experience the world in quite diverse

ways. In order to understand the meanings of a person's actions, we must become adept, through empathy, at seeing things from their point of view.

2. *Symbolic interactionism*. Symbolic interactionists emphasize that a social situation has meaning only in the way people define and interpret what is happening. That is, people do not react to 'objective' aspects of their environments, but rather their actions are guided by their personal interpretations of the situation. It follows that different people, on the basis of their past experiences and their particular social positions may come to interpret a specific situation in quite divergent ways, and act in conflicting fashions. For example, a male obstetrician might view childbirth in quite a different way from a female midwife, and in turn their views might be quite discordant with that of a woman giving birth. In social and health care settings, it is useful to explore different perceptions of events, as it is clear from the work of symbolic interactionists that 'shared perspectives' among people cannot be taken for granted.

3. *Ethnomethodology*. Ethnomethodologists study the processes associated with the way in which people perceive, describe and explain the world. Ethnomethodologists argue that the meanings of specific actions and events are not necessarily obvious to a person, but are in fact rather ambiguous and problematic. People select and apply specific rules and principles in order to define and give meaning to situations in which they find themselves and in order to justify their actions in a given situation. Research carried out by ethnomethodologists demonstrates that we take an enormous amount of cultural context, such as norms and rules, for granted in our everyday communications and social interactions, and we tend to 'bracket' this as obvious or common sense. It must be remembered, however, that when the cultural backgrounds of individuals diverge, the understanding of personal meaning becomes less obvious or commonsense.

Although taking somewhat different views of personal meanings, the above three approaches have common themes and have all contributed to

Table 8.1 Contrast between quantitative and qualitative methods

	Quantitative	Qualitative
Perception of the subject matter	Reductionistic;identification and operational definition of specific variables	Holistic; persons in the context of their social environments
Positioning of researcher	Objective; detached observation and precise measurement of variables	Subjective; close personal interaction with subjects
Database	Quantitative; interrelationships among specific variables	Qualitative; descriptions of actions and related personal meanings in context
Theories	Normative; general propositions explaining causal relationships among variables	Interpretive; providing insights into the nature and social contexts of personal meanings
Theory testing	Controlled; empirically supporting or falsifying hypotheses deduced from theories	Consensual; matching researcher's interpretations with those of subjects and other observers
Applications	Prediction and control of health related factors in applied settings	Interacting with persons in a consensual, value consonant fashion in health care settings

Adapted from McGartland & Polgar (1994). Copyright (1994) The Australian Psychological Society Ltd. Reproduced by permission

the development of qualitative field research. Table 8.1 shows key aspects of qualitative field research, in contrast to quantitative approaches.

DATA COLLECTION AND INTERPRETATION IN QUALITATIVE FIELD RESEARCH

The fundamental aim of planning and designing qualitative field research is to position the investigator close to the participants, so as to gain access to and describe personal experiences, and to interpret their meanings in specific social settings. The following subsection develops in more detail the corresponding points presented in Table 8.1. Illustrative examples will be discussed later when we review data collection strategies in Chapters 9, 10 and 11.

Perception of subject matter

Qualitative field research is carried out in a natural setting and there is no attempt made by the investigator to control for extraneous influences. Furthermore, there are no operational definitions provided for the dependent or independent variables, but rather the phenomenon being studied is perceived and described as a whole.

Strong preconceptions or fixed hypotheses are not advantageous for qualitative field research. This is a different situation from that in

quantitative research, where there are precisely defined hypotheses or aims guiding the research. Qualitative researchers do have general aims and theoretical notions pertaining to the phenomena being studied, but these are tentative and are open to modification as the data collection proceeds.

Qualitative field research focuses on the in-depth understanding of specific individuals, rather than studying the general characteristics of a large population of individuals across specific variables. It should be kept in mind, however, that some quantitative designs may address single cases, as we have seen in Chapter 7 in relation to $n = 1$ designs. The difference is that $n = 1$ designs address specific variables representing aspects of the individual's behaviour or clinical symptoms, rather than attempting to describe and understand the individual holistically in the context of their natural social settings. Such an approach is called 'idiographic' (describing a specific individual) as opposed to the 'nomothetic' (describing general phenomena) view of research in quantitative research.

Positioning of the researcher

As discussed in Chapter 12, accurate and replicable measurements are valued in quantitative research. The fundamental positioning of the researcher is 'objective', that is aiming to perceive and record events without any personal bias or distortion. The situation in qualitative field research is far more complex, as the researcher is more a part of the phenomenon being investigated than the detached observer in quantitative research (see in Ch. 11). It is argued here that to understand personal meanings and subjective experiences one has to become involved with the lives of the subjects being studied. That is, some degree of empathy must develop between the researcher and the subject. By empathy, we mean the ability to 'put ourselves in the other person's shoes' or to see things from their perspective(s).

A particular reason for the advancement of quantitative research has been the development of instrumentation that has enabled the collection and recording of data to be more precise. It has also given access to phenomena not naturally accessible to unaided human senses, as with for example the development of light and electronic microscopy. However, when standardized tests and measures are used to study a person, they become 'enframed' within the limitations of the instrument, and their possible unique self-expression remains outside the scope of the enquiry. The qualitative researcher may find a measurement instrument intrusive, one which might restrict and confine the possibilities of understanding of a person.

There are advantages to a human 'measuring instrument' which are exploited in qualitative research. After all, we are more adaptable and multi-purpose than even very sophisticated machinery and can observe subtle behavioural changes and verbal and nonverbal cues in our subjects. In addition, as the investigation progresses, the human 'instrument' becomes more aware of what is happening and thus the data collection becomes more accurate.

Data base

The data obtained in quantitative research consists of sets of measurements of objective descriptions of physical and behavioural events. These are summarized and analyzed in accordance with statistical principles outlined at an introductory level in Sections 4 and 5 of this book. The data in qualitative research is descriptive, a 'thick' or thorough description of what people said, their actions and activities, non-verbal behaviours and interactions with other people: 'The reality of the place should be conveyed through representation of its mundane aspects in a straight forward manner' (Lofland, 1971, p. 4). An important aspect of field research is keeping thorough, up-to-date field notes. These should be recorded as closely as possible to the time of occurrence of the phenomena under study. The field notes should contain direct quotations from the participants and the settings in which the statements and actions were recorded. Where possible (if this is not inappropriate or intrusive), the researcher may use audio and video recordings, as outlined in Chapter 10. This helps to record events, and improves accuracy in conveying what was said and done in a given setting, since it is possible to review the obtained information.

Although 'objectivity' does not mean remaining detached from the situation, it is essential in qualitative research that the reports of events should be truthful. The investigators should not allow ideological biases to distort or censor their observations, or deliberately lie to place their subjects in a good or bad light. This is a particularly important point, as given the close personal interaction with the subjects, one may be predisposed to report favourably. An extreme of this in anthrophological research is called 'going native', when one completely adopts the views of the subjects being studied.

By 'data base', we mean the overall empirical evidence that forms the basis for theory formation and specific applications for health care. In quantitative research, the data base will consist of the statistically treated data which will enable us to see how specific variables are interrelated. In terms of qualitative field research, the data base is essentially a narrative (or a story if you like) that reports what has happened to people, what they did or said in specific situations. This narrative should be adequately detailed so as to illuminate for the reader the personal meanings that the reported events had for the subjects.

Theories

Theories are representations of our current state of knowledge about the state of the world. Theories are abstract logical coherent explanatory systems which integrate a broad range of research findings (i.e. the facts). Theories may be constituted of premises stated in everyday language, with particular attention paid to the appropriate use of concepts and the logical development of the premises.

Theories based on quantitative evidence integrate patterns of findings concerning the interrelationships among variables. Such theories often contain 'models', which may be mathematical and/or systems representations of the patterns of findings. Models of anatomical and physiological processes, such as that of the circulatory or nervous systems are good examples of successful quantitative models.

Conversely theories integrating evidence from qualitative field research do not address facts about how objects are constituted and interact, but rather are interpretations of personal meanings emerging in specific social settings. In qualitative field research there are several different approaches to theory formation. We will discuss some of these further in Chapter 10, in the context of interpreting data arising from unstructured, in-depth interviews.

Some commentators (Guba & Lincoln 1983) argue that data collection and theory formation should be intrinsically integrated rather than being different stages of the research process. In addition, it is suggested that personal meanings should be seen as unique and idiosyncratic, and thus no attempt should be made to integrate systematically such diverse personal positions. Theory, from an idiographic position, is seen essentially as the accurate presentation of the situation from a particular person's perspective.

Other qualitative researchers approach theory formation by attempting to identify common 'themes' or categories of meanings emerging from the data. The important point here is that the theoretical categories are developed from evidence expressing personal meanings, rather than 'facts' derived from the statistical treatment of objective measurements concerning variables (Ch. 11). In this way, theory is said to be 'grounded' in the narratives of particular individuals.

Some researchers stress the broad, culture interpreting aspects of qualitative field research. The formation of **critical theory** explains how personal meanings and actions emerge and are influenced by the person's social and cultural milieu. Critical theories identify the extent to which individual's self-perception and freedom for action may become distorted and limited by the operation of power and coercion within society (e.g. Grundy 1987, pp. 15–19, 106–114).

Theory testing

Theories based on quantitative evidence lead to clear-cut, empirically testable predictions or hypotheses logically deduced from the theories (see Ch. 1). Theories are supported or falsified by empirical evidence collected under controlled conditions. Testing qualitative theories is somewhat different, as no causal mechanisms may be included in the theoretical framework. The simplest verification of qualitative interpretations is to go to the subjects themselves, in order to establish if the researcher's interpretations make sense to them. The extent to which a consensus develops between researchers and their subjects is one of the important indications of the truth of qualitative theories.

Applications in health care delivery

The applications of quantitative evidence and theories are essentially *technical*, providing mechanisms in terms of which we can predict and control specific health related variables. That is, we apply quantitative approaches for discovering the causes and progress of diseases and disabilities, for developing and validating assessment procedures and for evaluating the effectiveness of interventions (see also Ch. 1).

In contrast, qualitative field research provides evidence and theories that enable us to better understand our clients as human beings. This research discloses how illnesses, disability and health care delivery affects people's lives interpreted from their points of view. In the following subsection, we will examine some of the applications of qualitative field research for improving health care delivery.

QUALITATIVE FIELD RESEARCH IN HEALTH CARE

When there are significant differences in the cultural backgrounds and experiences of persons, the understanding of personal meanings becomes problematic. For example, an anthropologist might need to spend decades immersed in, and systematically studying, a different culture before they are in a position to interpret accurately the actions and traditions of the participants.

There are numerous areas of health care where research involving the interpretation of personal meanings is essential to ensure effective practices. The following three examples illustrate areas where qualitative field research is making strong contributions for clarifying personal meanings, in situations where 'shared perspectives' of health care issues can not be taken for granted.

1. *Understanding cultural differences between health workers and clients.* In countries such as Australia, Canada or the UK we live in multi-cultural societies. There is persuasive evidence that the way people experience their bodies, or events such as childbirth, pain or illness depends to a large extent on their cultural backgrounds. When health practitioners misconceive their clients' view concerning their illness or injury, the outcome may be erroneous diagnoses, useless interventions and an inappropriate treatment of clients. A particularly important area of qualitative field research is to clarify personal meanings of clients and therapist with regard to health care problems, in an attempt to improve communications and enhance treatment outcomes.

2. *Evaluating the effects of health care environments.* Health care institutions, such as general and mental hospitals, can be seen as 'subcultures' having strong influences on the lives of both staff and clients. Persons with chronic illnesses and disabilities requiring long-term care might come to view themselves and their life situations from an 'institutionalized' perspective. The development of critical theories in these areas is particularly relevant for understanding the influences of health care environments. Research findings in this area have been applied to devise strategies to empower people such as those with intellectual disabilities to live and participate in the community.

3. *Relating to people with neurological or psychiatric problems.* People diagnosed as suffering from problems such as schizophrenia, intellectual disability or brain disorders may, to some extent, experience themselves and the world in ways different from 'ordinary' people. How such persons experience aspects of their world is by no means obvious, as these clients may demonstrate severe information-processing impairments, such as delusions, hallucinations or memory problems, which may make it extremely difficult to establish empathic relationships. However, in order to ensure that persons with such severe impairments or disabilities are treated appropriately and with understanding, health professionals must learn to see things from their perspectives. Qualitative field research has provided evidence which has helped to clarify the personal perspectives of people with severe disabilities.

The above are some obvious examples where qualitative research is appropriate for clarifying personal meanings, and enhancing understanding and communication in health care settings. However, personal meanings are relevant to *all* health care situations, not only in the obviously difficult area discussed above. The following exemplify questions which are appropriately approached through field research strategies:

- What is it like to have a speech disorder; in what ways does it disrupt the person's life, from their points of view?
- How do caregivers interact with terminally ill patients? How do health professionals experience the death of a patient?
- How do health professionals break the news

of unfavourable diagnoses, such as heart disease, to their patients? How are such situations seen from the perspectives of the health professional or the patients?

Qualitative field research is particularly relevant in professional areas such as occupational therapy, nursing or family medicine where a personal closeness and understanding between the health professional and the client is an essential part of the therapeutic process. In other areas, such as surgery, radiography or pathology, the technical aspects of the practice are seen as more important and this is reflected in the predominance of quantitative approaches.

We are arguing that quantitative and qualitative field research should be seen as complementary; the former contributing to the technical development of practices and the latter defining the personal and social frameworks in which health care is delivered.

THE INTEGRATION OF QUANTITATIVE AND QUALITATIVE METHODOLOGIES

When used jointly, quantitative research tools can be particularly powerful. One of the authors has recently conducted a study of how people evaluate primary health services (Thomas et al 1993a). The first step in this process was to conduct focus group interviews (see Ch. 10) with 20 groups of eight participants specifically selected from a wide range of ethnic backgrounds, ages and sexes. The groups were conducted by a facilitator who presented nine questions concerned with knowledge and opinions of, and satisfaction with, health services. The discussions were recorded and transcribed.

One set of analyses of the transcripts involved consideration of everything that had been said about the health services with regard to satisfaction or dissatisfaction. This resulted in 39 separate categories or themes. These themes, therefore, were directly derived from the participants' own words and interpretations of their experiences.

The themes were then framed in the form of

questions that sought information from people about their satisfaction and dissatisfaction with health services. The questions were then incorporated into a questionnaire (see Ch. 9). When the questionnaire was piloted with a sample of 500 people who attended several doctors' surgeries over a period of 3 weeks, it was found that none of the participants nominated new factors that affected their satisfaction and dissatisfaction. Thus, the procedure used in developing the questionnaire had very effectively captured how people decided whether they were satisfied or dissatisfied with their health services. This study is an example of where qualitative and quantitative research methodologies can combine powerfully.

THE VALIDITY OF QUALITATIVE FIELD RESEARCH

It should be noted that the unstructured and descriptive nature of the data collection process in field research often sits uneasily with those favouring 'quantitative' research strategies. The major problem with the unstructured data collection techniques is that observer bias may cloud or distort the data being collected. As previously discussed, there are well-known observer effects such as the Rosenthal effect and the Hawthorne effect. Structured data collection methods are most likely to control for these effects, although there are no guarantees that they will be eliminated.

Furthermore, the sampling processes involved in qualitative field research are complex. Most social phenomena are profoundly affected by their participants. 'Real' situations may not reflect these biases. An important issue in understanding qualitative research is the specific culture dependence of the findings; what is true in one social setting may not be true in another.

Therefore, as in other types of research, qualitative field studies also have to confront problems of external and internal validity. Guba & Lincoln (1983) recommended a variety of strategies to ensure the validity and reliability of field studies. These strategies included:

- asking subjects if the observations about them are credible (believable)
- prolonged engagement by the observers to minimize distortions caused by their presence
- triangulations, which involved pitting against each other different data and theoretical interpretations to provide cross-checks of observations and interpretations.

Therefore, despite controversies in the area, qualitative field researchers pay considerable attention to methodological issues to ensure the adequacy (that is, validity and reliability) of their investigations. The situation is essentially no different from quantitative research, although qualitative researchers take somewhat different steps to ensure the accuracy and generalizability of their empirical findings.

SUMMARY

Qualitative field research strategies include data collection which is aimed at understanding persons in their social environments. Rather than generating numerical data supporting or refuting clear cut hypotheses, field research aims to produce accurate descriptions based on face-to-face knowledge of individuals and social groups in their natural settings. The role of the observer in this context is crucial and usually involves physical and social closeness between the subject and the observer. Data collection involves objective and accurate reporting of the activities and appearances of persons in their natural environments. As with other strategies of research, investigators must pay considerable attention to the external and internal validity of field research. We briefly looked at some ways in which field researchers can cross-check their descriptions in an attempt to ensure the validity of their reports and interpretations.

Different research designs may be used to generate evidence of the same processes, although from different perspectives. For instance, any complex clinical phenomenon, such as schizophrenia, may be studied using any of the research strategies outlined in Chapters 4–8. To understand the scope of the problems and the effectiveness of the appropriate treatments, it is desirable to use a variety of research strategies. Conversely, a comprehensive theory of a clinical problem should generate any number of hypotheses within the realm of the research strategies discussed in this book.

SELF ASSESSMENT

Explain the meaning of the terms:

> personal meaning
> qualitative field research
> quantitative research
> ethnomethodology
> critical theory
> phenomenology
> empathy

TRUE OR FALSE

1. Qualitative field researchers focus on individuals behaving in their natural environments.
2. According to Lofland (1971), the field researcher should maintain a 'distance' from subjects in a physical and social sense.
3. A problem with unstructured data collection techniques is the possible distortion of the evidence through observer bias.
4. The basic aim of qualitative field research is to test clearly defined hypotheses.
5. It is essential in qualitative field research to place disadvantaged or oppressed people in a 'good light', to further their needs or causes.
6. Qualitative field researchers need not concern themselves with issues of validity.
7. Qualitative field research generally involves the use of precision instruments to

measure specific subject variables.

8. Qualitative field research generally produces intimate, face-to-face knowledge of other individuals.
9. Phenomenologists are concerned with the understanding of the nature of human conscious experience.
10. Quantitative research produces data well suited to the formulation of causal models.
11. Quantitative research is most appropriate for interpreting personal meanings in social settings.
12. Quantitative research is best suited to discovering how biological systems work.

MULTIPLE CHOICE

1. Qualitative field research involves:

   a the testing of clear cut hypotheses by employing sophisticated measuring instruments.
   b empathy with subjects of view
   c structured data collection
   d carrying out of research in the open air.

2. Which of the following is not an example of qualitative field research?

   a A researcher studying nursing conditions in major hospitals spends a week working as a nurse aide at Prince Henry's Hospital.
   b An anthropologist goes to live with a New Guinea tribe to find out about their religious practices.
   c A psychologist studying therapeutic processes attends group therapy as a client.
   d A speech pathologist compares two rival methods of treatment for stuttering.
   e A physiotherapy student spends a day in a wheelchair and uses this experience

to write a report on some of the problems of the physically handicapped.

3. Which of the following disciplines would most likely employ qualitative designs?

   a nuclear physics
   b anatomy
   c genetics
   d sociology.

4. The medical model, as discussed in Chapter 1, is best supported by:

   a qualitative field research
   b quantitative research
   c philosophical speculation
   d all of the above.

5. Which of the following is *not* a characteristic of quantitative research?

   a A holistic approach to persons
   b Precise definition of variables being studied
   c Prediction and control of phenomena
   d Theories including causal models.

6. An important basis of qualitative field research is:

   a phenomenology
   b numerology
   c measurement theory
   d the medical model.

7. A psychiatrist is interested in research to identify the relationship between brain dopamine levels and the occurance of specific well defined abnormal behaviours. This research would be:

   a based on phenomenological principles
   b a project in an ethnomethodological framework
   c a quantitative project
   d best described as qualitative field research.

SECTION 3

Discussion, Questions and Answers

The health sciences clinical researcher has a rich variety of research designs from which he or she may choose; including the experimental, survey, single case and qualitative field approaches. Each approach has its unique strengths.

The experimental and single-case designs are particularly suited to studies of the effects of health interventions. These are studies that are concerned with the clinical impact of administering different types of interventions (or non-intervention) upon people. In the classical two-group experimental study, similar groups of people are administered with either an intervention or a non- intervention condition and their outcomes are compared. The use of non-intervention with people who are ill has moral and ethical implications. So, often the experimental method is used to study the relative effects of two or more different types of intervention. There has been an affinity between the professions where health interventions are the norm and a form of enquiry which also involves intervention (i.e. the experimental and single-case types of research design). However, much high-quality health sciences research involves other types of research design.

Sample surveys are frequently employed to study the opinions of large groups of people concerning health services and their experiences of health and illness. Epidemiological research, which is aimed at studying the distribution of health and illness and associated risk factors in populations, generally involves large-scale sample surveys. These surveys often draw upon hospital and other health agency records.

Qualitative field research involves the disciplined examination of the personal meanings of individuals' experiences and actions in the context of their social environment. The emphasis in such research is upon depth of interpretation rather than extent of sampling. Therefore such studies typically employ much smaller samples of participants than, for example, sample surveys.

It is useful to consider examples of the application of the various techniques to the same type of research questions.

Let us consider the situation of people with back injuries associated with manual labour. The major problem associated with back injuries is disability arising from pain. In countries such as the USA and Australia older workers who come from non-English speaking backgrounds are over-represented among people with these injuries. This is probably because such people are over-represented in jobs that have a greater risk of back injury and the effects are cumulative over a long period.

Experimental example

Let us consider an example of where a clinical researcher is interested in comparing the effectiveness of two alternate interventions for treatment of the back injury. There are two common approaches: a conservative approach, such as physiotherapy, and surgery. So, if we took 20 workers with back injuries and, after random allocation, 10 of them were treated with a conservative intervention, such as physiotherapy, and 10 were treated with surgery, we could compare their outcomes.

To achieve a true experimental design, the people need to be randomly allocated to surgery or physiotherapy. Incidentally, to implement this procedure in real life would require a lot of talking to the relevant ethics committees. All the participants would have to volunteer.

As far as the measurement of outcome is

Discussion, Questions and Answers

concerned, most experimental studies would employ a quantitative measure of outcome. For example, the workers could fill in a pain questionnaire, perhaps on several occasions after the intervention, in order to compare the outcomes for the two groups. The use of a written questionnaire, especially if it is provided in English only to people from a non-English speaking background, makes assumptions about the literacy of the participants which may not be valid.

Natural comparison example

If the clinical staff had chosen the interventions for the patients on a non-random basis, the study as described above would be a natural comparison study. Simply comparing groups does not mean we have an experimental design. Otherwise, the study could be structured in an identical fashion to the experimental example described above.

Single-case example

A single-case design involves the administration and withdrawal of interventions in a systematic fashion in order to observe their impact upon the phenomenon under study. The person in the single-case trial is usually challenged with varied interventions to compare the effects of each. This type of design closely approximates the natural clinical history of interventions with many patients, particularly those with chronic illness. However, the interventions in a single-case study are structured much more rigorously.

In the present context, while it would be possible to administer and withdraw physiotherapy and to have baseline phases of no treatment, the surgical intervention cannot be withdrawn. Once the surgery is done, it permanently and drastically changes the person's body. Therefore a single-case

example could involve the alternation of baseline (no treatment) and physiotherapy and then, as the last link in the chain of events, the surgery. This is not a methodologically strong design, as there could be carry-over effects from the previous interventions that interact with the surgery, and the order of the administration of the surgery could not be readily altered.

Survey example

An alternative way of conducting the study of workers with back injuries would be to select a large group of such people and survey them for the different types of interventions they have had for their injury. The outcomes for different groups could then be compared, because, as in a natural comparison study, we can compare groups in a survey design. For example, we could compare men and women respondents. We could even give them the same pain questionnaire as in the types of study previously discussed.

Surveys do not, of course, necessarily involve the use of questionnaires. One could bypass the patients and survey their medical records (with the necessary approvals) and use a coding schedule. Alternatively, the information could be collected in the form of a structured survey interview.

Qualitative field research example

An additional way of studying this issue would be to conduct in-depth interviews with a small number of injured workers to study their interpretations of their situation. Workers who had surgery, as well as those who had physiotherapy, could be interviewed. The interviews would normally be recorded verbatim, transcribed and then exhaustively analyzed for the theoretical constructs needed to describe the experiences of the participants.

Discussion, Questions and Answers

The use of checklists, survey inventories, etc., is normally avoided, although it is usual to have a list of issues to be introduced by the interviewer. The respondents typically describe their experiences and perceptions in their own natural discourse.

In studies which use questionnaires, there is limited interaction between the researcher and the respondent. As is suggested by their name, the respondents respond to the questions framed solely by the researcher. Such an approach can be useful in eliciting factual information in an economical manner. However, it places the respondent in a relatively passive role. If the researcher and the respondent do not share the same constructs, ideas, feelings and motives, the 'wrong' questions may be asked. Schatzman and Strauss (1973, p. 57) note that the researcher 'harbors, wittingly or not, many expectations, conjectures and hypotheses which provide him with thought and directives on what to look for and what to ask about'. The respondent in most questionnaire studies has very little opportunity to contribute to the research agenda. Generally, a token 'any other comments' section is the extent of the invitation for the respondent to contribute to this agenda.

Questions

1. What would be the 'best' design to study the impact of physiotherapy and surgery upon the pain of workers with back injuries?
2. If the participant has been measured frequently over an extended time period, what type of data analysis is required?
3. What type of research design does an epidemiologist typically employ?
4. What special arrangements should be made for participants in research studies with low literacy in English?
5. Is it possible to use an experimental design with in-depth interviewing techniques?

Answers

1. No doubt this question will generate much lively debate. The authors' view is that there is no single best method to conduct such investigations. Each of the methods listed has legitimate insights to offer, which provide a perspective different from that of the others, provided the study is conducted well.
2. This type of design requires an analysis method that can handle repeated measures data, i.e. this is a repeated measures design.
3. Although they may use a variety of different designs, the epidemiologist is likely to use large-scale surveys, often of clinical records. The goal of epidemiologists is to determine the patterns of distribution of illnesses and their relationship with risk factors. Although the modelling may be complex, the research design is simple. Do a large survey.
4. Clinical researchers who are often fluent in English frequently do not make appropriate arrangements for participants with levels of literacy in English lower than their own. Such arrangements could include the provision of interpreters, translated instructions and questionnaires, and interviewers to read the questions to the participants.
5. Yes it is possible to do so, however, it is very unusual. Experimenters typically employ quantitative outcome measures and researchers who use in-depth interviews tend to be disinclined to use experimental research designs. Perhaps both could learn from the other?

Data collection

There are numerous methods available for data collection. The appropriate methods are chosen depending on the aims, design and resources of the research project.

Questionnaires are commonly used with survey designs. In Chapter 9, we examine a number of ways in which we can draw up and validate questionnaires. There are different types of questionnaires ranging from highly structured, standardized scales to unstructured open-ended formats.

An interview (see Ch. 10) is, in a sense, a conversation between the interviewer and the person being interviewed. As they require the presence of an interviewer, this increases the cost and effort needed to obtain data. The presence of an interviewer may also influence the respondent's answers. Qualitative research studies often employ in-depth interviewing techniques which are preferably carried out in the 'natural' settings (homes, hospital, etc.) in which the respondents are living or receiving treatment.

Observational methods are also commonly used strategies for data collection. They may range from highly structured observational protocols, indicating precisely which behaviours or clinical signs should be recorded, to unstructured records of the experiences of participant observers, as used in qualitative research.

Depending on how the data is recorded and analyzed, interviews and observations may be used for both quantitative and qualitative research. However, the use of instrumentation to produce numerical data is most appropriate for quantitative research. A variety of standardized measurement instruments is now available for measuring biological and psychological functions (see Ch. 10).

Whatever data collection strategy is being used, we must ensure that it is reliable (replicable) and valid (accurate). Otherwise, as discussed in Chapter 12, the measurement error due to unreliable and invalid data collection strategies may prevent the researchers from achieving their goals.

9

Questionnaire design

INTRODUCTION

In research investigations, information can be collected through the application of a variety of techniques such as interviews, questionnaires, observation, direct physical measurement and the use of standardized tests. This chapter focuses on questionnaires and questionnaire design, since they are frequently used to collect data in health sciences research.

The specific aims of this chapter are to:

1. Introduce basic concepts in questionnaire design
2. Discuss the construction and administration of questionnaires.

QUESTIONNAIRE CONSTRUCTION

A questionnaire is a document designed with the purpose of seeking specific information from the respondents. Questionnaires are best used with literate people. The design of the questionnaire is crucial to its success. The process of design and implementation is usually termed questionnaire construction.

Questionnaire construction usually involves the following steps:

1. *The researcher defines the information that is being sought*. This may involve considerable thinking and discussion. Inspiration for selection of the required information comes from the investigator's research objectives, discussions with others, reading and other sources. At this stage, the document is

typically a list of information yet to be translated into specific question form.

2. *Drafting of the questionnaire*. The researcher next takes the list of information they wish to obtain from the respondent and attempts to devise draft questions. As is discussed later in this chapter, the phrasing and design of the questions and the overall design of the questionnaire are important for the validity of the obtained information. If the questionnaire is badly designed, then the responses may not accurately reflect the real situation for the respondents.

3. *Questionnaire pilot*. It is wise to pilot or trial a new questionnaire with a small group of the intended respondents and with clinical or research colleagues, in order to improve its clarity and remove any problems, before the main survey. The pilot respondents may be asked whether the questions were clear.

4. *Redrafting of the questionnaire*. If the pilot phase uncovers problems with the questionnaire, it will need to be redrafted in order to address these problems. If they are of a major nature, it is usual to repeat the pilot phase. If they are minor, the researcher may make the necessary changes and then proceed to administration of the questionnaire to the full sample of respondents.

5. *Administration of the questionnaire*. After the questionnaire has been developed, it is administered to the full sample of respondents. The responses are then analyzed in terms of the researcher's aims and objectives.

As with all research, the ethics of conducting surveys and designing questionnaires must be considered. For example, respondents should not be misled concerning the aims of a survey. A blatant example of unethical conduct is if one is asked to respond to a general 'market survey' and then to find a high-pressure salesperson on the doorstep. If the survey is said to be anonymous, then it is questionable practice by the investigator to secretly code the forms. The follow-up of non-responders can cause a dilemma; people choosing not to participate in a survey should not be pestered. However, forms are sometimes mislaid or forgotten and it is necessary to follow these up to ensure a representative sample.

In clinical research, the ethical issues relating to the possible effect of the contents of the questionnaire on the respondent must be taken into account. As an example, one of the present authors was involved in a survey aimed at establishing levels of knowledge of Huntington's disease and certain attitudes of people at risk with the condition (Telsher & Polgar 1981). Before the survey was undertaken, a pilot study was carried out to establish whether or not the questions were upsetting to the subjects. The actual subjects were randomly selected from a 'pedigree chart'. However, the questionnaires could not be sent out before it was clearly established that each of the prospective subjects already knew that they were at risk of developing the condition. It would have been appalling if a person learned from receiving this questionnaire that they were at risk of a severe genetic disorder.

QUESTION AND QUESTIONNAIRE FORMATS

Questions and questionnaires come in a variety of formats. The researcher must decide which is the most appropriate for the purpose of the study. Let us first consider the issue of the questionnaire format.

In some instances, researchers will not prepare a formal questionnaire to be filled in by the respondent, but will design an interview schedule to guide the interviewer who asks the questions. (Interviews are discussed in Chapter 10.) There are costs and benefits in both approaches, as shown in Table 9.1.

The interview schedule approach requires expert interviewers to administer the questions and this is expensive and time-consuming. Further, interviewer bias has been shown to influence responses, as respondents modify their responses to fit in with what they perceive to be the opinions of the interviewer. It is important to note that the structure and content of a questionnaire conveys a lot of information about

Table 9.1 Costs and benefits of interviews and questionnaires

	Costs	Benefits
Interview schedule administered by interviewer	Expensive to administer; requires expert help Responses much more susceptible to interviewer bias	Lower rejection rate More detailed responses can be elicited Greater control over filling out of response form
Self-administered questionnaire	Higher rejection rate Difficult to elicit detailed responses Less control over how response form is filled out	Cheap to administer Less susceptible to interviewer bias Can be administrated by mail

the researcher's agenda to the respondent. The respondent generally has little opportunity to influence the agenda. A questionnaire is not a conversation but a monologue from the researcher to which the potential respondent may or may not respond.

However, the self-administrated questionnaire approach is cheap, is less susceptible to interviewer bias and can be administered by mail. The disadvantages of this approach include higher rejection or refusal rates and much less control over how the response forms are filled out. Anyone involved in self-administered questionnaire analysis will attest to the sometimes remarkable talents of respondents in returning incomplete questionnaire response forms.

Having decided whether the questionnaire will be self-administered or administered by interviewers, the researcher must then decide upon the format for the individual questions.

Open-ended and closed-response formats

There are two major question formats, the open-ended and closed-response types. The distinction between the two is best illustrated by example (see Table 9.2).

Question 1 is an open-ended question whereas the second question is a closed-response question. In an open-ended question, there is no predetermined response schedule into which the respondent must fit their response. In a closed-response question, the respondent is supplied with a predetermined list of response options. The advantages and disadvantages of both question types are represented in Table 9.3.

Table 9.2 Open-ended and closed-response formats

Q1. How do you feel about the standard of the treatment you received while you were a patient at this hospital?

Q2. How would you rate the standard of the treatment you received while you were a patient at this hospital? (circle one number)

excellent	1
good	2
moderately good	3
fair	4
poor	5

Table 9.3 Costs and benefits of open-ended and closed-response formats

	Costs	Benefits
Open-ended	Less structured Responses difficult to encode and analyze using powerful statistical methods Greater time taken by respondent to answer Respondent may find writing an essay more difficult than circling a number	More detailed answers elicited
Closed response	Less 'depth' in answers May frustrate respondents	Tightly structured Responses easily encoded and analyzed Less time taken to collect responses

Although open-ended questions elicit more detailed responses, there are some possible disadvantages associated with this type of

Table 9.4 Questionnaire

Why did you choose XYZ Insurance to insure your car?
- ☐ Newspaper advertisement
- ☐ TV advertisement
- ☐ Personal recommendation
- ☐ Previous insurance with us

Table 9.5 Likert and forced-choice response formats

Q7. My medical practitioner always explains the chosen treatment to me (circle one number).

strongly agree	1
agree	2
undecided	3
disagree	4
strongly disagree	5

Q8. My medical practitioner always explains the chosen treatment to me (circle one number).

strongly agree	1
agree	2
disagree	3
strongly disagree	4

question. The responses generated by such questions require a large amount of effort to encode for data analysis and tend to give rise to categorical scales. These scales necessitate the use of less powerful statistical methods. Further, some respondents may take a long time to answer this type of question.

Of course, to a researcher employing qualitative orientation, these 'disadvantages' may not be seen as such. The opportunity to study the respondent's interpretations expressed in their own words might lead a qualitative researcher to advocate extensive use of open-ended questions. It is more likely that interview techniques rather than a written questionnaire would be employed. Questionnaires, particularly of the self-administered variety, are generally used for convenience and speed, not depth of analysis.

It is important that the lists of options for closed-response questions are carefully designed by the questionnaire designer. It is very easy to bias responses by restricting the range of answers in this type of question.

This brings to mind a short questionnaire distributed by an insurance company to one of the authors (see Table 9.4).

Two features are remarkable about this question. First, it does not allow for any answers other than the ones listed. Second, the range of available answers is very limited. What we wanted to say was that the insurers were cheap and reliable, i.e. were likely to pay up in the event of a claim. Clearly, the survey designer was a marketing person who had not satisfactorily trialled the questions with a non-marketing audience. While the designers may well have obtained the answers they wanted, the answers may not have been the ones the respondents wished to give. In the health sciences, there are often large differences in the ways in which health professionals and consumers approach

the same problems. In questionnaire design, it is vital that the researchers do not impose their own conceptualizations of the situations under investigation to the extent that validity is compromised.

A further example of this danger is provided by the results of a survey conducted at a major teaching children's hospital in Australia (Thomas et al 1989). The survey was designed to study why many parents chose to stay with their children in the hospital in order to plan better facilities and services. One of the questions asked of the respondents was 'Why did your child come to hospital today'? The investigators deliberately chose an open-ended response format for this question in order to tap into the parents' interpretations of the situation in their own words. What a treasure trove of answers! The answers provided considerable insight into the issues of importance to the parents, most of which we could not have predicted. Thus, the ways in which the questions are asked and the answers sought can have a major impact on the value of the information collected.

Likert and forced-choice response formats

In attitudinal questions, two possible response formats may be chosen, the traditional five- or seven-point Likert-type format, or the four-point forced-choice format. These are best illustrated by examples as shown in Table 9.5.

The first example is a conventional five-point Likert-type scale. The second is a four-

Table 9.6 Advantages and disadvantages of response formats

Response format	Advantages	Disadvantages
Likert-type	Allows middle 'undecided' response	Acquiescent response mode
Forced choice	Respondent forced to give either a positive or a negative response	'Undecided' response not allowed

point forced-choice type. The advantages and disadvantages are summarized in Table 9.6.

The forced choice format does not allow respondents to give a 'middle of the road' or undecided answer. This is to guard against respondents using an *acquiescent response mode*. Acquiescent response mode refers to the phenomenon that occurs when respondents give middle responses all the time. *Extreme response mode* occurs when a respondent never selects an intermediate point on the rating scale.

The wording and design of questions

The writing of good questions is an art, and a time consuming art at that. In order to obtain valid and reliable responses one needs well-worded questions. There are a number of pitfalls to be avoided:

1. *Double-barrelled questions.* This is where two questions are included in the one, 'Do you like maths or science?', for example. These questions should be separated so that it is perfectly clear to the respondent (and the researcher) which component is being answered.

2. *Ambiguous questions.* It is important to avoid vacuous words and terms that may mean different things to different people. For example, 'old people' may mean everyone above 30 years old to a teenager, but everyone above 60 to a 50-year-old.

3. *Level of wording.* It is important to tailor the level of wording of questions to accord with the intended respondents. Jargon is to be avoided, and it should be established in the pilot study that the respondents will understand the concepts. For instance, asking questions about 'Trisomy 21' might be inappropriate while 'mongolism' or 'Down syndrome' could be intelligible. Using double negatives should be avoided. In general, questions should be simple and concise.

4. *Bias and leading questions.* The wording of the question should not lead the respondent to feel committed to respond in a certain way. For example, the question 'How often do you go to church?' may lead the respondent to respond in a way that is not entirely truthful if they in fact never go to church. Not only can the wording of a question be leading but the response format may also be leading. For example, if a 'never' response were excluded from the available answers to the above question, the respondent would be led to respond in an inaccurate way. Bias might also arise from possible carry-over effects from answering a pattern of questions. For example, a questionnaire on health workers' attitudes to abortion might include the questions 'Do you value human life?' followed by 'Do you think unborn babies should be murdered in their mothers' wombs?'. In this case, the respondent is being led both by the context in which the second question is asked and the bias involved in the emotional wording of the questions. Surely, one would have to be a monster to answer yes to the second question, given the way it was asked.

Finally, it should be kept in mind that even a good questionnaire might be invalidly administered. For example, a survey on 'Attitudes to migration' might be answered less than honestly by respondents if the interviewer is obviously of immigrant background.

THE STRUCTURE OF QUESTIONNAIRES

Questionnaires may be structured in different ways, but typically the following components are included.

1. *Introductory statement.* The introductory statement describes the purpose of the questionnaire, the information sought and

how it is to be used. It also introduces the researchers and explains whether the information is confidential and/or anonymous.

2. *Demographic questions.* It is usual to collect information about the respondents, including details such as age, sex, education history, and so on. It is best to position these questions first as they are easily answered and serve as a 'warm-up' to what follows.

3. *Factual questions.* It is generally easier for respondents to answer direct factual questions, e.g. 'Do you have a driver's licence?', than to answer opinion questions. Often, this type of question is positioned early on in the questionnaire also to serve as a 'warm up'.

4. *Opinion questions.* Questions that require reflection on the part of the respondent are usually positioned after the demographic and factual questions.

5. *Closing statements and return instructions.* The closing statements in a questionnaire usually

thank the respondent for their participation, invite the respondents to take up any issues they feel have not been satisfactorily addressed in the questionnaire and provide information on how to return the questionnaire.

It is best to avoid complicated structures involving, for example, many conditional questions such as 'If you answered yes to Question 6 and no to Question 9, please answer Question 10'. Conditional questions usually confuse respondents and ought be avoided where possible.

SUMMARY

Questionnaires are frequently used for data collection in health sciences research. This chapter has reviewed the principles of questionnaire design, including issues arising from the selection of appropriate questions and response formats.

SELF ASSESSMENT

Explain the meaning of the following terms:

   acquiescent response mode
   bias
   closed response format
   extreme response mode
   forced response format
   Likert-type scale
   open-ended format
   piloting
   questionnaire

TRUE OR FALSE

1. The aim of survey research is to manipulate the attitudes or beliefs of the respondents.
2. A questionnaire is a measuring instrument which can be employed across a variety of research strategies.

3. If the draft questionnaire is well constructed, there is no need for 'piloting'.
4. As a questionnaire can cause no illness or pain, there is no need to worry about ethical issues when using this instrument.
5. The advantage of an interview schedule over a self-administered questionnaire is that interviews are generally cheaper and less time-consuming to administer.
6. Open-ended questions are easier to analyze and interpret than closed-response questions.
7. If we send out 100 copies of a well constructed self-administered questionnaire we can expect that at least 95 correctly filled-in forms will be returned.
8. A forced choice response format does not allow for 'undecided' responses.

9. 'Acquiescent response mode' refers to the phenomenon where respondents agree with only extreme points on a scale.

10. Survey research is more closely related to naturalistic designs than to true experimental designs.

MULTIPLE CHOICE

1. In which of the following ways is survey research similar to an experimental research design?

   a the selection of a representative sample from the population
   b the assignment of subjects into treatment groups
   c the manipulation of the independent variable by the investigator
   d a and c.

2. When a survey is employed as a research strategy:

   a the making of causal inferences from the data may be problematic
   b we must use a questionnaire for data collection
   c the respondents must be anonymous
   d the external validity of the investigation will be automatically assured.

3. Questionnaires:

   a might have ethical problems associated with their design and administration
   b are instruments for data collection
   c can be employed in experimental research
   d all of the above.

4. Redrafting a questionnaire involves:

   a eliminating questions which are not answered in the predicted direction

   b asking the 'pilot' subjects to write the questionnaire
   c rewriting the questionnaire on the basis of feedback from the 'pilot' administration
   d rewriting the questionnaire in such a way that 'pilot' subjects will select responses that are consistent with the investigator's predictions.

5. The question 'Do you attend gay parties?' is:

   a double-barrelled
   b leading
   c ambiguous
   d an acquiescent response.

6. The question 'Are you presently taking β-blockers?' is:

   a double-barrelled
   b ambiguous
   c biased
   d at the wrong level of difficulty.

7. The advantage(s) of an interview schedule approach over a self-administered questionnaire is that:

   a it is cheaper to administer
   b there is greater control over administration
   c observer bias is minimized
   d people who look a little odd need not be interviewed
   e all of the above.

Do you think it is important for undergraduate students in the health sciences to study statistics (circle one)?

Strongly agree
Agree
Undecided
Disagree
Strongly disagree.

SELF ASSESSMENT

8. The above is an example of:

   a an open-ended question
   b a Likert scale
   c a double-barrelled question
   d a leading question
   e none of the above.

9. The advantage of a closed-response format over an open-ended response format is that:

   a more 'in depth' responses can be elicited
   b there is a lower response rate
   c the responses are easily encoded and analyzed
   d it is more likely that the actual attitudes or feelings of the respondents will be revealed.

10

Interview techniques and the analysis of interview data

INTRODUCTION

An interview may be defined as a conversation between interviewers and interviewees with the purpose of eliciting certain information.

Interviews are a key tool for the clinician and the health researcher as a means of collecting information. However, interviews may vary substantially in their structure, content and the way in which the data are elicited and analyzed. This chapter is concerned with interviews and the analysis of interview data.

The specific aims of this chapter are to:

1. Distinguish between structured and unstructured interviews
2. Outline commonly used strategies for conducting interviews
3. Compare and contrast quantitative and qualitative strategies for conducting interviews.

STRUCTURED AND UNSTRUCTURED INTERVIEWS

Many researchers distinguish between structured and unstructured interviews. Sometimes the terms 'formal' and 'informal' or 'guided' and 'open-ended' are also used (see for example, Field & Morse 1985).

Denzin (1978, pp. 113–116) distinguishes between three forms of the interview: the schedule standardized interview in which 'the wording and order of all questions are exactly the same for every respondent', the non-schedule standardized interview where 'certain types of information are desired from all respondents but the particular phrasing of questions and their order are redefined' and the non-standardized interview in which 'no prescribed set of questions is employed'.

If one defines an interview as a conversation, then a schedule standardized interview is a very rigid form of conversation, almost like a play with a fixed script.

In its most structured form, a structured interview may involve the reading of a prepared questionnaire to a respondent and then filling in an answer form or response sheet for them on the basis of their answers. The questions are provided in a systematic order, with minimal or no deviation from the prepared script. In a structured interview, the role of the interviewer is to ask the questions and the role of the respondent is to provide the answers with minimal extraneous information. Conversely, an unstructured interview may involve the interviewer in asking no direct questions, but simply prompting the respondent to reflect on their current interests and concerns. Clearly, between these extremes lies a variety of different types of interview strategies and degrees of structure. The extent of 'structure' or 'formality' is determined by a number of factors, including the following:

1. *Whether there is a fixed set of questions or schedule.* In a structured interview, the interviewer has a preplanned set of questions or schedule. These questions may or may not be presented in a fixed order. In an unstructured interview, there may be particular 'themes' to be explored without a specific order required or specific question wordings.

2. *The way in which the information is recorded.* There are a number of ways in which interview information may be recorded. (This is discussed in detail in a later section of this chapter.) Structured interviews tend to employ pre-planned answer sheets or response schedules. Unstructured interviews have less expectations and restrictions on the answer formats of the respondents. The interviewer may record the interview or take free-form notes.

3. *The types of questions.* Structured interviews tend to employ more closed response questions, in which the valid answers have been preplanned, rather than open-ended questions. As discussed in the survey chapter of this text, with open-ended questions the respondents provide their answers in their own words, whereas closed response questions involve a choice of answers provided by the interviewer.

4. *The extent of control by the interviewer.* In a structured interview, the interviewer explicitly guides or directs the conversation (e.g. 'Now Mr. Smith, let's discuss how your family feels about your problem') rather than the respondent setting the agenda. In an unstructured interview, the respondent may assume a more active role in the conversation.

It is useful to consider some of the advantages and disadvantages of the different types of interview approaches. These are summarized in Table 10.1.

The appropriateness of the different interview approaches is determined by the objectives of the researcher. If the researcher simply wished to collect some basic symptom data, an unstructured interview would be inefficient. However, if the researcher wished to study people's conceptualization and interpretation of their illness, an unstructured interview may be quite suitable.

Table 10.1 Advantages and disadvantages of structured and unstructured interviews

	Advantages	Disadvantages
Structured interviews	May be less time consuming The same information is collected for all respondents	Responses may not be recorded in the respondents' own words
Unstructured interviews	Responses may be recorded in the 'own words' of the respondents, hence less bias through interpretation The respondent has some input into the research agenda	May be time consuming Not all the same information is collected for all respondents

Some clinical interviews such as history taking are highly structured whereas other clinical interviews, such as those involving management of a long-term problem, may be less so.

METHODS OF CONDUCTING INTERVIEWS

Since an interview is a conversation, there exist several possible methods for conducting it. The interview may be conducted in person ('face to face') or by remote means such as by telephone. There are a number of advantages associated with face to face interview. (These are also discussed in the survey chapter of this text.) Face-to-face interviews permit the non-verbal reactions of the respondent to be observed and perhaps the development of a closer rapport arising from the more 'natural' setting. The interviewer may use their observations of non-verbal cues to supplement the verbal information being provided and use their own non-verbal cues in a similar fashion. However, the face-to-face interview may require a substantial amount of participant travel time and hence higher costs than for a telephone interview. With certain interview objectives, however, telephone interviews may not be suitable. If the interviewer and their credentials are not well known to the interviewee, it is unlikely that participants in a telephone interview would provide valid and reliable personal information about personal topics. Conversely, if the interviewer is trusted, some people find disclosure of sensitive information to be easier by telephone. The face to face interview may be too confrontational or embarrassing for them.

THE INTERVIEW PROCESS

1. *Selection of interviewees.* One of the interviewer's first tasks is to select those to be interviewed. In qualitative research, techniques such as random sampling are used infrequently. Rather, the interviewer selects those who are most likely to provide the required insights into the situation or issue under study, i.e. the 'key informants'.

2. *Recruitment of interviewees.* The interviewer must then enlist the participation of the interviewees. Typically, the interviewer will contact the potential participant, explain the purposes of the interview and make a number of assurances. These assurances may include anonymity, the ability to vet materials based on the interview and the extent of time involvement of the interviewee. Often, the interviewer might write to the interviewee first and then contact them personally to be less 'confronting'.

3. *The interview.* The process of the interview varies substantially according to the methodology to be employed by the interviewer. The process of a structured interview is quite different from that of an unstructured interview. However, some basic goals are shared. The desirability of tapping the interviewee's views rather than reflecting those of the interviewer (i.e. maximization of validity) is paramount. To achieve this, interviewers need to be sensitive, non-evaluative, alert and skilled at delivering and sequencing their questions. In in-depth interviewing, multiple interviews may be required. In this type of approach, the emphasis is on depth of analysis with a smaller number of interviewees rather than the breadth of coverage of interviewees offered by a sample survey. Substantial practise and good interpersonal skills are required to achieve competence in interviewing.

Both video and audio recording of interviews have one large advantage over other methods of recording interview information. This is that the interviewer's interpretation of the interviewee's answers is open to independent scrutiny, because the primary materials are available for study by others.

4. *Use of response schedules/answer checklists.* When conducting an interview, the interviewer may record the information provided by the interviewee on a predesigned response schedule/answer checklist. For example, the schedule may contain information such as the sex and age of the respondent and areas for recording their answers to particular questions. Typically, the response sheet is completed during the interview, although it can be completed at some

time following the interview. Immediate recording is probably more valid and reliable, although, once again, the mere presence of a recording device may be of concern to the respondent. Unless the response sheet is well-designed, there is a major problem of handling novel or unexpected turns in the interview. The interviewer is interpreting, on the fly, the answers and information provided by the interviewee. If those do not conform to the assumptions designed into the response sheet, these interpretations may not be satisfactory or well considered. Telephone interviews may involve the use of computer assistance where the interviewer is prompted by, and records the responses on a computerized schedule.

5. *Free form (unstructured) notes.* This method of recording involves the interviewer making free- form notes to record information they believe to be salient, either during or following the interview. This method of recording is used extensively by clinicians in case notes. There are a number of advantages and problems with such recording; these result from the process whereby the interview is distilled into the notes. This process involves substantial judgment and interpretation on the part of the interviewer. Such distillations result in highly refined and reduced data, the validity of which, at least in terms of the interview, is inaccessible to scrutiny. Further, free-form note-taking may not result in the recording of the same type of data across interviewees. Often, when case audits from records are being performed, it is not possible to derive the required data from clinical notes because of this problem.

6. *Follow-up.* Having completed the interviews, the interviewer may wish to follow-up the participants. Some interviewers undertake to give the interviewees copies of their findings and may offer the right of vetting the materials based on the interview.

METHODS OF RECORDING INTERVIEW INFORMATION

Interviewers may use a number of different means of recording interview information, ranging from written summary notes of the interview to an actual video or audio taping of the live interview. These recording methods have a number of advantages and disadvantages, as discussed below.

1. *Video recording.* Video technology has reduced in cost and improved to such an extent that high-quality video recordings of interviews are well within the budgets of many organizations and individuals. Video recordings provide a wealth of information about the interview. It is possible to observe non-verbal communication channels as well as to construct audio transcripts of the interaction between the participants. However, some interviewees find the presence of the camera to be threatening. This may have a number of effects; one may be to refuse to participate, another may be to alter the normal flow of the interview. Some respondents may be unwilling to commit personal information and/or controversial views to tape, if they believe there is a risk that the interviewer might disclose the interview to others. The interviewee would find it difficult to deny their views when they have been videotaped expressing them. This is why the police in some countries videotape their interviews with suspects.

2. *Audio taping.* Many interviewers use audio recording of interviews in order to be able to prepare transcripts for later study. Many of the same issues that pertain to video recording are also relevant to audio recording. The use of audio recording may result in greater refusal rates and the 'sanitization' of the views expressed by participants for fear of reprisals arising from disclosure of the interview to others.

Qualitative research methodologists have developed systematic methods in note-taking and coding of interview information. For an excellent treatment of these issues, the reader is referred to Minichiello et al (1991).

Advantages and disadvantages of interview recording methods

The advantages and disadvantages of the

Table 10.2 Advantages and disadvantages of different ways of recording interview information

	Advantages	Disadvantages
Video recording	Full transcripts of interview possible Non-verbal data available Accessible to independent analysis	Intrusive Less disclosure Necessity for substantial, and costly, post interview analysis Potentially greater rates of refusal to participate
Audio recording	Full transcripts of interview possible Accessible to Independent analysis	Intrusive (but probably less than video) Reduced disclosure Necessity for substantial, and costly, post interview analysis Potentially greater rates of refusal to participate
Response sheets	Same data recorded for all interviews Little post-interview analysis required reducing costs	Unexpected answers may not be well handled Interviewer may bias data in its recording Inaccessible to independent analysis
Unstructured notes	Cheap and simple	Interviewer may bias data in its recording Some data may be omitted Inaccessible to independent analysis Necessity for some post interview analysis

various recording methods may be summarized in Table 10.2. Thus, video recording is intrusive, requires substantial post-interview analysis and may result in less disclosure, yet provides very rich information that can be independently analysed. The use of a recording method such as a response sheet requires great trust in the judgment and recording abilities of the interviewer. There is a potential for bias arising from the interviewer 'adjusting' the information provided by the interviewee to fit the recording method and/or expectations of the interviewer. Further, there is no opportunity for re-analysis.

So which information recording method for interviews is the most appropriate? The appropriateness of the method of recording interview information is determined by the needs of the person using the information. For example, if the information user simply wants some basic data such as the age, sex and symptom profile of a patient, it would be absurd to use video recording. This would be very time consuming. Each tape would have to be made then viewed again for analysis. In this instance, a simple response sheet or checklist would suffice. However, if the interviewer was interested in exploring reactions of interviewees to the death of a close relative, perhaps the use of audio or video recording would provide a richness of data suitable for that interest.

Although most interviews are conducted with one interviewer and one interviewee present, sometimes group interviews with many participants are conducted. The focus group, which is a form of group interview, involves a discussion among a small group of people, including a moderator or facilatator (Thomas et al 1992). The facilitators' role is to introduce the topics or questions for discussion and to facilitate the contributions of the group participants. Merton (1946) originally proposed the focused interview, which was the forerunner for the focus group.

Focus groups differ fundamentally from the individual interview in that the researcher is outnumbered and the participants may interact with each other, modify each others responses and ask questions of each other. The researcher is no longer at the centre of the process. Focus groups are now widely used in health research because they provide rich sources of insights and interpretations from the participants.

THE ANALYSIS OF INTERVIEW DATA

The manner in which interview data may be analyzed is determined in part by how the data have been recorded and in part, by the theoretical orientation of the researcher. In the previous section, we have seen that these formats include videotapes, audiotapes, completed response sheets and free-form summary interviewer notes.

The basis for many analyses of interview data is the interview transcript. The transcript of an interview is a verbatim written version of the conversation that took place between the participants. To provide an example, an excerpt from an interview transcript produced by Janet Doyle at La Trobe University follows. The transcript is of an interview between a clinician and a client, concerning the client's hearing loss.

Clinician:	Okay. So what are you noticing with your hearing?
Client:	Well in a crowded area I can't you know understand the other people.
Clinician:	Right, sound's a bit jumbled up.
Client:	And when I am in the next room I can't even hear the phone.
Clinician:	Right.
Client:	I am not bad, it is like I am not that bad but still at times.
Clinician:	Right.
Client:	There is a lot of times I can't hear it.
Clinician:	If people speak directly to you like this you are fairly good?
Client:	Yes I am alright.
Clinician:	But in a group have a bit of trouble?
Client:	Have trouble.
Clinician:	Right, does one ear seem better than the other ear?
Client:	Yes, this one seems better than this.
Clinician:	Right.
Clinician:	How long have you been noticing your difficulty?
Client:	Oh about 12 to 18 months I suppose.
Clinician:	Just gradual was it?
Client:	Yes.
Clinician:	Okay. Do you get any ringing or buzzing in your ears?
Client:	Oh now and again, very seldom though.
Clinician:	It doesn't bother you?
Client:	No.
Clinician:	Okay. Have you had medical trouble with your ears like infection or anything?
Client:	No, no.
Clinician:	Do you know of any family history of hearing loss?
Client:	No, only the older brother, he has got a hearing aid.
Clinician:	Right.
Client:	That's all.
Clinician:	Have you been exposed to excessive noise?
Client:	Yes.
Clinician:	…machinery or?
Client:	Yeah. I worked down the car plant you know with the heavy machinery.
Clinician:	The assembly line?

Client:	Right.
Clinician:	Were you doing that sort of work for a long time?
Client:	Oh yes, 30 years.
Clinician	Yeah, that's a fair…
Client:	I wasn't on the line all the time but.
Clinician:	Right.

And so the interview continued.

Let us consider some of the analysis options under the quantitative and qualitative headings.

Quantitative analysis of interview transcripts

A number of quantitative analyses possibilities are presented with interview transcripts. For example, the researcher might count the number of words spoken by each participant to obtain a quantitative measure of their relative contributions to the conversational process. Another possibility would be to count the number of questions asked by the clinician. These quantitative measures could then be used to test various hypotheses. Analyses of interview transcripts similar to the example shown above, in the study from which it was taken, have demonstrated substantial sex differences between the number of questions asked by male and female clients. It seems that the male clients asked many more questions than the females. Thus, the quantitative researcher might use interview transcripts to count and analyze certain features of the transcripts.

Qualitative analysis of interview transcripts

Under the qualitative heading there is a broad variety of approaches to the collection and analysis of interview data. Such approaches may, however, be broadly categorized as descriptive or theoretical.

A descriptive qualitative study is often termed an ethnography. They are often written from the perspective of the participant(s) in the first person. The purpose of the ethnography is to provide a detailed description of a particular set of circumstances and to encourage the reader to make their own interpretations. A celebrated example of such an ethnography is found in Bogdan & Taylor's (1976) description of Ed Murphy's life. Ed Murphy was a former resident of a home for the intellectually disabled in the USA.

Many qualitative studies, however, are theoretical in nature. That is, they attempt to develop theories and concepts and, often, to verify these concepts and theories.

A key approach to theoretical qualitative research is provided by Glaser & Strauss' (1967) grounded theory (see also Strauss 1987). Glaser & Strauss advocate two methods for the development of grounded theory: the constant comparative method in which the researcher codes and analyzes data to develop concepts and the theoretical sampling method in which cases are selected purposively to refine the 'theory' previously developed. Glaser & Strauss provide highly detailed examples of their analytic methods in the above references and the interested reader is referred to them for further detail.

Glaser & Strauss' approach is not universally accepted in that some qualitative researchers argue for the necessity to both develop and verify their theories. Taylor & Bogdan (1984) provide an extended discussion of these issues.

Notwithstanding these theoretical differences, many qualitative researchers share common analysis tools such as coding and thematic analysis.

Coding and thematic analysis

Coding is used to organize data collected in an interview and, for that matter, in other types of documents such as field notes. Different qualitative researchers advocate different approaches to coding but it typically involves the following steps. The researchers first study their materials, in this case transcripts, and develop a close familiarity with the material. During this process, all the concepts, themes and ideas are noted to form major categories. For example, in interviews of nursing home residents, some theme might include personal safety, autonomy and decision making, personal hygiene, and so on. Often, the researcher will then attach a number or label to each category and record their positions in the transcript. Coding is an iterative process, with the researcher coding and recoding, as the scheme develops. Some computer programmes are now available to assist with the coding analysis of machine-readable transcripts and these ease some of the clerical burden, although most qualitative researchers still employ manual coding methods. The researchers, having developed the codes and coded the transcripts, then attempt to interpret their meanings in the context in which they appeared. The reporting of this process typically involves 'thick' or detailed description of the categories and their context, with liberal use of examples from the original transcripts.

SUMMARY

Interviews may be defined as a conversation between interviewers and interviewees with the purpose of eliciting certain information. Structured interviews generally involve a fixed set of questions or schedule, the use of pre-planned response sheets, a greater proportion of closed response questions and direction from the interviewer. Unstructured interviews tend not to have these attributes, with less structure and control. Interviews may be conducted face to face or by telephone and both these methods have certain advantages and disadvantages. The focus group is a valuable alternative to the individual interview. Interview data may be recorded in a number of different ways, but the transcript is often used. Transcripts may be analyzed using quantitative or qualitative techniques.

SELF ASSESSMENT

Explain the meaning of the terms:

> interview
> structured interview
> unstructured interview
> coding
> response schedule
> transcript
> grounded theory
> ethnography

TRUE OR FALSE

1. A structured interview always involves a written questionnaire.
2. In an unstructured interview, the questions are asked in a fixed order.
3. In an interview, it is important for the interviewer to express their feelings.
4. In a response schedule, the interviewer records his/her interpretation of the interviewee's statements.
5. Coding is a method of qualitative analysis of interview transcripts.
6. An ethnography is generally written in the third person.
7. A transcript is a summary of the interviewer's interpretation of their questions.
8. Video recording of an interview may affect the honesty of the interviewee's answers.

MULTIPLE CHOICE

1. One of the problems with unstructured interviews is that:

   a the same questions may not be asked of all interviewees
   b the answers are recorded in the interviewee's own words
   c the questions are all asked in the same order
   d the interviews are too brief.

2. One of the problems with structured interviews is that:

   a the same questions may not be asked of all interviewees
   b the answers are not recorded in the interviewee's own words
   c the questions are all asked in the same order
   d the interviews are often too long.

3. One of the advantages of a face to face interview is that:

   a the interviewer can take an audio recording of the interview
   b non-verbal cues can be ignored
   c the interviewer can minimize their influence on the answers
   d the interviewer has more credibility than a telephone interviewer.

4. A qualitative analysis of an interview transcript is likely to include:

   a counting the number of words spoken by each participant
   b the use of a checklist
   c coding of recurrent themes and ideas
   d checks on the quality of the interviewer's speech.

5. A quantitative analysis of an interview transcript is likely to include:

   a the use of unstructured field notes
   b coding of recurrent themes and ideas
   c counting the number of words spoken by each participant
   d checks on the quality of the interviewer's speech.

6. To record the age, sex, height and weight of a patient, it would be best:

   a to use a video recorder
   b to use an audio tape recorder

SELF ASSESSMENT

c to use a transcript of the interview

d to use a response checklist.

7. An ethnography is:

a an interview with a non-English speaking person

b an interview with a foreign-born but English-speaking person

c a type of descriptive qualitative study of someone's experiences

d a type of quantitative study.

8. Coding is:

a a qualitative method of analysing interview data

b a method of keeping interview data confidential

c a quantitative method of analyzing interview data

d usually performed without a written transcript.

11

Observation

INTRODUCTION

Observation is a common method for data collection both in scientific and health care research, as well as in clinical practice. Observation involves being close to things, such that the observer is in a position to directly perceive and record specific aspects of the environment under study. The advantage of observational data collection over questionnaires and interviews in human research is that the researcher is in a position to see and hear how people actually act, rather than relying on their perhaps biased reports and justification of their actions.

The specific aims of the present chapter are to:

1. Outline different approaches to conducting observations and examine their relative advantages
2. Discuss the different roles observers may adopt
3. Examine observation in the context of qualitative and quantitative approaches.

OVERVIEW OF DIFFERENT APPROACHES TO OBSERVATION

Depending on the phenomenon being studied and the research questions being asked, one or more of a number of different observational approaches may be employed in the data collection. Each of these approaches have associated advantages and disadvantages. The basic issues are:

- who is to make the observations
- the settings in which the observations are made
- the use of instrumentation.

Self-observation or outside observer

When research involves the observation of human subjects, self-observation becomes possible and at times advantageous. As an example, consider the study of a phenomenon such as pain. Here the patients themselves are particularly well positioned to provide subjective evidence concerning the intensity and location of pain over a period of time. Figure 11.1 shows a typical chart for guiding self-recorded pain observations in chronic pain patients, which is used in both research and clinical assessment.

The self-observations of the patients provide data for understanding how patients' pain experiences change over time, events correlating with the onset and offset of the pain and also

evidence for evaluating the relative effectiveness of pain management strategies.

Given that the experience of pain may be expressed in the sufferer's overt behaviour, we may observe such pain-related behaviours when assessing pain. For instance, in a study involving comparison of pain behaviours of surgical patients with different cultural backgrounds, independent observers recorded pain-related behaviours in patients at agreed time intervals during physiotherapy treatments. Figure 11.2 is based on whether the observers recorded a yes or no for each category for each time interval in which the behaviours were sampled.

There are probable relative advantages and disadvantages to using self-observation or outside observers, as shown in Table 11.1.

Settings in which observation is conducted

Some disciplines, such as astronomy or geography,

	On average, what was your level of pain during today?										
Monday	0 no pain	1	2	3	4	5	6	7	8	9	10 very intense
Tuesday	0 no pain	1	2	3	4	5	6	7	8	9	10 very intense
Wednesday	0 no pain	1	2	3	4	5	6	7	8	9	10 very intense

Fig. 11.1 Typical chart for self recorded pain observations.

Behaviours	Time		
	t_1	t_2	t_3
Verbal complaint			
Vocalisation			
Protective response			

Fig. 11.2 Observation guide for recording pain behaviours.

Table 11.1 Advantages and disadvantages of using self-observation or outside observers

	Advantages	Disadvantages
Self-observation	Greater access to subjective experience (introspection) Less intrusive Less expensive	Greater bias Less likely to record accurately Less likely to carry out observation as agreed
Outside observer	Greater objectivity Less bias More likely to record accurately More likely to carry out observations as agreed	Cannot directly access subject's perceptions More intrusive More expensive and time consuming

Table 11.2 Advantages and disadvantages of laboratory and natural settings for making observations

	Advantages	Disadvantages
Laboratory setting	Better control over extraneous variables Observation aids and recording equipment available	Distortion of phenomena in artificial environments Problematic ecological validity
Natural setting	Increased ecological validity Observation of phenomenon as it occurs naturally	Little control over extraneous variables Observation aids and recording equipment may be more difficult to use

focus on phenomena which are best studied as they occur, in their natural settings. Other disciplines, such as anatomy or chemistry are more likely to be studied in a laboratory. In the broad range of health sciences research, phenomena are studied in either laboratory or natural settings, and observational data collection may be appropriate in both of these settings.

The general advantage of laboratory environments is that we can impose a considerable degree of control over extraneous variables which may systematically influence our observations. In addition, equipment for facilitating or recording observations is more readily available. For example, in the 1960s, Masters and Johnson began a series of studies to examine the physiology of the human sexual response. The controlled laboratory setting and the use of appropriate instrumentation enabled these researchers to observe and record previously undiscovered aspects of human sexual functioning. This work was thought to be fundamental for developing clinically useful interventions aimed at helping people with sexual dysfunctioning.

The disadvantage with laboratory settings is that the phenomenon being observed may change in an artificial setting. This is particularly true for human behaviour, where the social contexts are fundamental determinants of the behaviours and experiences. In other words,

laboratory research sometimes has problematic ecological validity. Table 11.2 summarises some of the relative advantages and disadvantages of laboratory and natural settings for making observations.

Unaided observation or the use of instrumentation

The accurate observation of a variety of phenomena is possible through the unaided senses; for example, observing aspects of human behaviour or clinical symptoms such as abnormal postures, discoloration of the skin, or abnormalities in patients' eye movements.

Other phenomena may be inaccessible to unaided observation such as, for example, very small objects and events, where we might need to use a microscope for accurate observations. Some events are also extremely complex and occur relatively quickly in relation to the observer. An example of this is human locomotion where recording the event using a device such as a video camera greatly enhances the accuracy of the observation. A fundamental reason for the advancement of science and clinical practice has been the development of sophisticated instrumentation.

There are, however, certain disadvantages associated with using instrumentation. These issues are discussed further in Chapter 12, when

Table 11.3 The advantages and disadvantages of using instruments for aiding observations

	Advantages	Disadvantages
Unaided observations	Less disruptive Best suited for observing human behaviour Relatively simple and inexpensive	Insufficient for observing some phenomena Insufficient accuracy and detail
Instrumentation	Access to events outside unaided human senses Increased accuracy and detail	May distort phenomena May be complex and expensive to use

we review instrumentation and measurement. We can note here, however, that the use of instruments may distort the event being observed: for example, the preparation of tissue for electron microscopy changes to some extent the internal organelles of a cell being observed. It requires considerable expertise to use more complex instruments, and a strong theoretical background to separate the artefacts from useful data and interpret the observations. Human subjects also react to being observed. The more intrusive the observer is with equipment and instruments the more likely that the subjects' behaviour will change.

The use and relative advantages and disadvantages of recording techniques were discussed in the context of interviewing techniques in Chapter 10. Table 11.3 represents the relative advantages and disadvantages of using instruments for aiding observations.

OBSERVER ROLES

Whether or not instrumentation is used, observation involves a person perceiving and recording an event. There are various positions observers may take in relation to observing human behaviour in health care settings. The fundamental issue is the extent to which the observer becomes involved or participates in the events being observed.

There are four main roles: complete participant, participant as observer, observer as participant and complete observer. These are discussed below.

The *complete participant* assumes the role of participant in the setting under investigation and does not normally disclose his or her intent to the other participants. Thus, the researcher actively participates in the setting without the knowledge or consent of the other participants. The purpose behind this approach is to minimize any changes in behaviour of the other participants as a result of their being observed. It can, however, border on the edge of unethical practice and must be used with caution.

An example of the use of the complete participant method is provided by Rosenhan's (1975) study of 'pseudo-patients' in psychiatric hospitals. Here, the observers posed as (and were admitted as) psychiatric patients in order to study the experiences of psychiatric patients. The pseudo-patients were not recognized as impostors by the staff or the institutions. In this way, they could make and record observations about the interpersonal interactions between the staff and patients. However, in order to be admitted, the observers deliberately misled the staff, who were in fact under study.

The *participant as observer* participates fully in the situation under study, but discloses his or her identity and purpose to the other participants. Examples of this can be seen in anthropological studies, where the observer attempts to participate as an active member of a cultural group.

The *observer as participant* makes no pretence of participation but interacts with the other participants. When using this method in a health setting, the observer obtains permission to record events and observe patients, while interacting with the staff and the patients. An example of this method is provided by a study recently performed by a PhD student with a nursing background, supervised by one of the authors. The student's objective was to investigate how psychiatric nurses working in the community make decisions to act in a crisis situation with a disturbed person. He accompanied the nurses on their crisis visits. While travelling to the crisis scene, he interviewed the nurses about their expectations. He observed the crisis scene and its participants and immediately following its conclusion interviewed the nurses about it.

The *complete observer* does not interact with the other participants at all and as with complete participation does not disclose his or her identity or purpose. As an example, one might investigate therapist–patient interactions by observing from behind a one-way mirror. Observers can, if they wish, use a structured schedule for making the observations.

The level of participation chosen involves a tension between the requirements of objective and independent analysis, and the proximity from which the social and clinical phenomena can be studied. Clearly, the participation of the observer introduces changes in the phenomenon under study. It is a question of whether these changes are so large as to negate the benefits obtained by closer observation afforded by actual participation. This is a vexed question and one that has had much discussion in the social and clinical sciences.

OBSERVATION IN QUALITATIVE FIELD RESEARCH

Observation data collection in the context of qualitative field research requires providing authentic pictures and reports of individuals functioning in their natural environments. Lofland (1971) outlined the following four features for approaching field research:

1. The investigator should establish proximity with the subjects in both a physical and a social sense. It is desirable that this involvement should be long term, both to enable understanding and to reduce the subjects' reactivity to the presence of the investigator.
2. The report should be truthful. The reporter should not allow ideological biases to distort or censor their observations or deliberately lie to place their subjects in a good or bad light.
3. The data should contain a large amount of 'pure description of action, people, activities and the like. The reality of the place should be conveyed through representation of its

mundane aspects in a straightforward manner' (Lofland 1971, p.4).
4. The data should contain direct quotations from the participants. Note-taking, audio and video recordings are appropriate for conveying the actual situation. The obtrusiveness of the data collection methods is a major factor. It would not do to assume the role of a complete participant and turn up with a movie camera, while denying any other motives.

Lofland (1971) suggested that when observing subjects in the context of field research, the investigator might focus on the following categories:

1. *Acts and activities*. These are actions constituting brief or major involvements of an individual:

All pseudopatients took extensive notes publicly. Under ordinary circumstances, such behaviour would have raised questions in the minds of observers, as, in fact, it did among patients. Indeed, it seemed so certain that the notes would elicit suspicion that elaborate precautions were taken to remove them from the ward each day. But the precautions proved needless. The closest any staff member came to questioning these notes occurred when one pseudo-patient asked his physician what kind of medication he was receiving and began to write down the response. 'You needn't write it', he was told gently. 'If you have trouble remembering, just ask me again.'

Rosenhan (1975)

2. *Meanings*. These are verbal productions, defining or explaining the subject's activities:

Holding her breath, standing still, sniffing, and coughing were all means of countering what she felt as her mother's impingements.

Mary:	I used to hold my breath because my mother used to go on so quick and (pause).
Interviewer:	Moving you mean?
Mary	Yes.
Interviewer:	You mean your mother was moving about the house quickly?
Mary:	Yes and everything.
Interviewer:	And what did you do?
Mary:	Sort of stand like that.
Interviewer:	Can you demonstrate to me—sitting in a chair?

Mary:	Yes. I just sort of (shows what she did).
Interviewer:	With your elbows?

Laing & Esterson (1970)

3. *Participation*. This describes the subjects' involvement in a particular setting:

The pseudopatient behaved afterward as he normally behaved. The pseudopatient spoke to patients and staff as he might ordinarily. Because there is uncommonly little to do on a psychiatric ward, he attempted to engage others in conversation. When asked by staff how he was feeling, he indicated that he was fine, that he no longer experienced symptoms. He responded to instructions from attendants, to calls for medication (which was not swallowed), and to dining-hall instructions. Beyond such activities as were available to him on the admissions ward, he spent his time writing down his observations about the ward, its patients, and the staff. Initially these notes were written secretly, but as it soon became clear that no one much cared, they were subsequently written on standard tablets of paper in such public places as the day- room. No secret was made of these activities.

Rosenhan (1975)

4. *Relationships*. These are descriptions of the nature of the interrelationships among several people:

Her absence of social life, her withdrawal, appears to be an unwitting invention of her parents that never seems to have been called into question.

Ruth:	Well the places I like to go to my parents don't like me to go to.
Mother:	Such as?
Ruth:	Eddie's club.
Mother:	Oh, goodness. You don't really—
Father:	?
Ruth:	I do.
Interviewer:	What is 'Eddie's'?
Mother:	It's a drinking club. She doesn't really drink. It's just that she likes to meet different types.
Interviewer:	She sounds as though the people that she does want to go out with are people she feels you disapprove of.
Mother:	Possibly.
Father:	Yes.
Mother	Possibly.

Her parents' attitude to the life Ruth actually leads involves both the negation of its existence and the perception of mad or bad behaviour on Ruth's part. Thus, she is said to drink excessively, while, simultaneously, she is said not to drink at all.

Laing & Esterson (1970)

5. *Settings*. These are descriptions of the entire setting for the investigation:

A stranger entering an ICU is at once bombarded with a massive array of sensory stimuli, some emotionally neutral but many highly charged. Initially, the greatest impact comes from the intricate machinery, with its flashing lights, buzzing and beeping monitors, gurgling suction pumps, and whooshing respirators. Simultaneously, one sees many people rushing around busily performing lifesaving tasks. The atmosphere is not unlike that of the tension-charged strategic bunker. With time, habituation occurs, but the ever-continuing stimuli decrease the overload threshold and contribute to stress at times of crisis.

As the newness and strangeness of the unit wears off, one increasingly becomes aware of a host of perceptions with specific stressful emotional significance. Desperately ill, sick, and injured human beings are hooked up to that machinery. And, in addition to mechanical stimuli, one can discern moaning, crying, screaming and the last gasps of life. Sights of blood, vomitus and excreta, exposed genitalia, mutilated wasting bodies, and unconscious and helpless people assault the sensibilities. Unceasingly, the ICU nurse must face these affect-laden stimuli with all the distress and conflict that they engender.

Hay & Oken (1977)

Observations of the above classes of behaviours and settings will provide a report representing individuals' experiences and their interactions in a natural setting.

OBSERVATION IN QUANTITATIVE RESEARCH

Research involving human subjects may be conducted using either qualitative or quantitative approaches. With non-human phenomena, quantitative approaches are obviously more relevant. The following are common features of observations in the context of quantitative research.

1. *Observer roles*. In quantitative research, the observer attempts to be as objective and detached as possible. Therefore, the observer as participant *or* the complete observer roles are most suited for quantitative approaches.

2. *Definition of relevant variables*. Considerable effort is made in quantitative research to specify precisely what aspect of an object, event or

human behaviour the investigator intends to study and observe. In studies where several observers are involved in data collection, it is appropriate to discuss and demonstrate that there is a substantial degree of agreement among the observers. The above issues will be discussed in more detail in the context of operational definitions, validity and reliability in Chapter 12.

3. *Observation and structure.* For quantitative studies, we prefer the maximum level of control and structure. Bailey (1987, p. 243) suggested that there were two types of 'structures' relevant for observational data collection. The first is the degree of structure in the environment in which the observations are made. We have examined this point earlier, where we compared laboratory and natural settings with laboratory settings having a higher degree of structure or predictability. The degree of structure for observation may be further increased by using explicit, previously prepared observation guides of protocols. This is quite similar to how degrees of 'structure' or 'formality' are determined in the context of interview techniques, as outlined in the previous chapters.

We have examined two different types of observation guides (shown in Figs 11.1 and 11.2). If they are to be useful for conducting observational data collection, considerable effort must be made in the design of such guides and in establishing their reliability and validity, as we shall see in the next chapter.

The advantages of an observation guide are that the recording of the observations is made simple, and the data are easily summarized and evaluated using descriptive and inferential statistics, as discussed in later chapters of this book. The disadvantage of highly structured observations (as with interview and questionnaire techniques) is that the spontaneity and uniqueness of certain events may be lost, to the extent that only predetermined categories are recorded.

SUMMARY

Data collection based on observation is appropriate for a wide range of research designs, ranging from laboratory-based experiments to qualitative field research. A basic issue is the extent to which a structure is imposed on the observer. Highly structured observational frameworks are most suited for quantitative research while more loosely structured participant observation is better suited for qualitative research. In general, when making observations involving human subjects, researchers attempt to minimize subject reactivity and enhance the accuracy of recording the evidence. When appropriate, instrumentation may be used to enhance or record observations. It is worth noting that data collection using questionnaires, interviews and observations may well be used in combination in both research and clinical case work.

SELF ASSESSMENT

Explain the meaning of the following terms:

> acts
> complete observer
> complete participant
> meanings
> natural setting
> observer as participant
> participation
> relationships
> settings

TRUE OR FALSE

1. By 'meanings' Lofland was referring to verbal explanations of a person's behaviours.
2. Of the variety of observer roles, the 'complete participant' is the least likely to create ethical problems.
3. In a study involving changes in sleep patterns, self-observation would be an appropriate data collection strategy.

SELF ASSESSMENT

4. Detailed personal diaries of life events and their personal implications are suitable for qualitative research.

5. In the context of modern health sciences research, researchers must use instrumentation to facilitate and record their observations.

6. Anatomic research is well suited for the participant observer role.

7. 'Settings' refers to the physical and social environment in which field observations are conducted.

8. The 'observer as participant' attempts to create interesting, novel situations in the setting in which they carry out field research.

9. Laboratory settings require minimal structure for observational data collection.

10. Observational and interview data collection may be carried out simultaneously in clinical case work.

MULTIPLE CHOICE

1. The advantage of observation over interview as a data collection technique is that:

   a observations may be recorded and scrutinized later

   b observations enable the recording of actual behaviours, rather than subjects' interpretations

   c observation is scientific, unlike interviews which necessarily involve personal interactions

   d observations are unbiased and do not elicit reactions in human subjects.

2. You design an investigation to examine therapist–patient interaction in a hospital setting. Your suggested data collection involves a peep-hole and a hidden microphone for observing specific interactions unknown to the subjects. This study:

   a may well be rejected on ethical grounds

   b involves participant observation

   c would probably maximize subject reactivity

   d both a and c.

3. In order to reduce subjects' reactivity in the context of qualitative observational studies, the researcher should:

   a use subjects who do not react to being observed

   b inform the subjects of the detailed aims of the study, to reduce ambiguity

   c carry out the observations over a prolonged period of time

   d use video-recording equipment to minimize reactivity.

4. Participant observation may be defined as:

   a the observation of participants in the study

   b the observation of the researcher's input to a study

   c participation in a group while studying it

   d the study of observational and clinical techniques.

5. One of the major problems associated with the use of participant observation as a research strategy is that:

   a it is more expensive than experimental approaches to implement

   b it does not allow 'in-depth' study of any phenomena

   c the results cannot be replicated

   d participation may alter the phenomena under study.

6. Observation in the context of qualitative field research:

   a involves the use of well designed and pre-defined observation guides
   b depends on the precise definition of the variables being observed
   c requires physical and social proximity with the subjects
   d both *a* and *b*.

7. The advantage of observational data collection in laboratory settings is that:

   a extraneous events disrupting observations are more easily controlled
   b the ecological validity of the study as a whole is improved
   c there is less distortion of the phenomena because of the improved structure

   d there is no need to use expensive equipment for recording observations.

8. Which of the following would represent an 'observer as participant' role?

   a A researcher pretends to be a non-English speaking migrant to observe doctors' responses to reports of low back pain
   b A physiotherapist carries out observations of patients while carrying out their normal clinical practice
   c A researcher is given permission to attend clinical sessions in order to observe doctor–patient interactions
   d A neurologist suffers a stroke and keeps detailed records of her observed cognitive and sensory changes.

12

Measurement and instrumentation

INTRODUCTION

The term *measurement* refers to the procedure of attributing qualities or quantities to specific characteristics of objects, persons or events. Measurement is a key process both in research and in clinical practice. If the measurement procedures in a study are poor, then the internal and external validity of the findings, and hence the usefulness of the study, will be severely limited. Similarly, the validity of diagnoses and treatment decisions can be compromised by inadequate measurement.

The specific aims of this chapter are to:

1. Discuss fundamental aspects of measurement procedures.
2. Establish the features of 'good' measurement in both research and clinical settings.
3. Evaluate and discuss the different types of measurement scales.

OPERATIONAL DEFINITIONS

Sometimes, researchers start off with rather vague views of how to measure the variables included in a study. For example, if researchers are interested in measuring 'levels of pain' experienced by patients, then the researchers must convert their notions of pain to a tightly defined statement of how this variable is to be measured. Depending on their theoretical interpretation of the concept of pain, and the practical requirements of the investigation, one of the many possible measures of pain is selected.

In general, the process of converting theoretical ideas to a tightly defined statement of how variables are to be measured is called *operationalization*. It is important that researchers give exact details of how the measures were taken in order that others may judge their adequacy and appropriateness. A study that is adequate in terms of design, sampling methods and sample size may have poor validity owing to poor measurement techniques. Let us first consider the issue of operationalization.

The **operational definition** of a variable is a statement of how the researcher in a particular study chooses to measure the variable in question. It ought to be unambiguous and have only one possible interpretation.

At the outset, let us note that there is no single best way of taking measurements, particularly in the case of social and clinical variables. For example, if a researcher claimed that their therapeutic techniques significantly increased 'motor control' in their sample of patients, the question that should immediately be asked is what was meant by 'motor control' and how it was measured. If our researcher replied that they were interested in motor control, as measured by the Plunkett Motor Dexterity Task scores, they have supplied their operational definition. Another researcher may challenge the adequacy of this definition and substitute their own, stating that patients' self ratings of control in various tracking tasks is a more appropriate definition.

A good operational definition will contain enough information to enable another investigator to replicate the measurement techniques, if so desired. Similarly, a good operational definition of a clinically relevant variable will enable a fellow professional to replicate the diagnostic or assessment procedures. An operational definition can be an unambiguous description, a photograph or diagram, or the specification of a brand name. In describing a piece of research, one must include operational definitions of the measuring apparatus and all procedures, so that readers are quite clear as to what has been done and to whom.

OBJECTIVE AND SUBJECTIVE MEASURES

A distinction is commonly drawn between objective and subjective measures, often with overtones of suspicion directed towards subjective measures. Let us make a much less value-laden distinction and define them as follows: objective measurements involve the measurement of physical quantities and qualities using measurement equipment whereas subjective measures involve ratings or judgements by humans of quantities and qualities.

One should not confuse the distinction between objective and subjective measures as corresponding to good or bad measurement techniques. Equipment might be improperly calibrated, complicated to use, or become damaged during an investigation. For example, a researcher might have an inaccurate weighing machine that gives results at variance with the correct measures. With the sophistication and complexity of much current measurement equipment, it is often difficult to calibrate the equipment. One case recently involved the overdosing of participants in a study with radioactive material due to the failure of the measurement equipment. This was not detected for some time after the trials. Just because a machine is involved in measurement does not mean that the results will be adequate. Furthermore, many quantities and qualities associated with persons and clinical phenomena are difficult to measure objectively, such as the personal attractiveness of individuals or aspects of patient–therapist relationships. In these instances, measurement of the variables might well call for subjective interpretations.

DESIRABLE PROPERTIES OF MEASUREMENT TOOLS

Measurement tools ought to yield measurements that are reproducible, accurate, applicable to the measurement task in hand and practical or easy to use. These properties correspond to reliability, validity, applicability and practicability. These properties will be reviewed in detail in the following sub sections. Test theory and method is concerned with the development of measurement tools that maximize these properties.

Before these specific test properties are reviewed, it is useful to review some basic concepts in test theory. In any measurement, we have three related concepts: the observed value or test score, the true value or test score and measurement error. Thus, if I could be weighed on a completely accurate set of weighing scales, my true score might be 90 kg. However, the scales that I use in my bathroom might give me a reading of 85 kg. The difference between the observed score and my true score is the measurement error. This relationship can be expressed in the form of an equation such that:

$$\text{Observed value} = \text{true value} \pm \text{error}$$

Thus, measurement tools are designed with a view to minimizing measurement error.

RELIABILITY

Reliability is the property of reproducibility of the results of a measurement procedure or tool. There are several different ways in which reliability can be assessed. These include test-retest reliability, interobserver reliability and internal consistency. Let us examine each.

Test-retest reliability

A common way to assess test reliability is to administer the same test twice. The results obtained from the first test are then correlated with the second test. Reliability is generally measured by a correlation coefficient (see Ch. 16) which may vary from − 1 to + 1 in value. A test-retest reliability of + 0.8 or above is generally considered to be quite sound, although the interpretation of this figure depends on the context in which the measures are to be applied. When the measurement process involves clinical ratings, e.g. a clinician's rating of the dependency level of a CVA patient, test–retest reliability is sometimes termed *intra-observer* reliability, i.e.

the same observer rates the same patients twice and the results are correlated.

Inter-observer reliability

A common issue in clinical assessment is the extent to which clinicians agree with each other in their assessments of patients. The extent of agreement is generally determined by having two or more clinicians independently assess the same patients and then comparing the results (also with a correlational statistical analysis). If the agreement is high then we have high *inter-observer* reliability.

Table 12.1 illustrates examples of both high and low interobserver reliability on ratings of patients on a five-point scale. Imagine that this scale measures the level of patient dependency and need for nursing support. As mentioned earlier, the degree of reliability is quantitatively expressed by correlation coefficients, which are examined in Chapter 16. However, by inspection you can see that in Table 12.1 there is a high degree of disagreement in the two observers' ratings in the 'Low reliability' column. Clearly, in this instance the clinical ratings would be unreliable and inappropriate to use in the research project. Conversely, the outcome shown in the 'High reliability' column in Table 12.1 shows a high level of agreement.

An example of a study of inter-rater and intra-rater reliability is provided by Coppleson et al (1970). Over an 11-month period, 29 biopsy slides with suspected Hodgkins disease were presented to three pathologists. The pathologists

Table 12.1 Interobserver reliability

| Subjects | Observers' ratings | | | |
| | Low reliability | | High reliability | |
	A	B	A	B
1	4	3	4	4
2	2	5	2	3
3	3	4	4	5
4	1	4	2	2
5	3	1	1	1
6	4	4	5	5

were asked to make a number of judgements about features of the specimens. The specimens were unlabelled and over the year of the study were presented on two occassions to each of the three observers. This permitted an assessment of the test-retest or intra-rater reliability of each observer. The three observers disagreed with themselves on seven, eight and nine occasions, respectively, out of the total number of specimens. Overall, inter-rater agreement was calculated at 76% or 54%, depending on the diagnostic classification system used by the observers.

Internal consistency

Measurement tools will often consist of multiple items. For example, a test of your knowledge of research methods might include 50 items or questions. Similarly, a checklist designed to measure activities of daily living might have 20 items. The internal consistency of a test is the extent to which the results on the different items correlate with each other. If they tend to be highly correlated with each other, then the test is said to be internally consistent. Internal consistency, is also measured by a form of correlation coefficient and is generally considered to be a desirable property for a test.

Thus, the reliability of an assessment or test can be determined in several different ways including the test-retest, intra-rater, inter-rater and internal consistency methods.

VALIDITY

Just because one keeps getting the same result upon repeated administrations, or agreement among independent observers, does not mean that all is well. For example, an unscrupulous foreman might place a foot on his side of the scales when fruit pickers come in to have their efforts weighed for payment. Although upon repeated weighings the same box of fruit would register the same result, the measurement error may be as large as, say, 20 kg.

Validity is concerned with the accuracy of a test or measure; in other words, the amount of measurement error. The concept of validity implies that we can know the true value of a test, that is, we have a 'gold standard'. In physical measurement, we usually do have gold standards and tests. For example, some sets of weighing scales such as beam balances have very high validity. We can time how long it takes people to walk 500 m to a very high degree of accuracy. However, in clinical measurement, we often do not have gold standards. (What is the gold standard for the measurement of depression, for example?) Fortunately, we have a number of types of procedures to assess validity that can cope without a gold standard.

A case study in clinical test validity

The early detection of breast cancer in women has been recognized as an important public health initiative in many countries. Common methods of detecting suspicious lumps include breast self-examination and mammography, an X-ray of the breasts. Mammography is a common screening procedure and some countries such as Australia have funded large-scale programmes to promote it.

However, commendable as these initiatives may be, there are some doubts about the validity of mammography as a diagnostic tool. Walker & Langlands (1986) studied the mammography results of 218 women, who, through the use of a gold standard diagnostic biopsy, were known to have breast cancer. Of the 218 women with cancer, 95 (43.6%) had recorded a (false) negative mammography test result. Of these patients, 47 had delayed further investigation and treatment for almost a year, no doubt relieved and reassured by their favourable test results. The delays in treatment, in all likelihood, seriously compromised the health and ultimate survival of these women. In this instance, the accuracy (or lack of it) of the test results has very important consequences for the people concerned. Measurement theory might sometimes sound boring, but test design is of profound importance in research and clinical practice, as is demonstrated by the above example.

Types of test validity

As with reliability, test validity may be assessed in a number of different ways. These include content validity, sensitivity and specificity and predictive validity.

Content validity. In many contexts it is difficult to find external measures to correlate with the measure to be validated. For example, an examination in a particular academic subject may be the sole measure of the student's performance available to determine grades. How can it be determined whether the tests administered will be valid or not? One way is to write down all the material covered in the course and then make sure that there is adequate sampling from the overall content. If this criterion is satisfied it can be said that the test has content validity.

Sensitivity and specificity. The concepts of sensitivity and specificity are most commonly applied to diagnostic tests, where the purpose of the test is to determine whether the patient has a particular problem or illness. There are four possible outcomes for a test result, as shown in Table 12.2.

Sensitivity refers to the proportion of people who test as positive who really have the disease (i.e. the proportion of true positives out of all positives). Specificity refers to the proportion of individuals who test as negative who really do not have the disease (i.e. the proportion of true negatives out of all negative test results). If a diagnostic test has sensitivity of 1.0 and specificity of 1.0 it is a perfectly accurate or valid test.

Predictive validity. Predictive validity is concerned with the ability of a test to predict values of it or other tests in the future. Some tests are designed to assist with prognostic decisions.

Let us examine an example of predictive validity. Say a researcher devises a rating scale, X, for selecting patients to participate in a rehabilitation programme. The effectiveness of the rehabilitation programme is assessed with rating scale Y and each rating scale involves assigning scores 1–10 to the patients' performance. Table 12.3 illustrates two outcomes: low predictive validity and high predictive validity.

Although the calculation of correlation coefficients is needed to indicate quantitatively the predictive validity of test X, it can be seen in Table 12.3 that in the 'Low predictive ability' column, the scores on X are not clearly related to the level of scores on Y. Conversely in the 'High predictive ability' column, scores on the two variables correspond quite closely. Within the limits of the fact that only six subjects were involved in this hypothetical study, it is clear that only the results in the 'High predictive ability' column are consistent with rating scale X being useful for predicting the outcome of the rehabilitation programme, as measured on scale Y.

At this point we should again refer to the concepts of internal and external validity. The concepts of predictive and content validity apply to the specific tests and measures a researcher or clinician uses. Internal and external validity refer to characteristics of the total research project or programme. Test validity ought not to be confused with other forms of research design validity such as external and internal validity.

External validity is concerned with the researcher's ability to generalize their findings to

Table 12.2 Possible outcomes of test results

Test result	Real situation	
	Disease present	Disease not present
Disease present	True positive	False positive
Disease not present	False negative	True negative

Table 12.3 Predictive validity

Subjects	Low predictive validity		High predictive validity	
	Score on X	Score on Y	Score on X	Score on Y
1	4	3	3	3
2	4	8	4	3
3	5	2	5	5
4	5	7	5	5
5	6	4	6	6
6	8	5	8	7

other samples and settings. It is affected by the sample size, the method of sampling, and the design characteristics and measures used in the study. If we say a study has high external validity, we mean that its findings generalize to other settings and samples outside the study. It does not make sense to talk about the external validity of a particular test.

Similarly, internal validity is concerned with the design characteristics of experimental studies. If a study is internally valid, any effects/changes or lack thereof in the dependent variable can be directly attributed to the manipulation of the independent variable. It is important not to confuse the meanings of these terms.

STANDARDIZED MEASURES AND TESTS

Because reliability and validity of measures are so important, many researchers have devoted considerable time and energy to the development of measuring instruments and procedures that have known levels of reliability and validity.

The development of measurement standards for physical dimensions, such as weight, length and time, has been fundamental for the growth of all areas of science. That is, we have standards for comparing our measurements of a variable and we can meaningfully communicate our findings to colleagues living anywhere in the world. There are a variety of clinical measures, such as the Apgar Tests for evaluating the viability of neonates, which represent internationally recognized standards for communicating information about attributes of persons or disease entities.

Furthermore, there are standards relevant to populations, in terms of which assessments of individuals become meaningful. For example, there are standards for the stages of development of infants, with levels of physical, emotional, intellectual and social development occurring as a function of age. The interpretation of these standards will be discussed further in Chapter 15.

Some tests have been trialled on large samples, and reliability and validity levels recorded. Tests which have been trialled in this way are known as standardized measures or tests. A large variety is available, particularly in the clinical and social areas. The classic book *Psychological Testing* (Anastasi 1976) is a very useful source of descriptions of such tests. Many American firms and cooperatives market standardized tests. However, many researchers use tests and measures that have not been standardized, and do not report levels of reliability in their literature. This is of particular concern in studies where subjective measures with incomplete operational definitions are employed.

MEASUREMENT SCALE TYPES

Measurement can produce different types of numbers, in the sense that some numbers are assigned different meanings and implications from others. For example, when we speak of Ward 1 and Ward 2, we are using numbers in a different sense from when we speak of infant A being 1 month old, and infant B being 2 months old. In the first instance, we used numbers for naming, in the second instance the numbers indicate quantities. There are four scale types, distinguished by the types of numbers produced by the measurement of a specific variable.

Nominal scales

The 'lowest' level of the measurement scale types is the nominal scale, where the measurement of a variable involves the naming or categorization of possible values of the variable (see Table 12.4). The measurements produced are 'qualitative' in the sense that the categories are merely different

Table 12.4 Some other examples of nominal scaling

Variable	Possible values
Patients' admission numbers	3085001, 3085002
Sex	Male, female
Religion	Catholic, Protestant, Jewish, Muslim, Hindu
Psychiatric diagnosis	Manic-depressive, schizophrenic, neurotic
Blood type	A, B, AB, O
Cause of death	Cardiac failure, neoplasm, trauma

from each other. If numbers are assigned to the categories they are merely labels and do not represent real quantities; for example Ward 1 and Ward 2 might be renamed St Agatha's Ward and St Martha's Ward without conveying any less information.

The only mathematical relationship pertinent to nominal scales is equivalence or non-equivalence, that is, A = B or A ≠ B. A specific value of a variable either falls into a specific category, or it does not. Thus, there is no logical relationship between the numerical value assigned to its category and its size, quantity, or frequency of occurrence. The arbitrary values of a nominal scale can be changed without any loss of information.

Ordinal scales

The next level of measurement involves rank ordering values of a variable. For example, 1st, 2nd or 3rd in a foot race are values on an ordinal scale. The numbers assigned on an ordinal scale signify order or rank (see Table 12.5).

With ordinal scales, statements about ranks can be made. Where A and B are values of the variable, we can say A > B or B > A. For example, we can say Mrs Smith is more cooperative than Mr Jones (A > B), or Mr Jones is more cooperative than Mr Krax (B > C). We cannot, however, make any statements about the relative sizes of these differences.

Table 12.5 Examples of ordinal scales

Variable	Possible values
Severity of condition	Mild = 1, moderate = 2, severe = 3, critical = 4
Patient's satisfaction with treatment	Satisfied = 1, undecided = 2, dissatisfied = 3
Age group	Baby, infant, child, adult, geriatric (in decreasing order)
Cooperativeness with nurse or patients in a ward	Mrs Smith, Mr Jones, Ms Krax

Interval scales

Examples of interval scales are shown in Table 12.6. For these scales, there is no absolute

Table 12.6 Some examples of interval scales

Variable	Possible values
Heat (Celsius or Fahrenheit)	−10°C, +20°C, +5°C, 10°F
Intelligence (IQ)	45, 100, 185

zero point, rather, an arbitrary zero point is assigned. For example, 0°C does not represent the point at which there is no heat, but the freezing point of water. An IQ of zero would not mean no intelligence at all, but a serious intellectual or perceptual problem in using the materials of the test.

The use of an interval scale enables identification of equal intervals between any two values of measurements: we can say A–B = B–C. For example, if A, B, and C are taken as IQ scores, and A = 150, B = 100, and C = 50 then it is true that A–B = B–C. However, we cannot say that A = 3C (that A is three times as intelligent as C).

Ratio scales

The zero is not arbitrary in ratio scales. For example, in the Kelvin temperature scale, 0 K represents an absence of heat, in that the molecules have stopped vibrating completely, whereas in Celsius 0°C is simply the freezing point of water. Thus K is a ratio scale and 0°C is an interval scale. Examples of variables measured on ratio scales are shown in Table 12.7.

Table 12.7 Variables measured on ratio scales

Variable	Possible values
Weight	10 kg, 20 kg, 100 kg
Height	50 cm, 150 cm, 200 cm
Blood pressure	110 mmHg, 120 mmHg, 160 mmHg
Heart Beats	10 per min, 30 per min, 50 per min
Rate of firing of a neurone	10 per ms, 20 per ms, 30 per ms
Protein per blood volume	2 mg/cc, 5 mg/cc, 10 mg/cc
Vocabulary	100 words, 1000 words, 30 000 words

Table 12.8 compares the characteristics of different scales or levels of measurement.

Table 12.8 Characteristics of levels of measurement

| Characteristic | Level of measurement | | | |
	Nominal	Ordinal	Interval	Ratio
Distinctiveness	●	●	●	●
Ordering in magnitude		●	●	●
Equal intervals			●	●
Absolute zero				●

Distinctiveness: different numbers assigned to different values of property.
Ordering in magnitude: larger values represent more of the property.
Equal intervals: same distance between points on a scale.
Absolute zero: zero value represents absence of property.

Interval and ratio scales produce quantitative measurements. A ratio scale is the 'highest' scale of measurement, in the sense that it involves all the characteristics of the other scales, as well as having an absolute zero. A measurement on a higher scale can be transformed into one on a lower level, but not vice versa, because the higher scale measurement contains more information and the values can be put to more use by permitting more mathematical operations than those on a lower scale.

A given variable might also be measured on one of several types of scales, depending on the needs of the investigator. Consider, for example, the variable 'height'. This variable could be measured on any of the four scales, as follows:

- *ratio scale*: the height of individuals above the ground, for example, 180 cm
- *interval scale*: the height of individuals above an *arbitrary* surface: for example 100 cm above the surface of a bench
- *ordinal scale*: the comparative heights of individuals, for example, rank ordered from tallest to shortest
- *nominal scale*: categorizing individuals as, for

example, 'Normal' or 'Abnormal' (giant or dwarf).

The different types of measurement scales are important when considering statistical analysis of data. Statistics are numbers with special properties from data. The type of measurement scale determines the type of statistic that is appropriate for its analysis. This issue is considered in Chapter 19.

SUMMARY

In previous chapters we examined how some measuring instruments such as questionnaires are constructed, and ways of collecting evidence in field research. This section extends issues in data collection by defining what constitutes good measurement and by examining and comparing types of numbers which measurement can produce.

The first step in measurement is to define concepts operationally so that other investigators can also carry out or assess the measurement procedure. Next, using correlations we can establish the reliability and validity of our measurements. A high degree of reliability and validity is necessary for minimizing measurement error. It was pointed out that subjective measures are not necessarily unreliable or invalid. However, tests are available for clinical measurement which have the advantage of known validity and reliability.

Four different scale types were discussed: nominal, ordinal, interval, and ratio. These scales have different characteristics, particularly in relation to the permissible mathematical operations. In subsequent sections, we shall see that the scale type involved in our measurements determines the descriptive and inferential statistics appropriate for describing and analyzing the data.

Explain the meaning of the terms:

> content validity
> interval scale
> interobserver reliability
> measurement
> nominal scale
> objective measures
> operational definition
> ordinal scale
> predictive validity
> ratio scale
> standardized measures
> standardized tests
> subjective measures
> test–retest reliability

TRUE OR FALSE

1. The term 'measurement' refers to the assignment of qualities or quantities to specific aspects of objects or events.
2. An operational definition of a variable entails an explicit statement of how the variable is to be measured.
3. An objective measure is produced by the use of a measuring instrument.
4. A reliable test or measure will tend to produce accurate results.
5. A test–retest reliability as indicated by a correlation coefficient of 0.9 indicates a rather low reliability.
6. When an instrument is valid, we mean that it is measuring the characteristic which it is supposed to be measuring.
7. To establish the predictive validity of a test, we correlate the scores of individuals on the test with scores on other relevant measures.
8. A high correlation for scores between a college entrance examination and the subsequent examination results of students indicates that the entrance examination lacks predictive validity.
9. One of the advantages of using a

standardized test is that its validity and reliability are already known.
10. Ordinal measures involve rank-ordering the values of a variable.
11. An interval scale has an absolute zero.
12. All arithmetical operations are permissible with measurements based on interval scales.
13. The levels of measurement which have the properties of distinctiveness, ordering of magnitude, and equal intervals are the ordinal and nominal scales.
14. The statement 'Anxiety is a feeling of impending injury' is an example of an operational definition.
15. 'Operationalization' is defined as a statement specifying how a variable should be measured.
16. For a general concept such as 'intelligence' only one operational definition is possible.
17. Subjective measures are necessarily unreliable.
18. Objective measures can be invalid and unreliable.
19. A correlation coefficient of 1.0 indicates an excellent test–retest reliability.
20. If a measurement is valid, then it is necessarily reliable.
21. A test may be highly reliable but invalid.
22. A low interobserver reliability implies that the observed scores for a set of subjects on repeated tests tend to be unrelated to one another.
23. High predictive validity necessarily implies high content validity.
24. With a nominal scale, we can only make statements about the distinctiveness of scores.
25. The mathematical statement A–B = B–C is in correct form, given an ordinal scale.
26. Nominal scales do not have the characteristic of 'distinctiveness'.
27. The variable 'motor functioning' could be measured on either an ordinal or a nominal scale.

SELF ASSESSMENT

28. The variable 'blood sugar level' could be measured on either an ordinal or a ratio scale.
29. Ordinal scales are generally preferable to interval scales.
30. Statements such as $y = zx$ can be made validly with ratio measures.

MULTIPLE CHOICE

1. Which of the following does not include an operational definition?

   a Patients were encouraged to eat healthy food.
   b Males under 60 who were currently in full-time employment were the population for study.
   c Anxiety was measured by the Spielberger Anxiety Scale.
   d Patients who did not return for a scheduled follow up appointment 4 weeks after initial treatment were classified as dropouts.
   e Students who get over half the test items correct will be classified as having passed.

2. Subjective measures:

   a are not operationally defined
   b are always less valid than objective measures
   c involve measuring physical attributes
   d are not reliable because everybody's subjective experience is different
   e none of the above.

3. Which of the following statements does not include an operational definition of the dependent variable?

   a In the present study, intelligence was measured on the Stanford Binet IQ test.
   b In the present study, intelligence was

measured in terms of the level of subjects' knowledge of their cultures.
   c In the present study, intelligence was measured by the number of hairs on the subjects' heads.
   d b and c
   e a and c.

4. Objective measures:

   a are always more valid and reliable than subjective measures
   b involve extensive human intuition for interpretation
   c are always more reliable, but not necessarily more valid, than subjective measures
   d are used in experimental, but not in non-experimental, investigations
   e involve the measurement of physical qualities and quantities using measuring equipment.

5. A test is assessed for its reliability and its predictive validity. Both these measures are expressed as correlation coefficients, with the reliability coefficient being 0.9 and the predictive validity coefficient being 0.2. This indicates that:

   a the test is not reliable
   b the test has face validity
   c the test is reliable but does not appear to measure the variable of interest
   d the test is reliable, so it must measure the variable of interest
   e the test is a good one.

6. If the test-retest reliability of a measure is low, then it follows that:

   a the scores for different people tend to be different
   b the validity must be high
   c the scores for different people tend to be the same

d the same person measured twice tends to produce different results.

7. If a test is valid then:

   a it might be reliable
   b it must be reliable
   c the reliability is unaffected
   d it must be unreliable.

8. The reading '64 kilograms' is a value on a(n):

   a ratio scale
   b interval scale
   c ordinal scale
   d nominal scale.

9. In a study of weight problems in a sample of pre-adolescent children, the relevant variable was expressed as 'percentage overweight' or 'underweight', given the child's height. This is an example of a(n):

   a ordinal scale
   b ratio scale
   c nominal scale
   d interval scale.

10. The gender of patients is an example of a(n):

   a ratio scale
   b nominal scale
   c ordinal scale
   d interval scale.

11. Which of the following variables has been labelled with an incorrect measuring scale?

   a The number of heart beats per minute: interval
   b Platform numbers at a railway station: nominal
   c Finishing order in a horse race: ordinal
   d Self-rating of anxiety levels on a five point scale: ordinal.

12. '10th' is a value on a(n):

   a ratio scale
   b interval scale
   c ordinal scale
   d nominal scale.

13. Response delay in milliseconds is an example of a(n):

   a ratio scale
   b ordinal scale
   c interval scale
   d nominal scale.

14. In a patient records system, patients are randomly assigned a unique identification number. These numbers represent a(n):

   a nominal scale
   b ratio scale
   c interval scale
   d ordinal scale.

Therapists assess levels of clients' 'independence' using the following scale:

   0: Totally dependent on assistance from other/s for the activity
   1: Maximum assistance from other/s; can assist in a limited way
   2: Minimum assistance from 1 person; contributes significantly in carrying out the activity
   3: Supervised by another person due to mental/physical limitations and/or to ensure safety
   4: Independent with aids. Safe and consistent; would need assistance/supervision without aids
   5: Independent. Safe and consistent without aids, supervision or assistance.

Questions 15–17 refer to this scale.

15. The above scale is:

   a ratio
   b interval

SELF ASSESSMENT

   c nominal

   d ordinal.

16. If the subjects are assigned scores by the therapist's clinical judgement, then the measurement process is:

   a subjective

   b objective

   c unreliable

   d invalid

   e *a* and *b*.

17. Given the following three independence scores for three clients A, B, and C:

   A 4

   B 2

   C 0

which of the following statements is (are) true?

   a Client A is twice as independent as B

   b The difference in independence between clients A and B is the same as that between clients B and C

   c Client A is more independent than either B or C

   d *b* and *c*.

18. Which of the following measures of the variable 'weight' is nominal?

   a Weight in kg

   b Weight as percentage overweight in relation to 'healthy' weight

   c Weight as obese/overweight/normal/underweight/grossly underweight

   d Weight as 'normal against pathological' (obese or grossly underweight).

19. If a variable is not defined operationally, then:

   a the investigation of the variable might be difficult to replicate

   b it might be difficult to explain how the variable was measured

   c *a* and *b*

   d neither *a* nor *b*.

20. The terms 'external' and 'internal' validity refer to:

   a complete investigations

   b specific measurements

   c measurement scales, as a whole

   d characteristics of standardized, objective measures.

SECTION 4

Discussion, Questions and Answers

The same research questions may be answered by the use of a variety of different research methodologies. There is no single 'correct' research method to answer a research question. Indeed the 'triangulation' of methods is sometimes used to try and answer the same research question, so that the answer can be demonstrated not to be an artefact of the method used. Just as in land surveying, in which several reference points are used to better fix the position of the object being surveyed, researchers may study the same question or phenomenon using a variety of research techniques. The results may then be compared to get a better 'fix' on the question. The use of a single reference point or methodology gives one perspective of the object under study.

To illustrate this point it is proposed to consider a research issue of some importance and much contention in modern health care: the allocation of donated organs to transplant recipients. Despite the advances in transplantation techniques, there is a chronic worldwide under-supply of donor organs, to the extent that, in some countries, over one-third of patients accepted for transplantation die while on the waiting list due to the unavailability of suitable organs. A consequence of the chronic under supply of donor organs is the necessity for transplantation teams to choose the most 'worthy' candidate to receive the donated organ from a panel of potential recipients. How these decisions are made and how they ought to be made has been the subject of substantial research.

Many transplantation units around the world use a points system to assist with decisions concerning the priority of their people on the waiting lists. The points are typically based on tissue and blood type match (methods of measuring donor–recipient compatibility), time on the waiting list, 'urgency' (the extent to which the patient can wait) and prognosis (the quality of the expected outcome). This is in addition to certain technical requirements that vary with the organ system being replaced. For example, the size of the donor's and recipient's organ systems is a factor in heart–lung transplants. However, in recent years many commentators have presented data that indicate that 'social' criteria (such as the age, sex, education, race and wealth of the potential recipient) as well as 'medical' criteria are highly influential in the allocation of organs to recipients. These findings have generated considerable controversy.

How might one discover what criteria are used in the allocation of organs? One method might be to conduct a survey of those people involved in the decisions. The survey could take the form of an individual or group interview, or a written questionnaire. Alternatively, one could examine the written policies of various transplantation units or examine the medical records of the potential recipients for transplantation in the units and follow up the actual outcomes for each candidate.

Let us consider the questions we may wish to ask of people involved in the organ transplant decisions. They might include:

- 'In your opinion, what criteria *should be used* in deciding who should receive an organ transplant?'
- 'In your opinion, what criteria *are actually used* in deciding who should receive an organ transplant?'

These questions could be asked directly of the respondents in person and their comments recorded on tape and/or in the form of notes for subsequent analysis. In other words, the

Discussion, Questions and Answers

respondents could be interviewed. Excerpts of typical responses to these questions when the authors have asked them of members of transplant teams include:

We have an unwritten policy that we won't transplant into patients over 60. We think they have had their turn. Also their prognosis is often poorer than younger patients.

A consequence of the HLA emphasis is that people with unusual tissue types never get a transplant. I have a problem with this. In my area, there is only slim evidence that it makes much difference. Fifteen per cent max (sic) between best and worst case match. Most people fall in the middle so the actual difference would be even smaller. This means a lot of people miss out. I think it should be a strict queue.

Another method of collecting the data would involve getting people to use a structured response question in a questionnaire. The following might be an example:

In your opinion, what criteria *should be used* in deciding who should receive an organ transplant'. Please circle as many as you like.

Age	Urgency of need
Sex	Prognosis
Education level	Whether recipient is a parent
Race	Citizenship status
Occupation	Other, please specify
Wealth	

Blood type match between donor and recipient
HLA match between donor and recipient tissues

A follow-up question might include something like:

When you have selected the criteria you consider should be used in allocating organs to recipients, please write a number alongside each one to indicate your opinion of its importance in the decision. For example, the one you consider the most important should have a '1' placed alongside it, the second a '2' and so on until you have exhausted all the ones you selected.

In this type of exploratory study, the use of fixed response questions may send a clear signal to the respondent as to what the researcher considers to be acceptable criteria. Therefore,

the respondent may not be inclined to reveal their true answer if it is not included in the list of available answers, because of fear of disapproval or perhaps disinclination for the effort to do so. Thus, before a structured response question is used, the clinical researcher needs to ensure that all possible and likely answers are included. The current authors advocate the use of unstructured questions with a small sample prior to the use of structured questions in a large-scale survey.

It is interesting to note that in a study of 310 Australian people from the general community recently conducted by the authors the respondents consistently nominated the age of the recipient, their prognosis, the length of time they spent on the waiting list and whether they had children as the four factors they considered ought be used to determine recipient priority in transplantation decisions.

Thus, the clinical researcher could use interview or questionnaire approaches in the conduct of their survey. A further approach would involve the auditing of potential recipient medical files over a period in the various transplantation units in order to check whether those who actually received the transplants were representative of the potential recipient pool. For example, if it were found that women were less likely to receive transplants than men, taking into account their relative proportions in the recipient pool, then this would be of major concern. Unfortunately, as mentioned above, there is strong evidence in the USA (where most such research has been performed) that social factors have an important impact upon the actual transplantation decisions. These findings reflect the situation in the delivery of health care in areas other than transplantation.

Questions

1. What are some of the possible

Discussion, Questions and Answers

disadvantages of using structured response questions when the researcher is unsure as to what answers respondents may want to use?

2. When are structured response questions best used?

3. If you wanted to study the outcomes of transplant patients at a hospital, how would you go about gaining access to the records?

4. In the case where a researcher uses a structured questionnaire, to what extent does the respondent have the opportunity to contribute to the research agenda?

5. How can a researcher avoid bias in designing a questionnaire?

Answers

1. If the researcher is unsure as to what answers the respondents wish to give, structured response questions will probably not do the job required; even an open-ended response written question will not do the job, if the answer is complicated, because people are often a lot more fluent in their speech.

2. If the questions being asked are straightforward, e.g. 'what is your sex?' or 'what is your age?' or 'how often did you go to the doctor last month?' then structured response questions will give structured data cheaply and quickly.

3. Access to confidential data requires a lot of work, although you may find that some of the data you require may be published in the annual report for the hospital or agency. Typically, one starts by contacting the head of the unit concerned and then progresses through the ethics committees and

procedures laid down by the agency. If access is granted at all, it can be many months before permission is given, as the rights of the patients to their data are now strictly enforced in most countries.

4. Most structured research questionnaires are designed wholly by the researcher, without input from the respondents to be studied. What questions are asked, how these are asked and what is not asked can send clear messages to the respondents about the researcher's agenda and assumptions. In this context, it is rare that respondents challenge the researcher, even if they believe that the researcher has missed the point. The typically low level of respondent input avoids anarchy (imagine every single respondent to a survey questionnaire designing their own questions!). However, if the researcher has a totally different understanding of the situation under study from the respondents, then they may ask the 'wrong' questions. The data may then be invalid because they do not reflect the true positions of the respondents.

5. It depends upon the type of bias. With adherence to principles of question design, problems such as the use of leading questions should be avoided. However, since the researcher selects their questions, which may number 30 or so, from a range of several billion possible, selection bias is unavoidable. Every study is not a study of the universe. Focus and selectivity is unavoidable and is inherent to the reductionist scientific process. A problem of 'bias' may arise when the researcher does not ask the questions the respondents believe they should be answering.

Descriptive statistics

Depending on the complexity of the research design and the number of measurements obtained during data collection, we will have generated a set of scores called 'raw data'. Section 5 is concerned with the principles of descriptive statistics, which include mathematical principles for organizing and summarizing the raw data.

In Chapter 13 we outline techniques used for tabulating and graphing data. These techniques enable us to visualize trends, and identify differences across levels of the independent variables. When the data has been appropriately organized, we may calculate statistics, such as the percentages and proportions of scores found in the groups being studied.

Another important use for descriptive statistics is to 'crunch' or condense data into typical values for representing scores. The statistics are discussed in Chapter 14 and include 'measures of central tendency' (mode, median and mean) and also measures of dispersal (range, semi-interquartile range and standard deviation). Using these statistics enables us to condense the raw data and to convey to the reader information about the research findings.

Statistics such as the mean and the standard deviation can be also applied to calculating standard scores. Standard scores are used to establish the position of a particular score relative to a population. In Chapter 15 we examine how the standardized normal distribution can be used to calculate the position of any specific score within a population and how to interpret the clinical implications of these scores.

In Chapter 16 we examine another important class of statistics called correlation coefficients. The correlation coefficient is used to express the degree and direction of association between two or more variables. For example, we could use correlation coefficients to demonstrate if there is an association between the variables 'level of exercise' and 'body weight'. The closer the calculated correlation coefficient is to 1.0 (the maximum value), the more precisely we may predict from one variable to the other. Although correlation coefficients are extremely important for showing how different variables are associated, they do not necessarily indicate causal relationships between the variables. Showing causal effects requires appropriate research designs, as we suggested in Section 3.

13

Organization and presentation of data

INTRODUCTION

The summary and interpretation of data from quantitative research entails the use of statistics. By *statistics*, we mean the way of organizing and interpreting observations and measurements. However, when we speak of *a statistic*, we mean a particular number obtained by the mathematical treatment of specific data.

Descriptive statistics describe specific characteristics of data, such as how many cases fall into a particular category of measurement, typical values and the degree of interrelationship or correlation among measurements.

In previous chapters we examined how interviews, observations and measurement are used to produce data in clinical or scientific investigations. It can be extremely difficult, however, to make sense of raw data when it consists of a large number of varied measurements. That is, before we can interpret or communicate the information provided by an investigation, the raw data must be organized and presented in a clear and intelligible fashion. The aim of this chapter is to outline methods used in descriptive statistics for the organization, tabulation and graphic presentation of data. We will also examine the use of some simple statistics directly derived from the tabulation of the data into frequency and cumulative frequency distributions.

The specific aims of this chapter are to:

1. Outline methods for organizing and representing data as in the form of frequency distributions, tables or graphs

2. Demonstrate how the measurement scale used for data collection influences the organization and presentation of the evidence
3. Discuss the calculation and use of some simple descriptive statistics, including percentages, ratios and rates.

THE ORGANIZATION AND PRESENTATION OF NOMINAL OR ORDINAL DATA

A fundamental consideration in selecting appropriate statistics is the question of whether the data are discrete or continuous. Nominal and ordinal data are necessarily discrete, so that the organization of the data involves counting the number (frequency) of cases falling into each category of measurement. Let us examine two simple examples as an illustration.

Organization of discrete data

Example 1: nominal data

We are interested in the sex of patients (nominal data) undergoing gall bladder surgery (cholecystectomy) at a public hospital over a period of 1 year. The raw data, indicating the sex (M or F) of the patients is simply read off the patients' records, as follows:

F, M, M, F, F, F, M, F, M, F, M, F, F, F, F, F, F, F, F, M, F, F, F, M, M, F, M, F, M

Grouping the above nominal data involves counting the number of cases (or measurements) falling into each category. The total is M = 10 F = 20. The data can be presented in tabular form. Table 13.1 shows the following conventions in tabulating data:

1. Tables must be clearly and fully labelled; both

Table 13.1 Frequency distribution of gender of patients undergoing cholecystectomy at a hospital over a period of 1 year

Gender	*f*
Males (M)	10
Females (F)	20
	n = 30

the table as a whole, and the categories; so that the readers can interpret unambiguously what they are observing.
2. *f* represents frequency of cases or measurements falling into a given category.
3. *n* represents the total number of cases or measurements in a *sample*.
4. *N* represents the number of cases in a population. (See Section 3 for difference between samples and populations.)

Example 2: ordinal data

Ordinal data are presented by counting the number of cases (frequency) of each ordered rank making up the scale.

An investigator intends to evaluate the effectiveness of a new analgesic versus placebo treatment. A post-test only control group design is used: the experimental group receives the analgesic and the control group the placebo. 20 patients are randomly assigned into each of the two groups. Pain intensity is assessed by the patients' pain reports 5 h after minor surgery, on the following scale:

- 5: Excruciating pain
- 4: Severe pain
- 3: Moderate pain
- 2: Mild pain
- 1: No pain

The raw data is:

- Experimental group:
  3,4,5,3,3,3,4,2,1,3,2,1,3,4,5,2,3,3,3,3
- Control group:
  5,4,4,4,5,3,4,3,2,4,4,2,4,5,3,4,4,4,5,5

After tallying the results, the above data can be presented as a frequency distribution, as shown in Table 13.2. This demonstrates that when the data have been tabulated, we can see the outcome of the investigation. Here, the pain reported by the experimental group is less than that of the control group.

Graphing discrete data

Once a frequency distribution of the raw data

Table 13.2 Reported pain intensity of patients following placebo and analgesic treatments

Pain intensity	Experimental group (analgesic) f	Control group (placebo) f
1	2	
2	3	2
3	10	3
4	3	10
5	2	5
	n = 20	n = 20

has been tabulated, a variety of techniques is available for the pictorial or graphical presentation of a given set of measurements. Frequency distributions of qualitative data are often plotted as bar graphs (also termed 'column' graphs), or shown pictorially as pie diagrams.

A bar graph involves plotting the frequency of each category and drawing a bar, the height of which represents the frequency of a given category. Figure 13.1 graphs the data given in Table 13.1.

Figure 13.1 demonstrates conventions in plotting bar graphs:

1. The y axis, also called the ordinate, is used to plot frequencies.
2. The x axis, also called the abscissa, is used to indicate the categories.
3. The bars do not touch each other, reflecting the discontinuity of the measurement categories.

It should be noted that considerable attention must be given to interpreting graphs, as the axes may be translated or compressed, causing a false visual impression of the data. Make sure that you inspect the values along the axes, so that you are not misled.

It is also acceptable to calculate the percentage of scores falling into each category and to plot the percentages instead of the frequencies. For example, graphing Table 13.2 as percentages will produce the graph shown in Figure 13.2.

It can be seen in Figure 13.2 that by presenting the data for the experimental and control groups on the same graph, the reader gains a visual impression of the possible effectiveness of the analgesic treatment, in contrast to that of the control treatment.

Nominal data can also be meaningfully presented as a pie diagram, where the percentage of each category is converted into a proportional part of a circle or 'pie'. For example, in a given hospital we have the hypothetical spending patterns shown in Table 13.3.

Figure 13.3 represents a pie diagram of the information. In constructing Figure 13.3, we converted the numbers into percentages and then into degrees (out of a total of 100% = 360°), that is each 1% of the total is represented by 3.6° in the circle.

ORGANIZATION AND PRESENTATION OF INTERVAL OR RATIO DATA

As we discussed in Chapter 12, interval and ratio scales of measurement produce real numbers,

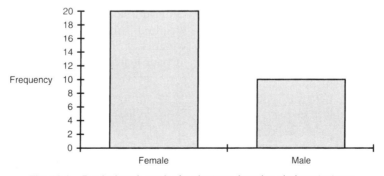

Fig. 13.1 Bar (column) graph of patients undergoing cholecystectomy.

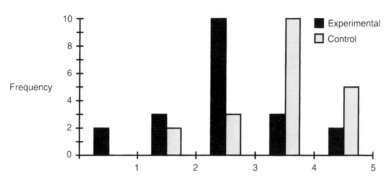

Fig. 13.2 Bar (column) graph of patients' pain intensity.

Table 13.3 Hypothetical spending patterns

Item	Cost ($)	Percentage of total
Wages and salaries	1 500 000	50.00
Medical supplies	500 000	16.67
Food and provisions	500 000	16.67
Administrative costs	500 000	16.67
Total	$3 000 000	100.00

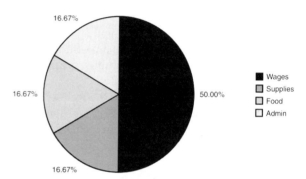

Fig. 13.3 Pie diagram of a hospital's spending pattern.

which can be processed according to the rules of arithmetic. Interval and ratio measurements often produce continuous data (such as weight, length, time, IQ), implying that increasingly accurate values of the variable are possible to obtain, depending on the sensitivity of the measurement. For example, the weight of a neonate could be measured as 4, 4.2, 4.18 or 4.183 kg.

Grouped frequency distributions

Often, when the continuous data are made up of a large number of varied measurements, it is useful to present the data as **grouped** frequency distributions.

When drawing up a grouped frequency distribution, the following conventions should be taken into account:

1. The table of grouped frequency distributions should have no more than 9 groups of values, otherwise it is too difficult to inspect. However, if too few groups are used, the meaning of the data is obscured, as varied measurements are combined into too few equivalent categories.

2. There should be equally sized class intervals, the *width* of which is represented by i.
3. Individual scores within a given class interval 'lose' their precise identity. The midpoint of each class interval is taken to represent the class interval.

Example

On admission to hospital, patients are routinely weighed. You are asked to summarize the weights of 50 male patients who were admitted in your ward over a period of time. The weights (raw data) are as follows (to nearest kg):

75, 67, 76, 71, 73, 86, 2, 77, 80, 75, 80, 96, 93, 75, 73, 83, 81, 82, 73, 92, 81, 87, 76, 84, 78, 79, 99, 100, 88, 77, 71, 76, 75, 83, 66, 79, 95, 85.77, 87, 90, 73, 72, 68, 84, 69, 78, 77, 84, 94

The steps in constructing a grouped frequency distribution are:

Table 13.4 Ordered array of data

Score	f	Score	f	Score	f	Score	f
100	1	91	0	82	1	73	4
99	1	90	1	81	1	72	2
98	0	89	0	80	2	71	2
97	0	88	1	79	2	70	0
96	1	87	2	78	2	69	1
95	1	86	1	77	4	68	1
94	1	85	1	76	3	67	1
93	1	84	3	75	4	66	1
92	1	83	2	74	0		

Table 13.5 Grouped frequency distribution of patients' weight in a given ward

Class interval	f
66–70	4
71–75	12
76–80	13
81–85	9
86–90	5
91–95	4
96–100	3
	$n = 50$

1. Organize data into an **ordered array**, and find the frequency of each score (see Table 13.4).
2. Find the **range** of scores. The range is the difference between the highest and lowest score plus 1. We add 1 to include the *real* limits for continous data (Figure 13.4). In this case the range is $100 - 66 + 1 = 35$.
3. Decide on the width (i) of the class intervals; i can be approximated by dividing the range by the number of groups or *class intervals*. In this instance, if we decide on seven classes, i will be $35/7 = 5.0$. When i is a decimal, it should be rounded up to the nearest whole number; here, $i = 5$. As stated earlier, the number of class intervals is arbitrary and will be chosen by the researcher, depending on the properties of the data. By convention, more than nine class intervals are rarely employed.
4. The next step is to determine the lowest class interval, and then list the limits of each class interval. Clearly, the lowest class interval

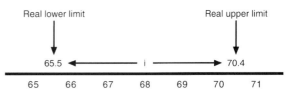

Fig. 13.4 Real limits of a class interval.

must include the lowest score in the distribution.
5. Then, the frequency of scores is determined from each class interval and tabulated, as in Table 13.3.

It is far easier to understand the data by inspecting Table 13.5 than by looking at the raw data. However, some precision in the data has been lost as somewhat different scores have been assigned into the same class intervals.

Graphing frequency distributions

The two common types of graphs used to graph frequency distribution of quantitative data are histograms and frequency polygons.

Histograms. A histogram resembles a bar graph but the bars are drawn to touch each other. The fact that the bars touch each other reflects the underlying continuity of the data. The height of the bars along the y-axis represents the frequency of each score or class interval plotted along the x-axis. With grouped data, the midpoint of each class interval becomes the midpoint of each bar, and the width of the bar corresponds to the real limits of each class interval.

For example, consider the lowest class interval 66–70 on Table 13.5. Because the data is *continuous*, the real upper and lower limits of the class interval are 65.5 and 70.4. Although all the weights are given as whole numbers of kilograms, these will in most cases be the result of rounding off by the nursing staff to the nearest whole number. Thus, someone who actually weighed 70.2 kg would have been recorded as weighing 70 kg and would fall into the 66–70 class. As Figure 13.4 shows, $i = 5$, and the midpoint of the class interval is 68.

Frequency polygons. Any data which can be

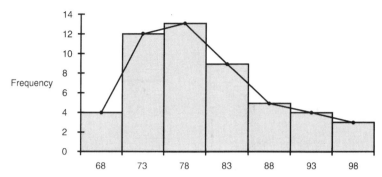

Fig. 13.5 Combined histogram and frequency polygon for the same data (see Table 13.5).

represented by a histogram can also be graphed as a frequency polygon. For this type of graph, a point is plotted over the midpoint of each class interval, at a height representing the frequency of the scores. Figure 13.5 represents a histogram and a frequency polygon for the data in Table 13.5.

Frequency polygons allow the reader to interpolate, that is, to estimate the frequency of values in between those actually measured or graphed. Of course, interpolation cannot be done for discrete data (for example, Fig. 13.1), as values between categories have no meaning. When a frequency polygon is plotted, it can take on a variety of shapes. The shapes which are of particular importance for frequency polygons are shown in Figure 13.6.

Figure 13.6A represents a bell-shaped, normal distribution. It is symmetrical, in the sense that one half is the same as the other. The curve indicates that most of the scores fell in the middle, with a relatively few scores towards either 'tail'. Figure 13.6B represented a negatively skewed distribution, with most of the scores being high and spreading out toward the lower end of the distribution. Figure 13.6C represents a positively skewed distribution, with most of the scores being low, but with some scores spreading out towards the upper end of the distribution.

An easy way to remember the direction of the skew is to consider the region where the 'tail' or portion of the graph with lower frequencies falls. For example, if it is toward the negative side of the x-axis, the graph is negatively skewed.

The significance of the skew or a symmetrical,

normal distribution will be discussed in subsequent sections.

SIMPLE DESCRIPTIVE STATISTICS

Once the data have been summarized in a frequency distribution, it is often useful to make comparisons concerning the relative frequencies of scores falling into specific categories. The following statistics are useful for understanding comparative trends in the data, and can be used for measurements on any scale; nominal, ordinal, interval, or ratio. A *statistic* is a number resulting from the manipulation of the raw data. The calculation of statistics is essential for 'crunching' the raw data into single numbers, which summarize the data.

Ratios

Ratios are statistics which express the relative frequency of one set of frequencies, A, in relation to another, B. The formula for ratios is:

$$\text{Ratio} = \frac{A}{B}$$

Therefore, the ratio of males to females for the data presented in Table 13.1 (p. 154) is:

$$\text{Ratio (males to females)} = \frac{10}{20} = 0.5$$

or

$$\text{Ratio (female to males)} = \frac{20}{.10} = 2.0$$

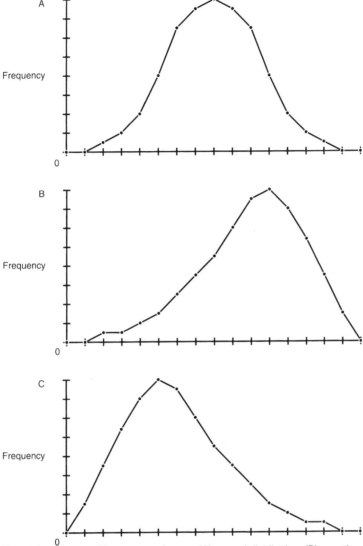

Fig. 13.6   Shapes of frequency polygons: (A) normal distribution; (B) negative skewing; (C) positive skewing.

Ratios are useful in the health sciences when we are interested in the distribution of illnesses or symptoms or the categories of subjects requiring or benefiting from treatment. The ratio calculated above tells us about the relative frequency of gall bladder surgery for males and females.

Proportions

Proportions are statistics which are calculated by putting the frequency of one category over that of the total numbers in the sample or the population:

$$\text{Proportion of } A = \frac{A}{A + B}$$

Therefore, the proportion of males in the sample represented in Table 13.1 (p. 154) is:

$$\text{Proportion of males} = \frac{f(\text{males})}{n} = \frac{10}{30} = 0.33$$

Percentages

Proportions can be transformed into percentages, by multiplying by 100. Of course, this is how we obtained the values of the y-axis for Figure 13.2 (p. 155). To illustrate, patients scoring 5 (excruciating pain) in the Control group:

$$\% \text{ scoring } 5 = 5/20 \times 100 = 25\%$$

The calculations for the values of the pie chart (Fig. 13.3, p. 156), also involved such calculations.

Rates

When summarizing the results of epidemiological investigations (Ch. 5), it is often useful to use this statistic to represent the level at which a disorder is present in a given population. The two rates which are commonly used in the health sciences are:

- *Incidence rates*, which represent the number of new cases of a disorder reported within a time period.

$$\text{Incidence rate} = \frac{\text{number of new cases of a disorder}}{\text{total population at risk of the disorder}} \times \text{base}$$

- *Prevalence rates* which represent the total number of cases suffering from a disorder.

$$\text{Prevalence rate} = \frac{\text{number of existing cases of a disorder}}{\text{total population at risk of the disorder}} \times \text{base}$$

Let us illustrate the above equation by applying it to hypothetical data. Let us consider the

Table 13.6 Incidence of herpes

Year	Incidence of herpes (per 1000)
1982	8
1983	15
1984	17
1985	16
1986	10

condition herpes, a nasty little condition associated with the virus herpes simplex which attacks various parts (lips, etc.) of the body. Assume that an epidemiologist is interested in the spread of the condition in a given community.

1. Assume that all the population above the age of 15 years ($N = 1\ 000\ 000$) is at risk of herpes.
2. In 1998, 5000 new cases were reported.
3. In 1998, there was a total (old and new active cases) of 15 000 known cases.

Here, substituting into the equation:

incidence rate for herpes = $5000/1\ 000\ 000 \times \text{base} = 0.005 \times \text{base}$

The statistic 0.005 is not seen as the best way to represent a rate.

Often, epidemiologists select a base to make the statistic more understandable. The base represents a number for transforming the rate. The base selected depends on the magnitude of the rate; conventionally a multiple of 10, such as 1000, 10 000 or 100 000 is selected. In this instance we select 1000 as the base. Therefore, substituting into the equation, we obtain:

Incidence rate for herpes simplex = $0.005 \times 1000/1 = 5$ per 1000

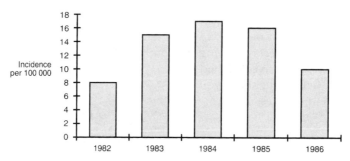

Fig. 13.7 Incidence rate of genital herpes 1982–1986.

Prevalence rate for herpes simplex:

$$= \frac{15\,000}{1\,000\,000} \times \frac{1000}{1} = 15 \text{ per } 1000$$

The above statistics can be graphed. For example, we may wish to represent pictorially the incidence of herpes simplex in the community over a period of 5 years. The (fictitious) evidence is shown in Table 13.6.

The graph of the time-series for the incidence over time (Fig. 13.7) gives us a visual impression of the incidence rate of the problem in question.

SUMMARY

We outlined several techniques for organizing, tabulating and graphically presenting both discontinuous (nominal, ordinal) and continuous (interval, ratio) data. It was shown that raw data can be organized and tabulated as a frequency distribution, by counting the number of cases falling into specific categories or class intervals. Data composed of a large number of highly varied measurements were shown to be best presented by grouping the scores into class intervals.

Several techniques of graphing data were discussed: bar graphs and pie charts for discontinuous data, and histograms and frequency polygons for continuous data. The possible shapes of frequency polygons were also examined. It was shown that data grouped in frequency distributions could be also represented as ratios, proportions, percentages or rates.

These statistics were obtained by the mathematical manipulation of the raw data, and were shown to be useful for summarizing the raw data. In the next section, we will examine further techniques of 'crunching' or condensing data by using appropriate descriptive statistics.

SELF ASSESSMENT

Explain the meaning of the terms:

    bar graph
    bell-shaped curve
    continuous data
    cumulative frequency
    discontinuous data
    frequency polygon
    frequency distribution
    histogram
    incidence rate
    negative skew
    ordered array
    pie diagram
    positive skew
    proportion
    rate
    ratio
    real limit

TRUE OR FALSE

1. The organization of nominal or ordinal data involves counting the number of scores falling into discrete categories.

2. Nominal and ordinal data are best graphed as histograms.
3. It is useful to organize interval or ratio data into ordered arrays before constructing frequency distributions.
4. Given a large number of varied scores, we can construct a grouped frequency distribution, usually with about seven class intervals.
5. The midpoint of a given class interval is i.
6. Frequency distributions of continuous data can be presented graphically as histograms or frequency polygons.
7. In a negatively skewed distribution most of the scores are low, with a few high scores spread along the x axis.
8. With a bell-shaped or normal distribution, most of the scores are located at the two extreme ends of the distribution.
9. 'Incidence rates' are statistics which represent the number of active cases of a disorder within a specific time period.
10. For a chronic condition like arthritis, we would expect the prevalence rates to be smaller than the incidence rates.

SELF ASSESSMENT

11. A 'base' represents a number for transforming a rate into a more easily understandable statistic.
12. The wider i, the more specific information is lost about the actual data.
13. A frequency polygon is appropriate for graphing continuously distributed variables.
14. The percentile rank of a score is equal to the frequency of the scores falling up to and including the score.
15. If a curve is negatively skewed, the distribution of the scores has a 'tail' towards the lower values of the variable.
16. The height of a bar (column) represents the frequency, rather than the value, of a variable.
17. A pie diagram is inappropriate for representing nominally scaled data.
18. Incidence rates represent the number of new cases of a disorder reported within a time period.
19. The 'base' for calculating incidence rates is always 10 000.
20. We cannot construct frequency tables for nominally or ordinally scaled data.
21. Ratios are the same as proportions.
22. We can only calculate proportions for nominally scaled data.

MULTIPLE CHOICE

1. Patients indicate their satisfaction with treatment by responding to a question with four options:

    (1) very dissatisfied
    (2) dissatisfied
    (3) satisfied
    (4) very satisfied.

    This is an example of a(n) (i) scale, and the resulting frequency distribution should be plotted as a (ii):
    a (i) nominal (ii) bar graph
    b (i) ordinal (ii) bar graph

    c (i) interval (ii) histogram
    d (i) ordinal (ii) histogram
    e none of the above.

2. Interval or ratio data should be graphed as a:

    a histogram
    b bar graph
    c frequency polygon
    d a and b
    e a and c.

3. Your class is asked to do an exam in theoretical physics. Given that only a few students know anything about this subject, the distribution of scores would be:

    a symmetrical
    b negatively skewed
    c positively skewed
    d bell-shaped
    e both a and b.

4. If a curve is symmetrical:

    a most of the scores fall at the higher values of the x-axis
    b most of the scores fall at the lower end of the x-axis
    c most of the scores fall at the higher end of the y-axis
    d most of the scores fall at the lower end of the y-axis
    e if folded in half, the two sides of the curves will coincide.

5. The percentile rank of a person's score on a test is 35. This means that:

    a the person got 35% of the items correct
    b the person performed better than 65% of the sample doing the test
    c both a and b
    d the person's score was equal to or better than 35% of the sample doing the test.

6. You are interested in calculating the incidence rate for Huntington's disease, which is a *very rare* disorder. Which of the following numbers would be your best 'base'?

  a 10
  b 100
  c 1000
  d 10 000

7. A continuous scale of measurement is different from a discrete scale in that a continuous scale:

  a is an interval scale, not a ratio scale
  b never provides exact measurements
  c can take an infinite number of intermediate possible values
  d never uses decimal numbers
  e *b* and *c*.

A researcher wished to study the effectiveness of a new treatment, A, upon the severity of migraine. A random sample of 50 subjects (*n* = 50) was selected from a group of migraine sufferers attending a pain clinic. Patients were randomly allocated to be treated either with A, or with a currently available biofeedback treatment, B. A pre-test/post-test experimental design was used. Level of pain was assessed using a standardized pain questionnaire, measuring pain responses on a scale between 1–100.

Questions 8–14 refer to the above information.

8. The independent variable in this study was:

  a the new treatment A
  b the type of treatment used
  c the migraine
  d the patients' scores on the pain questionnaire.

9. The dependent variable in the above study was:

  a the new treatment A
  b the type of treatment used

  c the migraine
  d the patients' scores on the pain questionnaire.

10. The scale of measurement used to assess the pain responses was:

  a nominal
  b ordinal
  c interval
  d ratio.

The data for the post-test pain scores for the two groups are summarized in the table below. Questions 11–14 refer to this table.

Pain ratings	Treatment A	Treatment B
31–40	1	1
41–50	2	2
51–60	3	–
61–70	10	3
71–80	4	4
81–90	3	10
91–100	2	5

11. What would be an appropriate way for this information to be graphed?

  a frequency polygon
  b histogram
  c bar graph
  d either *a* or *b*.

12. What are the real limits of the lowest category?

  a 31–40
  b 31.5–40.4
  c 30.5–40.4
  d 30.5–39.5

13. Which of the following statements is (are) true?

  a The post-test scores for Treatment B are skewed.

SELF ASSESSMENT

b i is equal to 9.

c 6% of Treatment A post-test scores are under 50.5.

d All of the above statements are true.

14. Which of the following statements is supported by the data, assuming that the pre-test scores were equivalent for the two groups?

a Treatment A appears to be more effective than B.

b Treatment B appears to be more effective than A.

c The two treatments appear to be equivalent.

d Treatment B appears to be harmful.

e a and d.

The total number of deaths reported in a hypothetical country for a given year was 120 000. The following lists deaths by cause as a percentage of all deaths:

Heart disease	35%
Cancer	25%
Cerebro-vascular disease	15%
Trauma	10%
Respiratory illness	5%
Infections	5%
Other causes	5%

Questions 15–20 refer to this data.

15. Data such as the above are compiled by asking hospitals, physicians, etc., to report deaths to a central agency. This type of information collection is best described as:

a a survey

b an experiment

c a mathematical model

d field research.

16. The variable 'cause of death' is measured on a(n):

a nominal scale

b ordinal scale

c interval scale

d ratio scale.

17. The above table should be graphed as a:

a frequency polygon

b histogram

c bar graph

d a and b.

18. The number of people who died of either heart disease or cancer was:

a 35 000

b 60 000

c 72 000

d 90 000.

19. Which of the following statements is false?

a The proportion of *all* deaths caused by cancer is 0.25.

b 5000 persons died of respiratory illnesses.

c Twice as many persons died of trauma than infections.

d 18 000 persons died of cerebro-vascular disease.

20. Of the people who died of trauma, the male:female ratio was 2:1. How many females died of trauma?

a 4000

b 8000

c 12 000

d Insufficient information to calculate answer.

21. Which of the following statements is true?

a A graph of continuous data enables the reader to interpolate.

b When constructing a frequency distribution for grouped scores, i should

SELF ASSESSMENT

be equal to the number of class intervals.

c A histogram is like a bar graph, except that with a histogram the bars do not touch each other.

d A bell-shaped curve is an example of a skewed distribution.

22. Descriptive statistics:

a are used to make inferences about populations from small samples

b are only appropriate in non-experimental designs

c summarize data about samples or populations

d are derived from probability theory.

A researcher has collected data concerning the amount of time in seconds that it took a group of normal and a group of brain-damaged subjects to complete a standard motor task. The data is shown below arranged in a grouped frequency distribution.

	Time in seconds	
Class interval	Normals	Brain-damaged
12–14	1	0
15–17	2	0
18–20	5	1
21–23	10	2
24–27	4	4
28–30	3	10
31–33	1	3

23. The total number of subjects used in this study was:

a 7

b 26

c 46

d 50.

24. The class interval width i is:

a 2

b 3

c 4

d 7.

25. The real limits for the class interval 15–17 are:

a 14.5–17.4

b 15 + 0.5

c 14–18

d 2.

26. The scale of measurement used for the dependent variable was:

a nominal

b ordinal

c interval

d ratio.

27. Which of the following statements is true?

a The distribution of scores for the normals approximates a normal distribution.

b The scores for the brain-damaged subjects was highly skewed.

c The above investigation should not be classified as an experiment.

d All the above are true.

28. On the basis of previous evidence, the score of 27.4 is taken as demonstrating adequate motor function, while longer times for completing the task demonstrate some motor impairment. The proportion of normals who scored under 27.4 is X while the proportion of brain-damaged who scored under this score was Y (insert values for X and Y).

a 4, 13

b 0.85, 0.35

c 0.80, 0.17

d 0.26, 0.20.

SELF ASSESSMENT

29. Assuming external validity, which of the following statements is supported by the evidence?

    a   Brain-damaged subjects take longer to complete the standard task.
    b   The greater the degree of brain damage, the slower the task completion.
    c   The task is valid for discriminating subjects with brain damage.
    d   *a* and *c*.

30. The selection of appropriate descriptive statistics for organising quantitative data is *most* influenced by the:

    a   Design of the research project.
    b   Scales of measurement used to collect data.
    c   The number of research participants.
    d   The expected magnitude of the differences among the groups.

14

Measures of central tendency and dispersion

INTRODUCTION

In the previous chapter we examined how raw data can be organized and represented in order to be easily communicated and understood. We might need to further condense our data, so that we can represent our finding in terms of only a few numbers (or statistics). The two statistics necessary for representing a frequency distribution are measures of central tendency and dispersion.

Measures of central tendency are statistics or numbers expressing the most typical or representative scores in a distribution. **Measures of dispersion** or variability are statistics or numbers expressing the extent to which scores are dispersed (or spread out) numerically.

The overall aim of this chapter is to examine the use of several types of measures of central tendency and dispersal commonly used in the health sciences. As quantitative evidence arising from investigations is commonly presented in terms of these statistics, it is essential to understand these concepts.

The specific aims of this chapter are to:

1. Discuss the selection and use of measures for central tendency
2. Discuss the selection and use of measures for dispersal
3. Outline the relationship between the skew of frequency distributions and the selection of appropriate descriptive statistics.

MEASURES OF CENTRAL TENDENCY

The mode

When the data are nominal, the appropriate measure of central tendency is the mode. The mode is the most frequently occurring score in a distribution.

Therefore, for the data shown in Table 13.1 (p. 154), the mode is the 'females' category. The mode can be obtained by inspection. It is the category with the largest frequency on a frequency table, the highest bar on a bar chart, or the largest segment of a pie graph. As we shall see later, the mode can also be calculated for data on higher scales of measurement.

The median

With ordinal, interval, or ratio scaled data, central tendency can also be represented by the median. The median is the score that divides the distribution into half; half of the scores fall under the median, and half above the median. That is, if scores are arranged in an ordered array, the median would be the middle score. With a large number of cases, it may not be feasible to locate the middle score simply by inspection. To calculate which is the middle score, we can use the formula $(n + 1)/2$, where n is the total number of cases in a sample. This formula gives us the number of the middle score. We can then count that number from either end of an ordered array.

In general, if n is odd, the median is the middle score; if n is even, then the median falls between the two centre scores. The formula $(n + 1)/2$ is again used to tell us which score in an ordered array will be the median. For example:

5, 8, 9, 10, 28.   Median = 9 (n is odd)
6, 17, 19, 20, 21, 27.   Median = 19.5 (n is even)

For a grouped frequency distribution, the calculation of the median might be a little more complicated. If we assume that the variable is continuous, (for example, time, height, weight, or level of pain) we can use a formula for calculating the median. This formula (explained in detail below) can be applied to ordinal data, provided that the variable being measured has an underlying continuity. For example, in a study of the measurement of pain reports we obtain the following data, where $n = 17$:

1, 1, 2, 2, 2, 2, 2, 3, 3, 3, 3, 4, 4, 4, 5, 5, 5

The above data can be represented by a bar graph. (Fig. 14.1).

Here we can obtain the mode simply by inspection. The mode = 2 (the most frequent score).

For the median, we need the ninth score, as this will divide the distribution into two equal halves (see Table 14.1). By inspection, we can see that the median will fall into category 3. Assuming underlying continuity of the variable and applying the previously discussed formula, we have:

$$Mdn \text{ (median)} = X_{L} + i \; \frac{(n/2) - cum f_{L}}{fi}$$

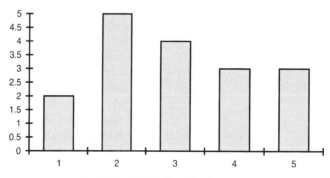

Fig. 14.1 Distribution of pain scores.

Table 14.1 Table of sample data

Score	Real class interval	f	cum f
1	0.5–1.4	2	2
2	1.5–2.4	5	7
3	2.5–3.4	4	11*
4	3.5–4.4	3	14
5	4.5–5.4	3	17
		n = 17	*class interval containing median

Table 14.2 Example data sets

A		B	
x	f	x	f
1	16	1	8
2	1	2	7
3	1	3	6
4	7	4	4
	n = 25		n = 25

Where X_L = real lower limit of the class interval containing the median, i = width of the class interval, n = number of cases, $cum\ f_L$ = cumulative frequency at the real lower limit of the interval and fi = frequency of cases in the interval containing the median.

Substituting into the above equation:

$$Mdn = 2.5 + 1\left[\frac{17/2 - 7}{4}\right]$$

$$= 2.5 + 1\left[\frac{1.5}{4}\right]$$

$$= 2.875$$

The mean

The mean, $\overline{X}$ or μ, is defined as the sum of all the scores divided by the number of scores. The mean is, in fact, the arithmetic average for a distribution. The mean is calculated by the following equations:

$$\overline{X} = \left[\frac{\Sigma x}{n}\right] \text{ (for a sample)}$$

$$\mu = \left[\frac{\Sigma x}{N}\right] \text{ (for a population)}$$

Where Σx = the sum of the scores, $\overline{X}$ = the mean of a sample, μ = the mean of a population, x = the values of the variable, that is the different elements in a sample or population and n or N = the number of scores in a sample or population.

The formula simply summarizes the following 'advice':

To calculate the average or mean of a set of scores ($\overline{X}$), add together all the scores (Σx) and divide by the number of cases (n).

Therefore, given the following sample scores:

2, 3, 5, 6, 7

To calculate the mean:

$$\overline{X} = \frac{\Sigma x}{n} = \frac{23}{5} = 4.6$$

When n or N are very large, the average is calculated with the formula above but usually with the assistance of computers.

COMPARISON OF THE MODE, MEDIAN, AND MEAN

The mode can be used as a measure of central tendency for any level of scaling. However, since it only takes into account the most frequent scores it is not a generally satisfactory way of presenting central tendency. For example, consider the following two sets of scores, A and B shown in Table 14.2.

It can be seen, either by inspection or by sketching a graph, that the two distributions A and B are quite different, yet the modes are the same, i.e. 1.

The median divides distributions into two equal halves, and is appropriate for ordinal, interval or ratio data. For interval or ratio data, however, the mean is the most appropriate measure of central tendency. The reason for this is that in calculating this statistic, we take into account *all* the values of the variable. In this way, it gives the best representation of the average score. Clearly, it is inappropriate to use the mean with nominal data, as the concept of 'average' does not apply to discrete categories. For example, what would be the average of 10 males and 20 females?

There is some justification for using the median as a measure of central tendency when the variable being measured is continuous. However this is controversial, and the mean should be preferred. Alternatively, when a distribution is highly skewed, the median might be more appropriate than the mean for representing the 'typical' score. Consider the distribution:

2, 2, 2, 5, 7, 8, 9
mode = 2
median = 5
$\overline{X}$ = 5
Let us change the 9 to 44:
2, 2, 2, 5, 7, 8, 44
mode = 2
median = 5
$\overline{X}$ = 10

Clearly, the median and the mode are less sensitive to extreme scores, while the mean is pulled towards extreme scores. This might be a disadvantage. For example, there are seven people working in a small factory, with the following incomes per week:

$100; $200; $200; $300; $400; $400; $1900
median = $300
$\overline{X}$ = $500

The distribution of wages is highly skewed, by the high income of the owner of the factory ($1900). The mean, $500, is higher than six of the seven scores; it is in no way typical of the distribution. In cases like this the median is more representative of the distribution.

Figure 14.2 illustrates the relationships between the skew of frequency distributions and the three measures of central tendency discussed in this chapter. We should remember that the mode will always be at the highest point, the median will divide the area under the curve into halves, and the mean is the average of all the scores in the distribution. Also, the greater the skew in distribution, the more the measures of central tendency are likely to differ.

MEASURES OF DISPERSAL

We have seen that a single statistic can be used to describe the central tendency of a frequency distribution. This information is insufficient to characterize a distribution; we also need a measure of how much the scores are dispersed or spread out. The dispersal of discrete data is of little relevance, as the degree of dispersal will be limited by the number of categories defined by

the investigator at the beginning of measurement.

Consider the following two hypothetical distributions representing the IQs of two groups of intellectually disabled children:

Group A: 45, 50, 55, 60, 60, 70, 80
Group B: 57, 58, 59, 60, 61, 62, 63

It is evident that although $\overline{X}_A = \overline{X}_B = 60$, the variability (or dispersal) of the scores of Group A is greater than that of Group B. In so far as IQ is related to the activities appropriate for these children, Group A will provide a greater challenge to the therapist working with the children.

The three statistics commonly used to indicate the numerical value of dispersal are the range, the variance and the standard deviation.

The range

The range is the difference between the highest and lowest scores in a distribution. As we mentioned, given the IQ data above, the ranges are:

Group A: 80 – 45 + 1 = 36
Group B: 63 – 57 + 1 = 7

Although the range is easy to calculate, it is dependent only on the two extreme scores. In this way, we are not representing the typical dispersal of the scores. That is, the range might be distorted by a small number of atypical scores or 'outliers'. Consider, for instance, the differences in the range for the data given. The example on the previous column shows that just one outlying score in a distribution has an enormous impact on the range ($1900 – $100 = $1800). Obviously, some measure of average dispersal would be a preferable index of dispersal.

The average deviation

A convenient measure of variability might be average deviation about the mean. Consider Group B shown previously. Here $\overline{X}$ = 60. To calculate average dispersal about the mean, we subtract the mean from each score, sum the individual deviations, and divide by n, the number of measurements (see Table 14.3).

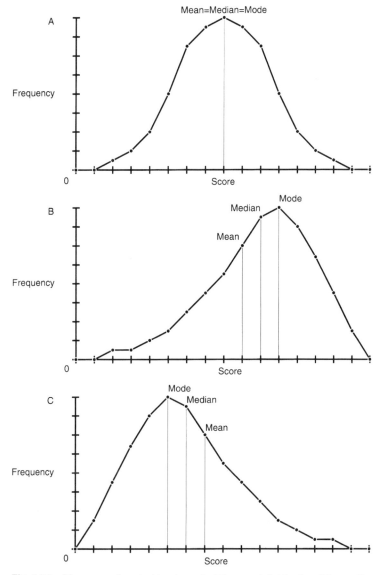

Fig. 14.2   Measures of central tendency in (A) normal distribution; (B) negative skewing; (C) positive skewing.

$$\text{Average deviation} = \frac{\Sigma(x - \overline{X})}{n}$$

Therefore: $\Sigma (x - \overline{X}) = (-3) + (-2) + (-1) + (0) + (1) + (2) + (3) = 0$

This is a general result; the sum of the average deviations about the mean is always zero. You can demonstrate this for the average deviation of Group A. The problem can be solved by squaring the deviations, as the square of negative numbers is always positive. This statistic is called the sums of squares (SS) and is always a positive number. This leads to a new statistic called the variance.

The variance

The variance (σ^2 or S^2) is defined as the sum of

Table 14.3 Average dispersal about mean for Group B

x	$x - \overline{X}$
57	-3
58	-2
59	-1
60	0
61	+1
62	+2
63	+3

Table 14.4 Calculation of variance

x	$x - \overline{X}$	$(x - \overline{X})^2$
57	-3	9
58	-2	4
59	-1	1
60	0	0
61	1	1
62	2	4
63	3	9
$\overline{X} = 60$		$\Sigma(x - \overline{X})^2 = 28$

the squared deviations about the mean divided by the number of cases.

$$\frac{\Sigma(x - \mu)^2}{N}$$

$\sigma^2 =$ (for a population)

$$\frac{\Sigma(x - \overline{X})^2}{n - 1}$$

$S^2 =$ (for a sample)

Divide by $n - 1$ when calculating the variance for a sample, when we use S^2 as an estimate of population variance. Dividing by n results in an estimate which is too small, given that a degree of freedom has been lost calculating $\overline{X}$.

For the IQ example shown above, the variance is calculated as shown in Table 14.4.

Substituting into the formula:

$$\sigma^2 = \frac{\Sigma(x - \overline{X})^2}{n - 1} = \frac{28}{6} = 4.67$$

The problem with variability as a measure of dispersal is that the deviations were squared. In this sense, we are overstating the spread of the scores. In taking the square root of the variance, we arrive at the most commonly used measure

of dispersal for continuous data: the standard deviation.

The standard deviation

The standard deviation (σ or s) is defined as the square root of the variance:

$$\sigma = \sqrt{\sigma^2} = \sqrt{\frac{\Sigma(X - \mu)^2}{N}}$$

$$s = \sqrt{s^2} = \sqrt{\frac{\Sigma(x - \overline{X})^2}{n - 1}}$$

Therefore, the standard deviation for Group B is:

$$s = \sqrt{s^2} = \sqrt{4.67} = 2.16$$

The size of the standard deviation reflects the spread or dispersion of the frequency distribution representative of the data. Clearly, the larger σ or s, the relatively more spread out the scores are about the mean in a distribution. Calculation of the variance or the standard deviation is extremely tedious for large n using the method shown above. Statistics texts provide a variety of calculational formulae to derive these statistics. However, the common use of computers in research and administration makes it superfluous to discuss these calculational formulae in detail.

The semi-interquartile range

We have seen previously that if we are summarizing ordinal data, or interval or ratio data which is highly skewed, then the median is the appropriate measure of central tendency. The statistic called *interquartile* and *semi-interquartile range* is used as the measure of dispersion when the median is the appropriate measure of central tendency for a distribution.

The interquartile range is the distance between the scores representing the 25th (Q1) and 75th (Q3) percentile ranks in a distribution.

It is appropriate to define what we mean by percentiles (sometimes called centiles). The percentile or centile rank of a given score specifies the percentage of scores in a distribution

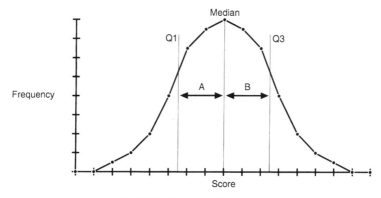

Fig. 14.3 Interquartile ranges.

falling up to and including the score. As an illustration, consider Figure 14.3, in which:

- 25% of cases fall up to and including Q1
- 50% of cases fall up to and including the median
- 75% of cases or scores fall up to and including Q3
- 25% of cases or scores fall above Q3.

The distances A and B represent the distances between the median and Q1 and Q3. When a distribution is symetrical or normal, the distances A and B will be equal. However, when a distribution is skewed, the two distances will be quite different.

The semi-interquartile range (sometimes called the quartile deviation) is half of the distance between the scores representing the 25th (Q1) and 75th (Q3) percentile ranks in a distribution. Let us look at an example. If we have a sample where $n = 16$ and the values of the variable are:

1, 5, 7, 7, 8, 9, 9, 10, 11, 12, 13, 15, 19, 20, 20, 20.

Clearly, a frequency distribution of this data is not even close to normal as the distribution is not symmetrical and the mode is at the maximum value. Therefore, the median is selected as the appropriate measure for central tendency, and we should use the interquartile range as the measure of dispersion.

Looking at the data, we find that:

| 1 | 5 | 7 | 7 | * | 8 | 9 | 9 | 10 | † | 11 | 12 |
| | 13 | 15 | ‡ | 19 | 20 | 20 | 20 |

where

* denotes 25th centile (first quartile, Q1), † denotes 50th centile: median (second quartile, Q2) and ‡ denotes 75th centile (third quartile, Q3)

The score which cuts off the first 25% of scores (25th centile) is the first quartile (Q1). Since we have $n = 16$, Q1 will cut off the first four scores (25% of 16 is 4).

$$\text{Thus: } Q1 = \frac{7+8}{2} = 7.5$$

The third quartile (Q3) is the score which cuts off 75% of the scores. As n = 16, Q3 will cut off 12 scores (75% of 16 is 12).

$$Q3 = \frac{15 + 19}{2} = 17.0$$

Therefore, the semi-interquartile range is:

$$\frac{Q3 - Q1}{2} = \frac{17.0 - 7.5}{2} = 4.75$$

The larger the semi-interquartile range, the more the scores are spread out about the median.

SUMMARY

In this section, we discussed two essential statistics for representing frequency distributions: measures of central tendency and dispersal. The measures of central tendency outlined were the mode and median for discrete data, and the mean for continuous data. Measures of dispersal or variability were shown to be the range, average deviation, variance, and standard deviation.

These statistics are appropriate for crunching the data together to the point that the distribution of raw data can be meaningfully represented by only two statistics. That is, the raw data representing the outcome of investigations or clinical measurements are expressed in this manner. We have seen that the mean and the standard deviation are most appropriate for interval or ratio data. The median and semi-interquartile range are used when the data was measured on an ordinal scale, or when interval or ratio data is found to have a highly skewed distribution. The mode represents the most frequent scores.

The contents of the section focused on the use and meaning of these concepts, rather than stressing calculations involved. These calculations are now made by computers. In Chapter 15, we discuss the application of the mean and standard deviation for relating specific scores to an overall distribution.

SELF ASSESSMENT

Explain the meaning of the following terms:

> central tendency
> descriptive statistics
> dispersion
> mean
> median
> mode
> range
> semi-interquartile range
> standard deviation
> statistic
> variability
> variance

TRUE OR FALSE

1. Inferential statistics are used to describe specific characteristics of the data.
2. With nominal data, the mean should be used as a measure of central tendency.
3. The mode represents the most frequently occurring score in a distribution.
4. With ordinal data, we can use both the mode and the mean as a measure of central tendency.
5. When the data are interval or ratio, we can use the mean as a measure of central tendency.
6. With continuous data, the median is the most appropriate measure of central tendency.
7. If a continuous distribution is highly skewed, the median might be the appropriate measure of central tendency.
8. When a frequency distribution is positively skewed, the mean is greater than the median or the mode.
9. Given a normal distribution, the three measures of central tendency are equivalent.
10. The range is the simplest indicator of variability.
11. The range is calculated by adding the lowest score to the highest score in a distribution.
12. Given nominal or ordinal data, we should use the standard deviation as a measure of dispersion.
13. The square root of the variance is called the standard deviation.
14. s and α indicate the extent to which scores are distributed about the mean.
15. When a distribution consists of very different scores, s or σ will be relatively large.
16. It is possible to have data with three different values for measures of central tendency.
17. The 50th percentile score and the median will always be the same value.
18. The median is less affected than the mean by extreme scores at one end of a distribution.
19. Central tendency describes the 'typical' value of a set of scores.

SELF ASSESSMENT

20. We use $n-1$ in the denominator of the equation for calculating the sample standard deviation, because it provides us with an accurate estimate of the population standard deviation.
21. If the number of raw scores is odd, the median is the score in the middle position.
22. The mean must have a value equal to one of the scores in the distribution.
23. 25% of the scores fall between Q1 and the median.
24. The distance between Q1 and the median is always different to the distance between Q3 and the median.
25. The semi-interquartile range is inappropriate to use with skewed distributions.

MULTIPLE CHOICE

1. Given a set of nominally scaled scores, the most appropriate measure of central tendency is the:

   a mean
   b mode
   c standard deviation
   d range.

2. Which of the following statements is true?

   a The mode is the most useful measure of central tendency.
   b The variance is the square root of the standard deviation.
   c The median and the 50th percentile rank have different values.
   d The mean is more affected by extreme scores than the median.

Questions 3–5 refer to the following data:

   2, 2, 3, 4, 6, 6, 7.

3. Σx is equal to:

   a 30
   b 40

   c 50
   d none of the above.

4. $(\Sigma x)^2$ is equal to:

   a 124
   b 128
   c 130
   d 900

5. The median is equal to:

   a 6
   b 5
   c 4
   d 3

6. The range for the above set of scores is:

   a 7
   b 5
   c 2
   d 1

A clinic had 50 patients attending in a month. The number of times each patient visited the clinic is given below in the form of frequency distribution.

No. of visits (X)	No. of patients (f)
7	3
6	6
5	6
4	10
3	21
2	0
1	4

Questions 7–9 refer to this information.

7. The total number of visits by the patients was:

   a 194
   b 28
   c 50
   d none of the above.

SELF ASSESSMENT

8. The mean number of visits by patients was:

   a   3.89
   b   3.50
   c   1.00
   d   3.88

9. The median number of visits per patient was:

   a   3.88
   b   3.50
   c   3.00
   d   4.00

10. The more dispersed, or spread out, a set of scores is:

    a   the greater the difference between the mean and the median
    b   the greater the value of the mode
    c   the greater the standard deviation
    d   the smaller the interquartile range.

11. The measure of central tendency which is most strongly influenced by extreme values in the 'tail' of the distribution is:

    a   the mean
    b   the median
    c   the mode
    d   the standard deviation
    e   none of the above.

12. The mean height of a student group is 167 cm. Assuming height is normally distributed this enables us to deduce that:

    a   approximately half of all students are taller than 167 cm
    b   being a student stunts your growth
    c   approximately half of all students are shorter than 167 cm
    d   a and c
    e   none of these.

13. If we subtract the value of the mean from every score in a set of scores the sum of the remaining values will be:

    a   impossible to determine
    b   equal to the mean
    c   a measure of the dispersion around the mean
    d   zero
    e   none of the above.

14. Given a normally distributed continuous variable the best measure of central tendency is the:

    a   mode
    b   median
    c   mean
    d   standard deviation
    e   none of the above.

15. If a distribution is negatively skewed, then:

    a   the median is greater than the mean
    b   the mode is greater than the median
    c   the mean is greater than the median
    d   both a and b are true
    e   none of the above are true.

16. In a normal distribution, the mean, the median and the mode:

    a   always have the same value
    b   the mean has the higher value
    c   the mean has the lower value
    d   have no particular relationship
    e   cannot take the same value.

17. The measure of central tendency which is the most frequently occurring score is:

    a   the mean
    b   the median
    c   the mode
    d   the standard deviation
    e   none of these.

18. Given the group of scores 1, 4, 4, 4 and 7, it can be said of the mean, the median, and the mode that:

  a the mean is larger than either the median or the mode
  b all are the same
  c the median is larger than either the mean or the mode
  d all are different
  e the mode is larger than either the median or the mean.

A nurse recorded the number of analgesic preparations taken by patients in a surgical ward. The resulting data were:

  5, 2, 8, 2, 3, 2, 4, 12.

Questions 19–23 refer to this data.

19. The mode for this distribution is:

  a 2
  b 3
  c 8
  d there is no mode.

20. The median is:

  a 2.00
  b 3.50
  c 3.00
  d 3.25

21. The mean is:

  a 3.52
  b 5.43
  c 4.75
  d 4.15

22. The range is:

  a 9
  b 10
  c 12
  d 2

23. The standard deviation is:

  a 3.04
  b 5.81
  c 2.28
  d 3.58

Questions 24–28 refer to this data:

  3, 3, 4, 5, 6, 7, 8, 9, 9, 10, 38, 60.

24. The median is:

  a 7.0
  b 7.5
  c 8.0
  d 3 or 9

25. Q1 is:

  a 4.5
  b 5.5
  c 8.0
  d 9.5

26. Q3 is:

  a 4.5
  b 6.0
  c 7.5
  d 9.5

27. The semi-interquartile range is:

  a 2.5
  b 4.5
  c 6.0
  d 9.0

28. The semi-interquartile range is preferred to the standard deviation as a measure of dispersal when:

  a the sample size is small
  b the distribution is standardized
  c the distribution is highly skewed
  d the range is small.

15

Standard scores and the normal curve

INTRODUCTION

In this chapter we will discuss the use of the mean and standard deviation for standardizing distributions. *Standard distributions* are useful for comparing different sets of measurements. Standard scores can specify the position of a score or measurement in relation to a population. In this way, standard scores can be applied to producing and understanding 'norms' in the health sciences.

That is, specific measurements relevant to health care are intelligible only against a background of how the population of scores are distributed. For example, how could clinicians make decisions about blood pressures being pathological without the background of how human blood pressures are generally distributed.

The specific aims of this chapter are to:

1. Define 'standard' scores.
2. Describe the characteristics of normal and standard normal curves
3. Show how standard normal curves can be used for calculating percentile ranks
4. Show how standard normal curves can be used to compare scores from different distributions.

STANDARD SCORES (z SCORES)

Consider this example: infant A walked unaided at the age of 40 weeks, while infant B is 65 weeks old but still cannot walk. What sense can we make of these measurements? Could infant B need further clinical investigation in case they have some neurological abnormality? The fact

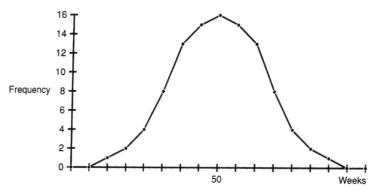

Fig. 15.1 Age at which children walk unaided.

that the infant B is unable to walk at the age of 65 weeks is not very informative in the absence of additional information about how this compares with norms for other children. However, say that it is known that the distribution of walking ages is such that $\mu = 50$ weeks, and $\sigma = 5$. Assuming that the frequency distribution is normal, the frequency polygon representing the population would look something like that shown in Figure 15.1.

In this instance, infant B's score is clearly above the mean. In fact, by inspection, we can see the infant's score at this point of time was three standard deviations (+3) above the mean (65 = 50 + (3 × 5)). In contrast, infant A began walking earlier than the mean, his score of 40 being two standard deviations below (–2) the mean. In general, any 'raw' score in a frequency distribution can be described in terms of its distance from the mean. The process of transforming a score into a measurement based on its distance from the mean in standard deviations is called **standardizing** the score. Such 'transformed' scores are called z scores or standard scores.

A z score represents how many standard deviations a given raw score is above or below the mean. The equation for transforming specific raw scores into z scores is given as:

$$z = \frac{x - \mu}{\sigma} \text{ (for a population)}$$

$$z = \frac{x - \overline{X}}{s} \text{ (for a sample)}$$

For the above equation, x is the raw score, $\overline{X}$ or μ is the mean of the distribution from which the score was drawn and s or σ is the standard deviation of the distribution. That is, when we know the mean and standard deviation of a distribution, we can transform any raw score into a z score. Conversely, when the z score is known, we can use the above equations to calculate the corresponding raw scores.

In the above example, the z scores corresponding to the infants' raw scores are:

$$\text{Infant A: } z = \frac{x - \mu}{\sigma}$$
$$= \frac{40 - 50}{5}$$
$$= -2$$

$$\text{Infant B: } z = \frac{x - \mu}{\sigma}$$
$$= \frac{65 - 50}{5}$$
$$= +3$$

These calculations correspond to our previous observations that A's score was two standard deviations below the mean and B's score was three standard deviations above the mean. In other words, A walked very early and B was a very late starter. The particular value of standardizing scores for understanding clinical or research evidence will be discussed in the context of the concepts of normal and standard normal distributions.

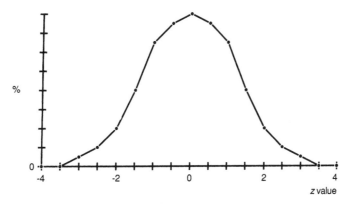

Fig. 15.2   Standard normal distribution.

NORMAL DISTRIBUTIONS

Many variables measured in the biological, behavioural and clinical sciences are approximately 'normally' distributed. What is meant by a normal distribution is illustrated by the normal curve (see Fig. 15.2) which is a frequency polygon representing the theoretical distribution of population scores. We assume here that the variable x has been measured on an interval or ratio scale and that it is a continuous variable such as weight, height or blood pressure.

The normal curve has the following characteristics:

1. It is symmetrical about the mean, so that equal numbers of cases fall above and below the mean (mean = median = mode).
2. Relatively few cases fall into the high or low values of x. Most of the cases fall close to the mean. (For the theoretical normal distribution, the arms of the curve do not intersect with the x-axis, allowing for a few extreme scores).
3. The precise equation for the normal curve has been worked out by the mathematician Gauss, so that it is sometimes referred to as a Gaussian curve.

We need not worry about the actual formula. Rather, the point is that given that the functional relationship between f and x is known, integral calculus can be used to calculate areas under the curve for any value of x. All normal curves have the same general mathematical form; whether we are graphing IQ or weight the same bell-shape will appear. The only differences between the curves are the mean value and the amount of variation. This is why the mean and the standard deviation provide us with important information about any particular normal distribution. Note that it is unlikely that any real data are precisely normally distributed. Rather, the normal distribution is a mathematical model which is useful for *representing* real distributions.

The standard normal curve

If we transform the raw scores of a variable into z scores and then plot the frequency polygon for the distribution, we will have a standard curve. If the original distribution was normal, then the frequency polygon will be a standard normal curve. Standard normal curves are identical regardless of the nature of the original variables.

By transforming raw scores into z scores, we are getting rid of differences in means and standard deviations, which are the only things which distinguish between non-standardized normal curves (Fig. 15.2).

The standard normal curve has the following additional properties:

1. The mean is always 0 (zero). For the previous example, the z score corresponding to $\mu = 50$ (as in the 'infants' walking age' example) is:

$$z = \frac{50 - 50}{5} = 0$$

2. The mean = median = mode, as the curve is symmetrical,
3. The standard deviation of z scores is always 1 (one). For instance, the z score for 55 (which is one standard deviation above the mean) is:

$$z = \frac{55 - 50}{5} = 1$$

4. It is assumed that the *total area under the curve adds up to 1.00*. Since the normal curve is symmetrical, 0.5 of the area falls above $z = 0$ and 0.5 falls below $z = 0$. This is another way of saying that 50% of the total cases fall below the mean, and 50% of the cases fall above the mean (which is equal to the median).
5. More generally, we can use appropriate *statistical tables* to estimate the area under the standard normal curve for any given z scores. These areas are available in table form (see Appendix A) so that for any value of z we can read off the corresponding area.
6. The area under the curve between any two points is directly proportional to the percentage of cases falling above, below or between those two points. We can use the standard normal curve to calculate the percentage of scores falling between any specified two scores.

In the next subsection, we will examine the use of the table of areas under the standard normal curve to understand the meaning of measurements in relation to distributions.

CALCULATIONS OF AREAS UNDER THE NORMAL CURVE

We have already examined the concept of percentile or centile ranks. The normal curve is useful for evaluating the percentile rank of scores in normal distributions. Appendix A gives the proportion of areas under the standard normal curve which lies:

- between the mean and a given z score
- beyond the z score

Since normal distributions are symmetrical, the same proportions are true also for the area between the mean and any negative z score. Only the positive values are given in Appendix A.

Let us see how we can use this information to estimate the percentile ranks of the two infants' walking ages. We have shown previously that for infant A, $z = -2$. Let us now turn to Appendix A. In going down the column of z scores, we find that the area corresponding to $z = 2.0$ is 0.4772 (between) and 0.0229 (beyond).

We know that the area A1 under the curve in Figure 15.3 must be:

Shaded portion = 0.5000 − 0.4772
= 0.0228 (as half the scores fall under the mean)

This proportion can be expressed as a percentage, so that 2.28% of the cases in the distribution fall

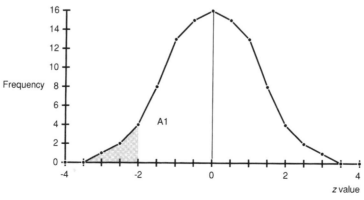

Fig. 15.3 Area (A1) corresponding to $z = -2$.

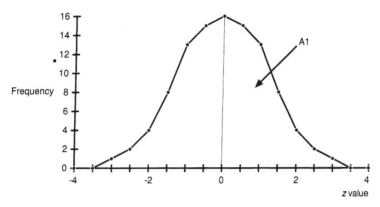

Fig. 15.4   Area (A1) corresponding to $z = 3$.

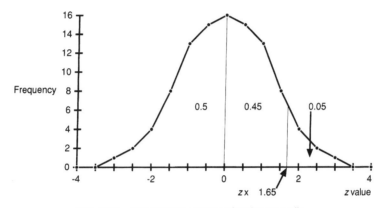

Fig. 15.5   Determining z score of 95th percentile.

below $z = -2$. We have defined percentile rank for a score as the percentage of cases in a distribution falling up to and including a specific score. Therefore, the percentile rank for infant A's walking is 2.28%. Of all children, only 2.28% learn to walk as early as or earlier than infant A. Clearly, he is doing well.

What then is the percentile rank for infant B's performance? As you remember, $z = +3$. Looking up the area corresponding to $z = 3$ in Appendix A we find the area (A1 in Fig. 15.4) is equal to 0.4987. Therefore, the proportion of scores falling up to and including $z = +3$ is $0.5 + 0.4987 = 0.9987$.

Expressing this finding as a percentage, we find that 99.87% of children learn to walk by the age of 65 weeks. As we said earlier, infant B still

is not walking. Perhaps further clinical tests are indicated, although we should keep in mind that an unusual or extreme score is not necessarily indicative of pathological states.

Critical values

We can work the other way by determining the raw scores corresponding to areas under the normal curve in Appendix A. For example, say that the slowest 5% of infants are offered some special exercises in learning to walk. What would be the age at which the exercises should be offered, should the child not be walking? The key here is to determine the score that corresponds to the 95th percentile of the distribution. This can be represented as shown in Figure 15.5.

From Figure 15.5 we can see that we need to discover the z score that corresponds to an area of 0.45 above the mean. By consulting the normal distribution table (see Appendix A), it can be seen that the corresponding z score is $z = 1.65$. This is a critical value for the statistic in defining an area.

Given the z score, we can calculate the corresponding raw score from the formula:

$$z = \frac{(x - \mu)}{\sigma}$$

Therefore $1.65 = \dfrac{x - 50}{5}$

$$x = (5 \times 1.65) + 50$$
$$= 58.25$$

That is, if the slowest 5% are thought to be in need of help, then children somewhat over 58 weeks old and not still walking would be recommended for the remedial exercises. Of course, we can use the tables for reading off the z scores corresponding to *any* specified area or percentage.

STANDARD NORMAL CURVES FOR THE COMPARISON OF DISTRIBUTIONS

One of the uses of standard distributions is that we can compare scores from entirely different distributions. For example, if a student scored 63 on test A, and 52 on test B, on which test did the student do better? If we define 'better' as solely in terms of raw scores, then clearly the student did better on test A. However, test A might have been easier than test B, so that if the overall performances of all students on the tests are taken into account, the student's relative performance might be better on test B.

Say test A, $\overline{X} = 65$ and $s = 8$

test B, $\overline{X} = 40$ and $s = 8$

Therefore, using the formula for calculating z scores, and looking up the corresponding areas in Appendix A (do this yourself) we obtain the results shown in Table 15.1. Thus, the student performed better on test B, by scoring higher than 93% of other students sitting for the test.

Table 15.1 Scores for example in text

Raw scores	z scores	Percentile ranks
$x = 63$	−0.25	40.1
$x = 52$	+1.50	93.3

Table 15.2 Blood Cholesterol

	Mean blood cholesterol (mg/cc)	Standard deviation
Meat eaters	0.6	0.15
Vegetarians	0.4	0.1

This example illustrates that in some circumstances the meaning of specific scores have to be interpreted against 'standards'.

Another use of standard distributions is in interpreting the meaning of the results of investigations in the health sciences. Let us examine the following hypothetical example. An investigator measured levels of blood cholesterol in a sample of 300 adults who are meat eaters, and 100 adults who are vegetarians. The results of the investigation are summarized in Table 15.2.

Now, imagine that you are a clinician working with patients with cardiac disorders and you are interested in the following questions:

1. Approximately what per cent of vegetarians had blood cholesterol levels greater than the average meat eater?
2. Approximately what per cent of meat eaters had blood cholesterol levels lower than that of the average vegetarian?

The percentage of cases of vegetarians with blood cholesterol greater than 0.6 (the mean for the meat eaters) is represented by area A1 in Figure 15.6.

$$z = \frac{0.6 - 0.4}{0.1} = 2$$
Area A1 = 0.0228

Therefore, approximately 2.3% of vegetarians had blood cholesterol levels higher than the average for meat eaters.

Figure 15.7 demonstrates the area (A2) corresponding to the percentage of meat eaters with

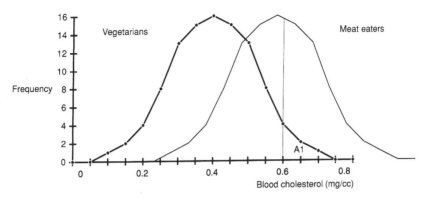

Fig. 15.6   Area A1 corresponds to the percentage of vegetarians with blood cholesterol higher than 0.6 mg/cc.

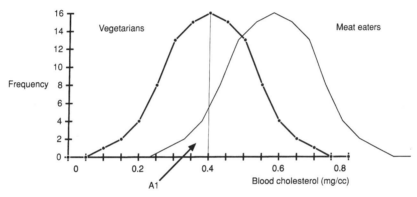

Fig. 15.7   Area A1 corresponds to the percentage of meat eaters with lower blood cholesterol than the mean for vegetarians.

lower blood cholesterol than the average vegetarian.

$$z = \frac{0.4 - 0.6}{0.15} = 1.33$$
$$\text{Area A2} = 0.0918$$

Therefore, approximately 9.2% of meat eaters had lower blood cholesterol levels than the average vegetarian.

SUMMARY

We found that if the mean and standard deviation for a given distribution have been calculated, then we can transform any raw score into a standard (or z) score. The z score represents how many standard deviations a specific score is above or below the mean. We described how to calculate this transformed score for a population or a sample. Also, we outlined the essential characteristics of the normal and the standard normal curves.

It was pointed out that if the original frequency distribution was approximately normal, then the table of normal curves (Appendix A) could be used to calculate percentile ranks of raw scores, or the percentage of scores falling between specified scores. Also, z scores were shown to be useful in comparing scores arising from two or more different normal distributions.

The above information is applicable to clinical practice, for example in interpreting the significance of an individual's assessment in relation to known population norms.

SELF ASSESSMENT

Explain the meaning of the following terms:

> normal curve
> probability
> standard score
> standard normal curve
> transformed score
> z score

TRUE OR FALSE

1. z scores express how many standard deviations a particular score is from the mean.
2. Negative z scores are further from the mean than positive z scores.
3. Even when the distribution of raw scores is skewed, the standardized distribution will be normal.
4. The mean of a standard normal distribution is always 1.0.
5. The total area under the standard normal curve is 1.0.
6. The area of a normal curve between any two designated z scores expresses the proportion or percentage of cases falling between the two points.
7. The greater the value of $\bar{X}$ and s the greater the value of the z scores in corresponding standard distributions.
8. About 10% of scores fall 3 standard deviations above the mean.
9. A standardized distribution has the same shape as the distribution from which it was derived.
10. Notwithstanding the level of skewness in a distribution, the standard normal curve is useful for determining the percentile rank of a score.
11. In a normal distribution, the higher the z score, the higher will be the frequency of the corresponding raw score.
12. 50% of scores fall between $z = 0.5$ and $z = -0.5$.

13. In a normal curve, approximately 34% of the scores fall between $z = 0$ and $z = -1$.
14. A percentile rank represents the number of cases falling above a particular score.
15. Given a bimodal distribution of raw scores, the standard normal curve is inappropriate for calculating percentile ranks.
16. $z = -2.58$ has a percentile rank of 98 in a normal distribution.
17. $z = 1.28$ cuts off the highest 10% of scores in a normal distribution.
18. Numerous human characteristics are distributed approximately as a normal curve.
19. If 20% of scores fall into a given class interval, then the percentile rank of the upper real limit of the class interval is 20.
20. The percentile rank of $z = 0$ is always 50.

MULTIPLE CHOICE

1. Which of the following statements is true?

    a A z score indicates how many standard units or deviations a raw score is above or below the mean.
    b The mean of a standard normal distribution is always 0 (zero).
    c The distribution of z scores takes the same shape as that of the raw scores from which they have been derived.
    d All the above statements are true.

2. In an anatomy test, your result is equivalent to a standard or z score of 0.2. What does this z score imply?

    a You performed poorly when compared to others.
    b You performed very well when compared to others.
    c Your result was slightly above average.
    d Your result was slightly below average.

SELF ASSESSMENT

3. The z scores of three persons X, Y and Z in a statistical methods test were +2.0, +1.0 and 0.0, respectively. In term of the original raw scores, which of the following statements is true?

   a The raw score difference between X and Y is greater than the raw score difference between Y and Z.
   b The raw score difference between X and Y is less than the raw score difference between Y and Z.
   c The raw score difference between X and Y is equal to the raw score difference between Y and Z.
   d No precise statement can be made about the relationships between the differences of the raw scores of X and Y and of Y and Z.

A group of patients has a mean weight of 80 kg, with a standard deviation of 10 kg. Questions 4–5 refer to this data.

4. What is the standard score(z) for a patient whose weight is 50 kg?

   a $z = +3$
   b $z = +2$
   c $z = -2$
   d $z = -3$

5. You are told that a patient's weight is two standard deviations below the mean. What is their weight?

   a 60 kg
   b 55 kg
   c 50 kg
   d 45 kg

6. We develop a new method of treating spastic hemiplegia by giving weekly ultrasound massages to the affected muscles. In a consecutive study of 200 children treated by this method we find that the average number of weeks to full recovery is 8, with a standard deviation of 2 weeks. Therefore we conclude that (given a normal distribution):

   a treatment may be stopped after 8 weeks
   b half of all children will need treatment for longer than 8 weeks
   c 90% of children will be fully recovered after 12 weeks of treatment.
   d a and c.

7. A percentile rank:

   a represents the frequency of occurrence of a particular category
   b tells you whether or not a distribution is skewed
   c can be used to estimate the range of distribution
   d tells you what percentage of scores fall at or below a particular score.

Use this information in answering questions 8–12: a normally distributed set of scores has a mean of 40 and a standard deviation of 8.

8. A raw score of 24 corresponds to a z score of:

   a 3.0
   b –3.0
   c 1.5
   d –1.5
   e –2.0

9. A z score of 1.25 corresponds to a raw score of:

   a 50
   b 10
   c 30
   d 56.4
   e 40

10. The percentile rank of a raw score of 48 is:

   a 34.13
   b 15.87

SELF ASSESSMENT

c 84.13

d 65.87

e incalculable from information given.

11. The percentage of scores between 32–44 is:

    a 68.26

    b 53.28

    b 53.28

    c 46.82

    d 32.74

    e 43.32

12. The raw score which cuts off the lowest 5% of the population (rounded to the nearest whole number) is:

    a 38

    b 13

    c 27

    d 53

    e 42

Questions 13–16 refer to a standard normal distribution.

13. The percentage of cases falling above $z = 0.35$ is:

    a 16.8%

    b 34.1%

    c 84.1%

    d 36.3%

14. The percentage of cases falling between $z = -1$ and $z = +1$ is:

    a 16.8%

    b 33.6%

    c 34.1%

    d 68.3%

15. The percentage of cases falling between $z = -0.5$ and $z = +2$ is:

    a 85.0%

    b 66.9%

c 28.6%

d 68.2%

16. The percentage of cases falling either below $z = -2$ or above $z = +2$ is:

    a 95.5%

    b 68.2%

    c 47.7%

    d 4.6%

The following information should be used in answering questions 17–20: a test of reaction times has a mean of 10 and a standard deviation of 4 in the normal adult population.

17. A person scores 8. That person's z score is:

    a 2

    b –2

    c –0.5

    d –1

18. What percentage of the population would have scores up to and including 14 on this test?

    a 84.13

    b 15.87

    c 65.87

    d 34.13

19. What is the percentile rank of a score of 8 on this test?

    a 19.15

    b 30.85

    c 80.85

    d 53.28

20. What score (to the nearest whole number) would cut off the highest 10% of scores?

    a 1

    b 14

    c 15

    d 18

Questions 21–25 refer to the following data: the mean for a population is 500, with a standard deviation of 90; the scores are normally distributed.

21. The percentile rank of a score of 667 is:

 a 4.14
 b 92.7
 c 3.22
 d 96.86

22. The proportion of scores which lie above 650 is:

 a 0.4535
 b 0.9535
 c 0.0475
 d 0.885

23. The proportion of scores which lie between 460 and 600 is:

 a 0.4394

 b 0.5365
 c 0.4406
 d 0.4635

24. The raw score which lies at the 90th percentile is:

 a 615.20
 b 384.80
 c 616.10
 d 383.90

25. The proportion of scores between 300–400 is:

 a 0.3665
 b 0.4868
 c 0.8533
 d 0.1203

16

Correlation

INTRODUCTION

A fundamental aim of scientific and clinical research is to establish relationships between two or more sets of observations or variables. Finding such relationships or covariations is often an initial step for identifying causal relationships.

The topic of correlation is concerned with expressing quantitatively the degree and direction of the relationship between variables. Correlations are useful in the health sciences in areas such as determining the validity and reliability of clinical measures (Ch. 12) or in expressing how health problems are related to crucial biological, behavioural or environmental factors (Ch. 5).

The specific aims of this chapter are to:

1. Define the terms correlation and correlation coefficient.
2. Explain the selection and calculation of correlation coefficients.
3. Outline some of the uses of correlation coefficients.
4. Define and calculate the coefficient of determination.
5. Discuss the relationship between correlation and causality.

CORRELATION

Consider the following two statements:

1. There is a positive relationship between cigarette smoking and lung damage.
2. There is a negative relationship between being overweight and life expectancy.

You probably have a fair idea what the above two statements mean. The first statement implies that there is evidence that if you score high on one variable (cigarette smoking) you are likely to score high on the other variable (lung damage). The second statement describes the finding that scoring high on the variable 'overweight' tends to be associated with low measures on the variable 'life expectancy'. The information missing from each of the statements is the numerical value for degree or magnitude of the association between the variables.

A *correlation coefficient* is a statistic which expresses numerically the magnitude and direction of the association between two variables.

In order to demonstrate that two variables are correlated, we must obtain measures on both variables for the same set of subjects or events. Let us look at an example to illustrate this point.

Assume that we are interested to see whether scores for anatomy examinations are correlated with scores for physiology. To keep the example simple, assume that there were only five ($n = 5$) students who sat for both examinations (see Table 16.1)

To provide a visual representation of the relationship between the two variables, we can plot the above data on a *scattergram*. A scattergram is a graph of the paired scores for each subject on the two variables. By convention, we call one of the variables x, and the other one y. It is evident from Figure 16.1 that there is a positive relationship between the two variables. That is, students who have high scores for anatomy (variable X) tend to have high scores for physiology (variable Y). Also, for this set of data we can fit a straight line in close approximation of the points on the scattergram. This line is referred to as a line of 'best fit'. This topic is discussed in statistics under 'linear regression'. In general, a variety of relationships is possible between two variables; the scattergrams on Figure 16.2 illustrate some of these.

Figure 16.2A and B represents a linear correlation between the variables x and y. That is, a straight line is the most appropriate representation of the relationship between x and y. Figure 16.2C represents a non-linear correlation, where a curve best represents the relationship between x and y.

Figure 16.2A represents a *positive* correlation, indicating that high scores on x are related to high scores on y. For example, the relationship between cigarette smoking and lung damage is a positive correlation. Figure 16.2B represents a

Table 16.1 Examination scores

| Student | Score (out of 10) | |
	Anatomy (*X*)	Physiology (*Y*)
1	3	2.5
2	4	3.5
3	1	0
4	8	6
5	2	1

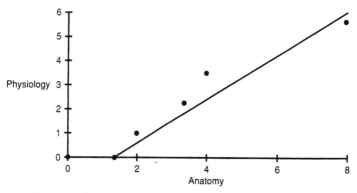

Fig. 16.1 Scattergram of students' scores in two examinations.

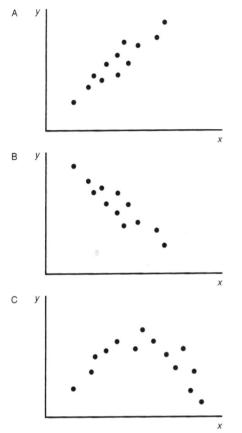

Fig. 16.2 Scattergrams showing relationships between two variables: (A) positive linear correlation; (B) negative linear correlation; (C) non-linear correlation.

negative correlation, where high scores on x are associated with low scores on y. For example, the correlation between the variables 'being overweight' and 'life expectancy' is negative, meaning that the more you are overweight, the lower your life expectancy.

CORRELATION COEFFICIENTS

When we need to know or express the numerical value of the correlation between x and y, we calculate a statistic called the correlation coefficient. The correlation coefficient expresses quantitatively the magnitude and direction of the correlation.

Selection of correlation coefficient

There are several types of correlation coefficients used in statistics. Table 16.2 shows some of these correlation coefficients, and the conditions under which they are used. As the table indicates, the scale of measurements used determines the selection of the appropriate correlation coefficient.

All of the correlation coefficients shown in Table 16.1 are appropriate for quantifying *linear* relationships between variables. There are other correlation coefficients, such as η (eta) which are used for quantifying non-linear relationships. However, the discussion of the use and calculation of all the correlation coefficients is beyond the scope of this text. Rather, we will examine only the commonly used Pearson's r, and Spearman's ρ (rho).

Regardless of which correlation coefficient we employ, these statistics share the following characteristics:

1. Correlation coefficients are calculated from pairs of measurements on variables x and y for the same group of individuals.
2. A positive correlation is denoted by + and a negative correlation by –.
3. The values of the correlation coefficient range from + 1 to –1; where +1 means a perfect positive correlation, 0 means no correlation, and –1 a perfect negative correlation.
4. The square of the correlation coefficient represents the **coefficient of determination**.

Table 16.2   Correlation coefficient

Coefficient	Conditions where appropriate
φ (phi)	Both x and y measure on a nominal scale
ρ (rho)	Both x and y measure on, or transformed to, ordinal scales
r	Both x and y measure on an interval or ratio scale

CALCULATION OF CORRELATION COEFFICIENTS: PEARSON'S *r*

We have already stated that Pearson's *r* is the appropriate correlation coefficient when both variables *x* and *y* are measured on an interval or a ratio scale. Further assumptions in using *r* are that both variables *x* and *y* are normally distributed, and that we are describing a linear (rather than curvilinear) relationship.

Pearson's *r* is a measure of the extent to which paired scores are correlated. To calculate *r* we need to represent the position of each paired score within its own distribution, so we convert each raw score to a *z* score. This transformation corrects for the two distributions *x* and *y* having different means and standard deviations. The formula for calculating Pearson's *r* is:

$$r = \frac{\Sigma Z_x Z_y}{n}$$

where z_x = standard score corresponding to any raw *x* score, z_y = standard score corresponding to any raw *y* score Σ = sum of standard score products and *n* = numbers of paired measurements.

Table 16.3 gives the calculations for the correlation coefficient for the data given in the example on page 192.

$$\text{Therefore: } r = \frac{\Sigma z_x z_y}{n} = \frac{3.94}{5} = 0.79$$

(The *z* scores are calculated as discussed in Ch. 15.)

This is a quite high correlation, indicating that the paired *z* scores fall roughly on a straight line.

Table 16.3 Example calculations for correlation coefficient

Student	Raw scores		z scores		
	x	*y*	z_x	z_y	$z_x z_y$
1	3	2.5	−0.22	−0.04	+0.01
2	4	3.5	+0.15	+0.39	+0.06
3	1	0	−0.96	−1.12	+1.08
4	8	6	+1.63	+1.46	+2.38
5	2	1	−0.59	−0.69	+0.41
	$\overline{X}$ = 3.6	$\overline{Y}$ = 2.6	$\Sigma z_x z_y$ = 3.94		
	S_x = 2.7	S_y = 2.33			

In general, the closer the relationship between the two variables approximates a straight line, the more *r* approaches +1. Note that in social and biological sciences correlations this high do not usually occur. In general, we consider anything over 0.7 to be quite high, 0.3 to 0.7 to be moderate, and less than 0.3 to be weak. The scattergrams in Figure 16.3 illustrate this point.

When *n* is large, the above equation is inconvenient to use to calculate *r*. Here we are not concerned with calculating *r* with a large *n*, although appropriate formulae or computer programmes are available. For example, Coakes & Steed (1999, Chapter 5) described how to use the program 'SPSS' for calculating correlation coefficients. The printouts provide not only the value of the correlation coefficients but also the statistical significance of the associations (see Section 5).

Assumptions for using *r*

It was pointed out earlier that *r* is used when two variables are scaled on interval or ratio scales and when it is shown that they are linearly associated. In addition, the sets of scores on each variable should be approximately normally distributed.

If any of the above assumptions is violated, then the correlation coefficient might be spuriously low. Therefore, other correlation coefficients should be used to represent association between two variables. A further problem may arise from the truncation of the range of values in one or both of the variables. This occurs when the distributions greatly deviate from normal shapes. The higher scale can be readily reduced to an ordinal scale.

If we measure the correlation between examination scores and IQs of a group of health science students, we might find a low correlation because, by the time students present themselves to tertiary courses, most students with low IQs are eliminated. In this way, the distribution of IQs would not be normal but rather negatively skewed. In effect, the question of appropriate sampling is also relevant to correlations, as it was outlined in Chapter 3.

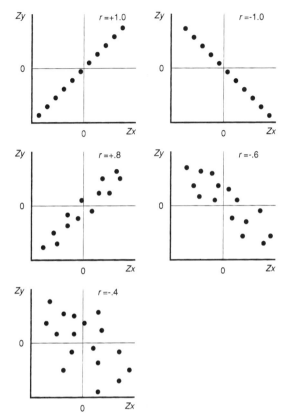

Fig. 16.3 Scattergrams and corresponding approximate *r* values.

discussed here. The 6 is placed in the formula as a scaling device; it ensures that the possible range of ρ is from –1 to +1 and thus enables ρ and *r* to be compared. Let us consider an example to illustrate the use of ρ.

If an investigator is interested in the correlation between socioeconomic status and severity of respiratory illness, and assuming that both variables were measured on, or transformed to, an ordinal scale, the investigator rank-orders the scores from highest to lowest on each variable (Table 16.4).

Table 16.4 Rank-ordering of scores

Patient	Socioeco-nomic status (rank)	Severity of illness (rank)	d (difference between ranks)	d^2
1	6	5	1	1
2	7	8	–1	1
3	2	4	–2	4
4	3	3	0	0
5	5	7	–2	4
6	4	1	3	9
7	1	2	–1	1
8	8	6	2	4
				$\Sigma d^2 = 24$

CALCULATION OF CORRELATION COEFFICIENTS: SPEARMAN'S ρ

When the obtained data are such that at least one of the variables *x* or *y* was measured on an ordinal scale and the other on an ordinal scale or higher, we use ρ to calculate the correlation between the two variables. The higher scale can be readily reduced to an ordinal scale.

If one or both variables were measured on a nominal scale, ρ is no longer appropriate as a statistic.

$$\rho = 1 - \frac{6\Sigma d^2}{n^3 - n}$$

where *d* = difference in a pair of ranks and *n* = number of pairs

The derivation of this formula will not be

Therefore, $\rho = 1 - \dfrac{6\Sigma d^2}{n^3 - n}$

$$= 1 - \frac{6 \infty 24}{8^3 - 8} = 0.71$$

Clearly, the association among the ranks for the paired scores on the two variables becomes closer, the more ρ approaches +1. If the ranks tend to be inverse, then ρ approaches –1.

USES OF CORRELATION IN THE HEALTH SCIENCES

Prediction

When the correlation coefficient has been calculated it may be used to predict the value of one variable (*y*) given the value of the other variable (*x*). For instance, take a hypothetical example that the correlation between cigarette

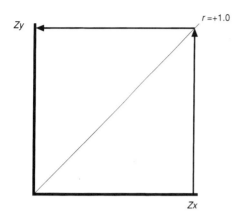

Fig. 16.4 Hypothetical relationship between cigarette smoking and lung damage. $r = +1.0$.

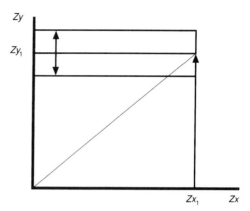

Fig. 16.5 Hypothetical relationship between cigarette smoking and lung damage. $r = +0.7$. With a correlation of <1.0 the data points will cluster around rather than exactly on the line and may vary between the range of values shown for any given values of X or Y and their corresponding z scores.

smoking and lung damage is $r = +1$. We can see from Figure 16.4 that given any score on x, we can transform this into a z score (z_x) and then using the graph we can read off the corresponding z score on y (z_y). Of course, it is extremely rare that there should be a perfect ($r = +1$) correlation between two variables. In this case, the smaller the correlation coefficient, the greater the probability of making an error in prediction. For example, consider Figure 16.5, where the scattergram shown represents a hypothetical correlation of approximately $r = 0.7$. Here, for any transformed value on variable x (say z_x) there is a range of values of z_y that correspond. Our best guess is z_y the *average value*, but clearly a range of scores is possible, as shown on the figure.

That is, as the correlation coefficient approaches 0 the range of error in prediction increases. A more appropriate and precise way of making predictions is in terms of regression analysis, but this topic is not covered in this introductory book.

Reliability and predictive validity of assessment

As you will recall, reliability refers to measurements using instruments or to subjective judgements remaining relatively the same on repeated administration (Ch. 12). This is called test–retest reliability and its degree is measured

Table 16.5 Assessment of disability (%) by observers X and Y

Patient	Observer X	Observer Y	Rank X	Rank Y
1	85%	98%	1	1
2	75%	86%	2	2
3	74%	80%	3	3
4	72%	79%	4	4
5	69%	70%	5	5

by a correlation coefficient. The correlation coefficient can be used also to determine the degree of interobserver reliability.

As an example, assume that we are interested in the interobserver reliability for two neurologists who are assessing patients for degrees of functional disability following spinal cord damage. Table 16.4 represents a set of hypothetical results of their independent assessment of the same set of five patients.

Observer Y clearly attributes greater degrees of disability to the patients than observer X. However, as stated earlier, this need not affect the correlation coefficient. If we treat the measurement as an ordinal scale, we can see from Table 16.5 that the ranks given to the patients by the two observers correspond, so that it can be shown that $\rho = +1$.

Clearly, the higher the correlation, the greater

the reliability. If we had treated the measurement as representing interval or ratio data, we would have calculated Pearson's r to represent quantitatively the reliability of the measurement.

Predictive validity is also expressed as a correlation coefficient. For example, say that you devise an assessment procedure to predict how much people will benefit from a rehabilitation programme. If the correlation between the assessment and a measure of the success of the rehabilitation program is high (say 0.7 or 0.8), the assessment procedure has high predictive validity. If, however, the correlation is low (say 0.3 or 0.4), the predictive validity of the assessment is low, and it would be unwise to use the assessment as a screening procedure for the entry of patients into the rehabilitation programme.

Estimating shared variance

A useful statistic is the square of the correlation coefficient (r^2) which represents the proportion of variance in one variable accounted for by the other. This is called the **coefficient of determination**.

If, for example, the correlation between variable x (height) and variable y (weight) is $r = 0.7$ then, the coefficient of determination is $r^2 = 0.49$ or 49%. This means that 49% of the variability of weight can be accounted for in terms of height. You might ask, what about the other 51% of the variability? This would be accounted for by other factors, say for instance, a tendency to eat fatty foods. The point here is that even a relatively high correlation coefficient $(r = 0.7)$ accounts for less than 50% of the variability.

This is a difficult concept, so it might be worth remembering that 'variability' (see Ch. 15) refers to how scores are spread out about the mean. That is, as in the above example, some people will be heavy, some average, some light. So we can account for 49% of the total variability of weight (x) in terms of height (y) if $r = 0.7$. The other 51% can be explained in terms of other factors, such as somatotype. The greater the correlation coefficient, the greater the coefficient of determination, and the more of the variability in y can be accounted for in terms of x.

CORRELATION AND CAUSATION

In Chapter 4, we pointed out that there were at least three criteria for establishing a causal relationship. Correlation or covariation is only one of these criteria. We have already discussed in Chapter 6 that even a high correlation between two variables does not necessarily imply a causal relationship. That is, there are a variety of plausible explanations for finding a correlation. As an example, let us take cigarette smoking (x) and lung damage (y). A high positive correlation could result from any of the following circumstances:

1. x causes y.
2. y causes x.
3. There is a third variable, which causes changes in both x and y.
4. The correlation represents a spurious or chance association.

For the example above, (1) would imply that cigarette smoking causes lung damage, (2) that lung damage causes cigarette smoking, and (3) that there was a variable (e.g. stress) which caused both increased smoking and lung damage. We need further information to identify which of the competing hypotheses is most plausible.

Some associations between variables are completely spurious (4). For example, there might be a correlation between the amount of margarine consumed and the number of cases of influenza over a period of time in a community, but each of the two events might have entirely different, unrelated causes. Also, some correlation coefficients do not reach statistical significance, that is, they may be due to chance (see Chs 18 and 19).

Also, if we are using a sample to estimate the correlation in a population, we must be certain that the outcome is not due to biased sampling or sampling error. That is, the investigator needs to show that a correlation coefficient is statistically significant and not just due to random sampling error. We will look at the concept of statistical significance in the next chapter.

While demonstrating correlation does not establish causality, we can use correlations as a source for subsequent hypotheses. For instance, in this example, work on carcinogens in cigarette tars and the causes of emphysema has confirmed that it is probably true that smoking does, in fact, cause lung damage (x causes y). However, given that there is often multiple causation of health problems, option (3) cannot be ruled out.

Techniques are available which can, under favourable conditions, enable investigators to use correlations as a basis for distinguishing between competing plausible hypotheses. One such technique, called path analysis involves postulating a probable temporal sequence of events and then establishing a correlation between them. This technique was borrowed from systems theory and has been applied in areas of clinical research, such as epidemiology.

SUMMARY

In this chapter we outlined how the degree and direction between two variables can be quantified, using statistics called correlation coefficients.

Of the correlation coefficients, the use of two were outlined: Pearson's r and Spearman's ρ. Definitional formulae and simple calculations were presented, with the understanding that more complex calculations of correlation coefficients are done with computers.

Several uses for r and ρ were discussed: for prediction, for quantifying the reliability and validity of measurements, and by using r^2 in estimating amount of shared variability. Finally, we discussed the caution necessary in causal interpretation of correlation coefficients. Showing a strong association between variables is an important step towards establishing causal links but further evidence is required to decide the direction of causality.

As with other descriptive statistics, caution is necessary when correlation coefficients are calculated for a sample and then generalized to a population. The question of generalization from a sample statistic to a population parameter will be discussed in the following chapters.

SELF ASSESSMENT

Explain the meaning of the following terms:

> correlation
> correlation coefficient
> curvilinear correlation
> linear correlation
> negative correlation
> coefficient of determination
> positive correlation
> shared variance
> zero correlation

TRUE OR FALSE

1. Correlation is defined as the relative difference between two variables.
2. The association between two variables can be plotted on a scattergram.
3. If the distribution of paired scores is best represented by a curve, the relationship is non-linear.
4. When we speak of a positive (+) relationship, we mean that high scores on one variable are associated with high scores on the other variable.
5. In a negative (−) relationship, low scores on one variable are associated with low scores on the other.
6. There are several types of correlation coefficients, the selection of which is determined by the level of scaling of the two variables.
7. When both variables are measured on an interval or ratio scale, Pearson's r is the most appropriate correlation coefficient.
8. When both variables are measured on, or converted to, ordinal scales, we must use φ (phi) to express correlation.

9. For two variables measured on nominal scales, we use ρ (rho) to express correlation.

10. Pearson's r is calculated by a formula where $\Sigma z_x z_y$ stands for the sum of the z score pairs multiplied together.

11. When calculating Spearman's ρ, Σd^2 is the sum of the square of the differences between the means.

12. When we use Pearson's r, we assume that both variables are continuous and normally distributed.

13. The calculated values of correlation coefficients range between 0 and –1.

14. When there is no linear association between two variables, r or ρ will be close to zero.

15. A correlation coefficient of –1 represents a very low linear correlation.

16. Where there is a correlation of $r = +1$ between two variables, then the z scores of variable x will be equal to the z scores of variable y.

17. The coefficient of determination is the square of the correlation coefficient.

18. If $r = 0.3$, then the coefficient of determination will be 9.0.

19. If $r^2 = 0.36$ for a set of data, this implies that 36% of the variability of y is explained in terms of x.

20. As the correlation coefficient approaches zero, the possible error in linear prediction increases.

21. The closer the correlation coefficient is to zero, the greater the predictive validity of a test.

22. If a correlation coefficient for the test–retest reliability of a test is close to 1, then the test is unreliable.

23. Given a –1.00 correlation coefficient for two variables, a raw score of 50 on the first variable must be accompanied by a score of –50 on the second variable, for a given case.

24. Even a high correlation is not necessarily indicative of a causal relationship between two variables.

25. As the value of r increases, the proportion of variability of y that can be accounted for by x, decreases.

26. Eta (η) is the appropriate correlation coefficient to use when two variables are nominally scaled.

27. If the relationship between two variables is non-linear, the value of the correlation coefficient must be negative.

28. Spearman's ρ is used where one or both variables are at least of interval scaling.

29. A scattergram is used to help to decide if the relationship between two variables is linear or curvilinear.

30. If the correlation between variables A and B is high, then there must be a direct causal relationship between A and B.

MULTIPLE CHOICE

1. Which of the following statements about correlations is false?

   a Spearman's ρ (rho) is appropriate to use when the relationship between two variables is non-linear.

   b A correlation coefficient of –0.8 represents a higher degree of association between two variables than a correlation coefficient of +0.6.

   c The construction of a scattergram is useful for evaluating whether a relationship between two variables is linear or curvilinear.

   d In a perfect positive correlation between two quantitatively measured variables, each individual obtains the same z scores on each variable.

   e Negative correlation implies that high scores on one variable are related to low scores on another variable.

2. A scattergram:

   a is a statistical test

SELF ASSESSMENT

b   must be linear
c   must be curvilinear
d   is a graph of x and y scores
e   is none of the above.

3. If the relationship between variables x and y is linear, then the points on the scattergram:

a   will fall exactly on a straight line
b   will fall on a curve
c   must represent population parameters
d   are independent of the variance
e   are best represented by a straight line.

4. If the relationship between x and y is positive, as variable y decreases, variable x:

a   increases
b   decreases
c   remains the same
d   changes linearly
e   varies.

5. In a 'negative' relationship:

a   as x increases, y increases
b   as x decreases, y decreases
c   as x increases, y decreases
d   both a and b
e   none of the above.

6. The lowest strength of association is reflected by which of the following correlation coefficients?

a   0.95
b   −0.60
c   −0.33
d   0.29
e   none of the above, as it cannot be determined.

7. The highest strength of association is reflected by which of the following correlation coefficients:

a   −1.0

b   −0.95
c   0.1
d   0.85
e   none of the above, as it cannot be determined.

8. Which of the following statements is false?

a   In a perfect positive correlation, each individual obtains the same z score on each variable.
b   Spearman's ρ is used when one or both variables are at least of interval scaling.
c   The range of the correlation coefficient is from −1 to +1.
d   A correlation of $r = 0.85$ implies a stronger association than $r = −0.70$.

9. We can calculate the correlation coefficient if given:

a   the top scores from one test and lowest scores from another test
b   at least two scores from the same tests
c   two sets of measurements for the same subjects
d   either a or b.

10. The correlation between two variables x and y is −1.00. A given individual has a z score of $z_x = 1.4$ on variable x. We predict their z score on y is:

a   1.4 above the mean
b   −1.4
c   between 1.4 and −1.4
d   −1.00

11. Professor Shnook demonstrated a correlation of −0.85 between body weight and IQ. This means that:

a   obesity decreases intelligence
b   heavy people have higher IQs than light people
c   people with high IQs are likely to be light

d malnutrition damages the brain

e none of the above.

12. A correlation coefficient of +0.5 was found between exposure to stressful life events and incidence of stress-induced disorders. A correlation of this direction and magnitude indicates that:

a a high level of exposure to stressful life events causes a high level of stress-induced disorders.

b a high level of stress-induced disorders causes a high likelihood of exposure to stressful life events.

c either or both of *a* and *b* may be correct—we cannot be sure.

d the levels of stress-induced disorders and of exposure to stressful life events are not causally related in any way.

13. You are told that there is a high inverse association between the variables 'amount of exercise' and 'incidence of heart disease'. A correlation coefficient consistent with the above statement is:

a *r* = 0.8

b *r* = 0.2

c *r* = −0.2

d *r* = −0.8

14. Of the following measurement levels, which is at a minimum required for the valid calculation of a Pearson correlation coefficient?

a nominal

b ordinal

c interval

d ratio

15. Of the following measurement levels, which is required for the valid calculation of the Spearman correlation coefficient?

a nominal

b ordinal

c interval

d ratio

16. You are told that there is a high, positive correlation between measures of 'fitness' and 'hours of exercise'. The correlation coefficient consistent with the above statement is:

a 0.3

b 0.2

c −0.8

d −0.3

e none of these.

You are interested in selecting a test suitable for client assessment in a clinical situation. You find 4 tests in the literature, tests P, Q, R, and S. Each of these tests has been validated against a clinically relevant variable. The test–re-test and predictive validity of the four hypothetical tests are:

Test–re-test reliability (*r*)	Validity *r*
P 0.8	0.50
Q 0.9	0.18
R 0.5	0.40
S 0.2	0.03

Questions 17 and 18 refer to the above information.

17. Which test would you choose for clinical assessment?

a P

b Q

c R

d S

18. Which test has the best test-retest reliability?

a P

b Q

SELF ASSESSMENT

c R
d S

An investigation aims to establish for a sample of subjects the relationship between blood cholesterol levels (in mg/cc) and blood pressure (in mmHg). Questions 19–20 refer to this investigation.

19. The correlation coefficient appropriate for establishing the degree of correlation between the two variables (assuming a linear relationship):

    a is determined by the sample size
    b depends on the direction of the causality
    c is Spearman's ρ
    d is Pearson's *r*
    e both *b* and *c*.

20. Say that the correlation coefficient is calculated to be +0.7. A correlation of this direction and magnitude indicates that:

    a high blood pressure causes high blood cholesterol
    b high blood cholesterol causes high blood pressure
    c there might be a third variable which causes both high blood pressure and high blood cholesterol
    d none of the statements *a*, *b* or *c* is consistent with the evidence
    e any of the statements *a*, *b*, or *c* might be correct; we cannot be sure from the available evidence.

21. When deciding which measure of

correlation to employ with a specific set of data, you should consider:

    a whether the relationship is linear or non-linear
    b the type of scale of measurement for each variable
    c *a* and *b*
    d neither *a* nor *b*.

22. The proportion of variance accounted for by the level of correlation between two variables is calculated by a:

    a $\bar{X}$
    b r^2
    c Σx
    d you cannot calculate this proportion under any circumstances.

23. If the correlation between two variables A and B is 0.36, then the proportion of variance accounted for is:

    a 0.13
    b 0.06
    c 0.60
    d 0.64

24. We find that the correlation coefficient representing the outcome for the predictive validity of a test is $r = 0.2$. Such a finding would indicate that the test had:

    a Low predictive validity
    b Acceptable predictive validity
    c High predictive validity
    d 20% predictive validity

SECTION 5

Discussion, Questions and Answers

Descriptive statistics are an integral part of everyday life and an important aspect of clinical practice. They are used to describe the essential characteristics of measurements for a sample of cases. Some descriptive statistics are quite familiar to the lay person. The mean or average is frequently used in discussions of public policy. For example, the question 'What has happened to the average household income in the UK over the last year?' uses this concept as does a question such as 'What is the average length of stay in hospital for an orthopaedic patient with a fractured neck of femur in this ward?'. Descriptive statistics are shorthand ways of conveying information about a sample of cases.

In recent years in the UK, Australia, Canada and the USA, there has been a growing preoccupation with the effectiveness and efficiency of health services, in particular, and government services in general. Economic conditions have resulted in the reduced availability of tax revenues and this has led to increased scrutiny of spending. Hospital services are an expensive component of health services in these countries. Much statistical information is collected concerning stays in hospital. The use of statistical information concerning case costs is heavily used to determine funding of hospitals by agencies such as government and insurers.

A key component of hospital costs is the length of time spent by the patient in the hospital. Each 'bed day' is very costly and most hospital services are under pressure to reduce the length of stay for their patients. However, one cannot reduce the length of stay for each patient too far, as this might be dangerous. Patients can come back unexpectedly because they require further hospitalization following discharge. This is termed an 'unplanned' readmission. Thus, the goal is to reduce lengths of stay but not increase unplanned readmissions.

Obviously, the expected length of stay for a woman giving birth ought to be much shorter than a man recovering from serious internal injuries and multiple compound fractures following a motor vehicle accident. How can these cases be compared without some adjustment for their differences? There is a large literature concerning how different types of patients might be compared. Comparability of types of patients is often achieved by the use of Diagnosis Related Groups (DRG) where patients of the same type are categorized together. This grouping enables hospitals and their funding agencies to compare how efficient and effective different hospitals are in treating the same types of patient.

Table D16.1 shows some data for patients admitted to an orthopaedics ward in a hospital.

Table D16.1   Details of patients admitted to an orthopaedics ward

Patient name	Diagnostic group	Length of stay in hospital (days)	Unplanned readmission within 14 days?
Jones	Fractured neck of femur	15	No
Ng	Fractured neck of femur	10	Yes
Thomas	Fractured neck of femur	19	No
Evans	Fractured neck of femur	12	No
Valperri	Fractured neck of femur	14	No
Hart	Fractured neck of femur	14	No
Elmahdy	Fractured neck of femur	13	No
Smith	Fractured neck of femur	11	Yes
Cairns	Fractured neck of femur	12	No
Eisenberg	Fractured neck of femur	12	No

Discussion, Questions and Answers

Table D16.2 Lengths of stay and readmission rates for 30 consecutive patients with a fractured neck of femur at five hospitals

Hospital	Number of cases (n)	Length of stay in hospital Average $\bar{x}$	Standard deviation (s)	Rate of unplanned readmissions per 100
A	30	13.0	2.6	6.7
B	30	12.3	2.4	10.0
C	30	13.4	2.8	6.7
D	30	14.4	3.3	3.3
E	30	14.8	3.0	3.3

All the cases with the same diagnostic category have been included.

For this sample of cases, the average length of stay was 13.2 days (standard deviation 2.5). The minimum stay was 10 days and the maximum stay was 19 days. The rate of unplanned re-admissions within 14 days was 2 in 10 or 20%.

If one was to take larger samples of cases from a variety of hospitals (say a consecutive series of 30 cases for each, then it would be possible to compare their lengths of stay and the rate of readmissions. This has been done in Table D16.2, with hypothetical data from five hospitals.

Although the differences in average numbers of days spent in hospital between the five hospitals may not appear to be great, a difference of 2.5 days for example, between hospital B and E may represent over £500 for each case. In a busy hospital department, this would soon run into large sums of money. However, it is worrying that the hospital with the shortest period of stay also seems to be the one with the highest rate of readmissions within 14 days. Perhaps they are discharging some of their patients too soon? With such a small sample of hospitals, (i.e. only five) and such a small number of readmissions (only three out of the 30 in the worst case), it would be difficult to conclude whether there is such a relationship. However, if these data were collected from a large number of hospitals with a larger number of cases, it would be possible to correlate these two variables to study the size of the relationship between them.

Correlation coefficients measure the size and direction of the statistical relationship between two variables. Following on from the above discussion, we might hypothesize that there is a negative correlation between the average length of stay and rate of readmission to hospital. In other words, we might expect that a shorter average stay in a hospital could result in a greater rate of readmission. The graph in Figure D16.1 shows the association between length of stay and rate of readmission for 30 hospitals, based on their 1993–1994 discharges for all their patients with a fractured neck of femur.

Each of the dots in the graph represents a different hospital. The graph shows that there is a tendency towards those hospitals with longer average lengths of stays for their patients to have lower readmission rates.

The Pearson correlation between these variables is −0.52, which indicates a moderately sized negative correlation between average length of stay and readmission rate for the 30 hospitals.

Evidence such as discussed above is being continually collected by health administrators and the results of these analyses impacts on

Discussion, Questions and Answers

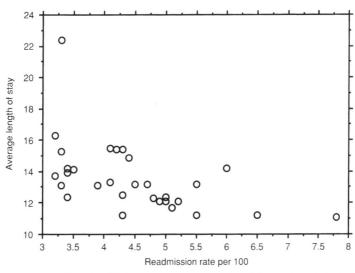

Fig. D16.1   Relationship between average lengths of stay and readmission rates for patients with fractured neck of femur at 30 hospitals.

the funding of your workplace and your opportunities for looking after your patients.

Questions

1. In Table D16.1, how many patients had a length of stay in hospital that was above the average of 13.2 days?
2. If a patient had a length of stay of 14 days, given that the sample mean was 13.2 days and the standard deviation 2.5, what would be their standard or z score?
3. Is it appropriate to compare hospital lengths of stay for patients with different diagnoses?
4. From Figure D16.1, what is the longest average length of stay for this sample of hospitals? What is the shortest?
5. Why is the correlation between average length of stay and readmission rate negative in sign?

Answers

1. Four: Jones, Thomas, Valperri and Hart.

2. The standard score is calculated using the following formula:

$$z = \frac{x - \bar{x}}{s}$$

Substituting into the equation, we find that:

$$z = \frac{14 - 13.2}{2.5} = 0.32$$

3. It is like comparing apples with oranges. It is quite reasonable to expect that an uncomplicated birth may involve a hospital stay of 3–4 days, whereas this would be quite unreasonable for a heart transplant. Thus it does not make sense to compare the lengths of stays of different types of patients, because the averages or means are quite different. However, it would make sense to compare standard scores for different types of patients.
4. About 22.5 days; About 11 days.
5. Because an increase in average length of stay is associated with a decrease in readmission rate.

Inferential statistics

The statistical analysis of the data is an essential stage in the process of quantitative research. The principles of inferential statistics, as introduced in this section, must be applied to data analysis, before we can decide if the data obtained shows the differences and patterns we set out to demonstrate in the population. This is true for descriptive, predictive and causal research, if we are using sample data to make inferences concerning populations.

Quantitative research in the health sciences mostly involves working with samples drawn from populations. In order to generalize our findings, we must draw generalizations and inferences from sample statistics (e.g. $\bar{X}$, s) to the population parameters (e.g. μ, σ). Inferences are always probabilistic, because even with random samples there is always the chance of sampling error. The finite probability of sampling error implies that the differences or patterns identified in our sample data represent random variations or chance patterns, rather than 'real' ones which are true for the population as a whole.

As an illustration, imagine that we have collected data in a study aimed at identifying age-related differences in the use of sedatives and tranquillizers in a given population. Our participants ($n = 200$) kept diaries over a period of 1 year, recording each time they had taken a sedative or tranquillizer. Assume that the following hypothetical data was obtained:

Sedative and tranquilliser consumption			
Age group	n	$\bar{X}$	s
20–39	100	20	5
40–59	100	30	5

Two important and interrelated issues are raised in Section 6 concerning sample data such as shown in the above table.

1. Even if we used an adequate sampling procedure (see Ch. 3) how confident are we to infer that the true population parameters (μ) are the same as, or are at least close to $\bar{X}$? For example, is it true that the mean tranquillizer intake for the 20–39 age group is $\mu = 20$?
2. It appears that there is a large difference between the two sample means; but is this difference also true for the populations? In other words is this difference 'real' or significant, or is it simply due to sampling error?
3. What we are inferring is that μ older > μ younger. In other words, are we justified in concluding that the mean sedative/tranquilizer intake for the older age group is greater than for the younger one?

We cannot eliminate sampling error, even with large and well-chosen samples but, as outlined in Section 6, we can apply the principles of inferential statistics to calculate the probability of error. We then use this information to minimize the probability of making errors when we generalize from sample statistics to population parameters.

In Chapter 17 we examine how sampling distributions are derived and used for calculating the probability of obtaining a given sample statistic. This information can be applied to the calculation of confidence intervals, which represents a range of scores which contains, the true population parameter (at a given level or probability).

In Chapter 18 we outline the logic of hypothesis testing, using single sample z and t tests as exemplars. Hypothesis testing is a procedure used to decide if a difference or pattern identified in our sample data is statistically significant. If the outcome of our analysis is significant, then we are in a position to decide that the patterns or differences found in our data may be generalized to the populations from which the samples were obtained.

There are numerous statistical tests available for analyzing the significance of our data. In Chapter 19, we discuss basic criteria for selecting an appropriate statistical test, including (i) scale of measurement used to collect the data, (ii) the number of groups being compared and (iii) the dependence or independence of measurements. We will use the χ^2 (chi-squared) test to demonstrate how statistical tests are selected and used to analyze the data.

Ultimately, statistical decision making is probabilistic, implying that the possibility of making decision errors can not be eliminated. Decisions may be correct, or involve what are called Type I and Type II errors. In Chapter 20, we examine how these errors may influence our interpretation of the obtained data in relation to the aims or hypotheses guiding our research, and we will examine strategies which can be employed to reduce the probability of making such errors.

17

Probability and sampling distributions

INTRODUCTION

Sample statistics (such as $\bar{X}$, s) should be seen as estimates of the actual population parameters. Even where adequate sampling procedures are adopted, there is no guarantee that the sample statistics are the exact representations of the parameters of the population from which the samples were drawn. Therefore, inferences from sample statistics to population parameters necessarily involve the possibility of sampling error. As stated in Chapter 3, sampling errors represent the discrepancy between sample statistics and true population parameters. Given that investigators usually have no knowledge of the true population parameters, inferential statistics are employed to estimate the probable sampling errors. That is, while sampling error cannot be eliminated completely its probable magnitude can be calculated using *inferential statistics*. In this way investigators are in a position to calculate the probability level of their estimations of the actual population parameters.

The aims of this chapter are to examine how probability theory is applied to generating sampling distributions and how sampling distributions are used for estimating population parameters. Sampling distributions can be used for specifying confidence intervals, as discussed in this chapter, as well as for testing hypotheses, as further discussed in Chapter 18.

PROBABILITY

The concept of probability is central to the

understanding of inferential statistics. Probability is expressed as a proportion between 0 and 1, where 0 means an event is certain not to occur, and 1 means an event is certain to occur. The probability of any event (say event A) occurring is given by the formula:

$$p(A) = \frac{\text{number of occurrences of A}}{\text{total number of possible occurrences}}$$

Sometimes the probability of an event can be calculated a priori (before the event) by reasoning alone. For example, we can predict that the probability of throwing a head (H) with a fair coin is:

$$p(H) = \frac{\text{number of occurrences of H}}{\text{total number of possible occurrences}}$$

$$= \frac{H}{H + T \text{ (tails)}} = \frac{1}{2} = 0.5$$

Or, if we buy a lottery ticket in a draw where there are 100 000 tickets, the probability of winning first prize is:

$$p(\text{1st prize}) = \frac{1}{100\,000} = 0.00001$$

This is true only if the lottery is fair; if all tickets have an equal chance of being drawn by random selection.

In some situations, there is no model which we can apply to calculate the occurrence of an event a priori. For instance, how can we calculate the probability of an individual dying of a specific condition? In such instances, we use previously obtained empirical evidence to calculate probabilities a posteriori (after the event).

For example, if it is known that the percentages (or proportions) for causes of death are distributed in a particular way, then the probability of a particular cause of death for a given individual can be predicted. Table 17.1 represents a set of hypothetical statistics for a community.

Given the data in Table 17.1, we are in a position to calculate the probability of a selected individual of over 65 dying of any of the specified causes. For example, the probability of a given individual dying of coronary heart disease is:

Table 17.1 Causes of death for persons over 65

Cause of death	Percentage of deaths
Coronary heart disease	50
Cancer	25
Stroke	10
Accidents	5
Infections	5
Other causes	5

$$p(\text{dying of heart disease}) = \frac{\begin{array}{c}\text{percentage of cases dying}\\ \text{of heart disease}\end{array}}{100\%}$$

$$= \frac{50\%}{100\%} = 0.5$$

This approach ignores individual risk factors and assumes that the environmental conditions under which the data were obtained are still pertinent. However, the example illustrates the principle that once we have organized the data into a frequency distribution, we can calculate the probability of selecting any of the tabulated values. This is true whether the variable was measured on a nominal, ordinal, interval or ratio scale. Here, we will examine how to calculate the probability of values for normally distributed, continuous variables.

We can use the normal curve model, as outlined in Chapter 15, to determine the proportion or percentage of cases up to, or between, any specified scores. In this instance, probability is defined as the proportion of the total area cut off by the specified scores under the normal curve. The greater the proportion, the higher the probability of selecting the specified values.

For example, say that on the basis of previous evidence we can specify the frequency distribution of neonates' weight. Let us assume that the distribution is approximately normal, with the mean ($\bar{X}$) of 5.0 kg and a standard deviation (s) of 1.5. Now, say that we are interested in the probability of a randomly selected neonate having a birth weight of 2.0 kg or under. Figure 17.1 illustrates the above situation.

The area A under the curve in Figure 17.1 corresponds to the probability of obtaining a score of 2 or under. Using the principles outlined in Chapter 15 to calculate proportions or areas

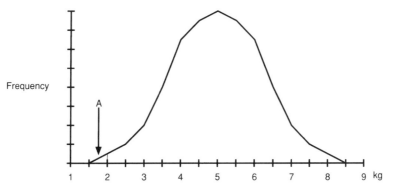

Fig. 17.1 Frequency distribution of neonate birth weights. Area A corresponds to z ≤ −2.

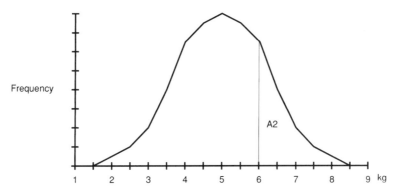

Fig. 17.2 Frequency distribution of neonate birth weights. Area A2 corresponds to probability of weight being between 6–8 kg.

under the normal curve, we first translate the raw score of 2 into a z score.

$$z = \frac{x - \overline{X}}{s} = \frac{2 - 5}{1.5} = -2$$

Now we look up the area under the normal curve corresponding to $z = -2$ (Appendix A). Here we find that A is 0.0228. This area corresponds to a probability, and we can say that 'The probability of a neonate having a birth weight of 2 kg or less is 0.0228'. Another way of stating this outcome is that the chances are 2 in 100, or 2%, for a child having such a birth weight.

We can also use the normal curve model to calculate the probability of selecting scores between any given values of a normally distributed continuous variable. For example, if we are interested in the probability of birth weights being between 6 and 8 kg, then this can be represented on the normal curve. (Area A2 on Figure 17.2). To determine this area, we proceed as outlined in Chapter 15. Let $s = 1.5$.

$$z_1 = \frac{6 - 5}{1.5} = 0.67$$

$$z_2 = \frac{8 - 5}{1.5} = 2.0.$$

Therefore: the area between z_1 and $\overline{X}$ is 0.2486 (from Appendix A) and the area between z_2 and $\overline{X} = 0.4772$ (from Appendix A). Therefore, the required area A2 (Figure 17.2) is:

$$A2 = 0.47720 - 0.2486 = 0.2286$$

It can be concluded that the probability of a randomly selected child having a birth weight between 6 and 8 kg is $p = 0.2286$. Another way of saying this is that there is a chance of 23 in 100 or a 23% chance that the birth weight will be between 6 and 8 kg.

The above examples demonstrate that if the mean and standard deviation are known for a normally distributed continuous variable, this information can be applied to calculating the probability of any set of events related to this distribution. Of course, probabilities can be calculated for scores not in a normal continuous distribution, but this requires integral calculus which is beyond the scope of this text. In general, regardless of the shape or scaling of a distribution, scores occurring within ranges of a high level of frequency are more likely to be selected than those occurring within ranges of a low level of frequency. Obviously, scores which are common or 'average' are more likely to be selected than those which are unusually high or low.

SAMPLING DISTRIBUTIONS

Probability theory can be applied also to calculate the probability of obtaining specific samples from populations.

Consider a container with a very large number of identically sized marbles. Imagine that there are two kinds of marbles present, black (B) and white (W), and that these colours are present in equal proportions, so that $p(B) = p(W) = 0.5$.

Given the above population, say that samples of marbles are drawn randomly and with replacement. (By 'replacement' we mean the samples are put back into the population, in order to maintain as a constant the proportion of $B = W = 0.5$.) If we draw samples of four (that is, $n = 4$) then the possible proportions of black and white marbles in the samples can be deduced a priori as shown in Figure 17.3.

Ignoring the order in which marbles are chosen, Figure 17.3 demonstrates all the possible outcomes for the composition of samples of $n = 4$. It is logically possible to draw any of the samples shown in Figure 17.3. However, only one of the samples, (2B) is representative of the true population parameter. The other samples would generate incorrect inferences concerning the state of the population. In general, if we know or

Possible outcomes	Number black	Number white	Proportion black
● ● ● ●	4	0	1.00
● ● ● ○	3	1	0.75
● ● ○ ○	2	2	0.50
● ○ ○ ○	1	3	0.25
○ ○ ○ ○	0	4	0.00

Fig. 17.3 Characteristics of possible samples of $n = 4$, drawn from a population of black and white marbles.

assume (hypothesize) the true population parameters, we can generate distributions of the probability of obtaining samples of a given characteristic.

In this instance, when attempting to predict the probability of specific samples drawn from a population with two discrete elements, the binomial theorem can be applied. The expansion of the binomial expression, $(P + Q)^n$, generates the probability of all the possible samples which can be drawn from a given population. The general equation for expanding the binomial expression is:

$$(P + Q)^n = P^n + \frac{n}{1}P^{n-1}Q + \frac{n(n-1)}{2}P^{n-2}Q^2 + \ldots Q^n$$

P is the probability of the first outcome, Q is the probability of the second outcome and n is the number of trials (or the sample size).

In this instance, P = proportion black (B) = 0.5; Q = proportion white (W) = 0.5; n = 4 (sample size). Therefore, substituting into the binomial expression:

$$(B + W)^4 = B^4 + 4B^3W + 6B^2 W^2 + 4BW^3 + W^4$$

Note that each part of the expansion stands for a probability of obtaining a specific sample. For the present case:

Sample 1 $p(4B0W) = B^4$ = $(0.5)^4$ = 0.0625
Sample 2 $p(3B1W) = 4B^3W$ = $4 \times (0.5)^3(0.5)$ = 0.2500
Sample 3 $p(2B2W) = 6B^2W^2$ = $6 \times (0.5)^2(0.5)^2$ = 0.3750
Sample 4 $p(1B3W) = 4BW^3$ = $4 \times (0.5)^3(0.5)$ = 0.2500
Sample 5 $p(0B4W) = W^4$ = $(0.5)^4$ = 0.0625

The calculated probabilities add up to 1, indicating that all the possible sample outcomes have been accounted for. However, the important issue here is not so much the mathematical

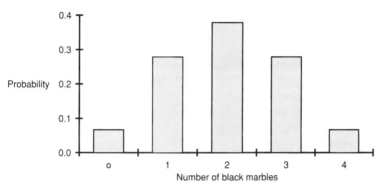

Fig. 17.4 Sampling distribution of black marbles; $n = 4$.

details, but the general principle being illustrated by the example. For a given sample size (n) we can employ a mathematical formula to calculate the probability of obtaining all the possible samples from a population with known parameters. The relationship between the possible samples and their probabilities can be graphed, as shown in Figure 17.4.

Taking the statistic 'number of black marbles in the sample' the graph in Figure 17.4 shows the probability of obtaining any of the outcomes. The distribution shown is called a 'sampling distribution'. In general, a **sampling distribution** for a statistic indicates the probability of obtaining any of the possible values of a statistic.

Therefore, having obtained our sampling distribution, we can see that some sample outcomes are quite improbable while others are highly likely. Although there is a finite chance of obtaining a sample such as 'all blacks', the probability of this happening is rather small ($p = 0.0625$). Conversely, a sample of 2B2W, which is equal to the true population proportions, is far more probable ($p = 0.375$). Generating sampling distributions for calculating the probability of given sample statistics is a basic practice in inferential statistics. The sampling distributions enable researchers to infer (with a determined level of confidence) the population parameters from the sample statistics.

SAMPLING DISTRIBUTION OF THE MEAN

The binomial theorem is appropriate for generating sampling distributions for discontinuous, nominal data. However, when measurements are continuous, the mean and standard deviations are appropriate as sample statistics and are measured on interval or ratio scales. The sampling distribution of the mean represents the frequency distribution of sample means obtained from random samples drawn from the population. The sampling distribution of the mean enables the calculation of the probability of obtaining any given sample mean ($\overline{X}$). This is essential for testing hypotheses about sample means (Chapter 18).

In order to generate the sampling distribution of the mean, we use a mathematical theorem called the *central limit theorem*. This theorem provides a set of rules which relate the parameters (μ, σ) of the population from which samples are drawn to the distribution of sample means ($\overline{X}$).

The central limit theorem states that if random samples of a fixed n are drawn from any population, as n becomes large the distribution of sample means approaches a normal distribution, with the mean of the sample means ($\overline{X}_{\overline{x}}$ or, $\mu_{\overline{x}}$) being equal to the population mean (μ) and the standard error of estimate ($s_{\overline{x}}$ or $\sigma_{\overline{x}}$) being equal to $\sigma/\sqrt{n}$. The standard error of the estimate is the standard deviation of the distribution of sample means.

Let us follow the above step by step.

1. Imagine we have a population of continuous scores or measurements with a mean of μ and a standard deviation of σ.

2. We select a very large number of random samples, each sample being of a size n.

3. Having obtained our samples, for each sample we calculate the sample mean ($\bar{X}_1, \bar{X}_2,$ … and so on).

4. Each sample mean, $\bar{X}$, is a number. The sampling distribution of the mean is a frequency distribution representing the large number of sample means.

5. The central limit theorem predicts theoretically the shape (normal for large n), mean $\bar{X}_{\bar{x}}$ or $\mu_{\bar{x}}$) and standard deviation ($s_{\bar{x}}$ or $\sigma_{\bar{x}}$) of a large number of sample means.

It should be noted that:

1. The sampling distribution of the mean is a frequency distribution of a large number of sample means of size n drawn from a given population. When n increases, the sampling distributions approach normal.

2. The mean of the sample means ($\mu_{\bar{x}}$ or $\bar{X}_{\bar{x}}$) is the mean of the distribution of sample means. $\bar{X}_{\bar{x}}$ and, $\mu_{\bar{x}}$ are equal to μ the population mean.

3. The standard error of the mean ($s_{\bar{x}}$ or $\sigma_{\bar{x}}$) is the standard deviation of the frequency distribution of sample means drawn from a population. The magnitude of $s_{\bar{x}}$ or $\sigma_{\bar{x}}$ is equal to $\sigma/\sqrt{n}$; the population standard deviation divided by the square root of the sample size.

4. $\mu_{\bar{x}}$ and $\sigma_{\bar{x}}$ are used in reference to a sampling distribution based on all the possible samples drawn from a population (a population of samples, would you believe?); while $\bar{X}$ and $s_{\bar{x}}$ are used when the sampling distribution is based on a 'sample' of samples.

Let us have a look at an example. Assume for a hypothetical test of motor function that $\mu = 50$ and $\sigma = 10$. What is the probability of drawing a random sample from this population with $\bar{X} = 52$ or greater (i.e. $\bar{X} \geq 52$) given that $n = 100$? The central limit theorem predicts that when we draw samples of $n = 100$ from the above population, the sampling distribution of the means will be as follows:

• The shape of the sampling distribution will be approximately normal.

• The mean of the sampling distribution will be equal to μ:

$$\mu_{\bar{x}} = \mu = 50$$

• The standard error of estimate ($\sigma_{\bar{x}}$) will be:

$$\sigma_{\bar{x}} = \frac{\sigma}{\sqrt{n}} = \frac{10}{\sqrt{100}} = 1$$

(We can show this as in Figure 17.5.)

Previously, we saw how we can use normal frequency distributions for estimating probabilities. Using the same principles as in Chapter 15, we can calculate the z score corresponding to $\bar{X} = 52$, and look up Appendix A to find out the area representing the probability in question:

$$z = \frac{\bar{X} - \mu_{\bar{x}}}{\sigma_{\bar{x}}} = \frac{52 - 50}{1} = 2$$

That is, $\bar{X} = 52$ is two standard error units above $\mu_{\bar{x}}$ the population mean for the sample means.

You may have noticed that the distribution of $\bar{X}$ is far less dispersed than X (i.e. the raw scores), as $\sigma_{\bar{x}} = 1$ and $\sigma = 10$.

Using Appendix A for establishing the probability, we find that the area representing $p(\bar{X} \geq 52)$, that is area A1 in Figure 17.5B, is:

$$p(\bar{X} \geq 52) = 0.5000 - 0.4772 = 0.0228$$

Therefore the probability of drawing a sample of $\bar{X} \geq 52$ is 0.0228). We will apply this notion to hypothesis testing in Chapter 18.

APPLICATION OF THE CENTRAL LIMIT THEOREM TO CALCULATING CONFIDENCE INTERVALS

Let us assume that you are asked to estimate the weight of a newborn baby. If you are experienced in working with neonates, you should be able to make a reasonable guess. You might say 'The baby is 6 kg'. Someone might ask 'How certain are you that the baby is exactly 6 kg?' You might then say 'Well, the baby might not be exactly 6 kg, but I'm very confident that it weighs somewhere between 5.5 and 6.5 kg'. This statement expresses a confidence interval—a range of values which probably include the true value. Of course, the

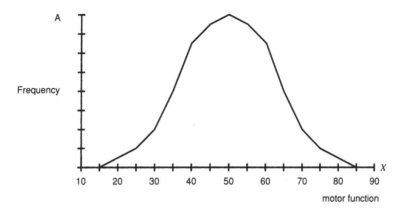

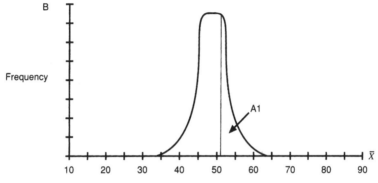

Fig. 17.5 Relationship between original population and sampling distribution of the mean, where $\mu = 50$ and $\sigma = 10$; (A) original population, (B) sampling distribution of the mean.

more certain or confident you want to be of including the true value, the bigger the range of values you might give: you are unlikely to be wrong if you guess that the baby weighs between 4 and 8 kg.

We have seen previously that if we know the population parameters we can estimate the probability of selecting from that population a sample mean of a given magnitude. Conversely, if we know the sample mean we can estimate the population parameters from which the sample might have come, at a given level of probability. Let us take an example to illustrate this point.

A researcher is interested in the systolic blood pressure (BP) levels of smokers of more than 10 cigarettes per day. They take a random sample of 100 10+ smokers in their district and find that the mean BP = 148 for the sample, with a standard deviation of $s = 10$.

They want to generalize to the population of smokers of more than 10 cigarettes/day in their district. The best estimate of μ (the population parameter) is 148, but it is possible that, because of sampling error, 148 is not the exact population parameter. However they can calculate a confidence interval (a range of blood pressures that will include the true population mean at a given level of probability).

A confidence interval is a range of scores which includes the true population parameter at a specified level of probability. The precise probability is decided by the researcher and indicates how certain they can be that the population mean is actually within the calculated range. Common confidence intervals used in statistics are 95% confidence intervals, which offer a probability of $p = 0.95$ for including true population mean, and 99% confidence intervals, which include the true population mean at a probability of $p = 0.99$.

Calculating the confidence interval requires the use of the following formula:

(lower confidence limit) $\bar{X} - zs_{\bar{x}} \leq \mu \leq \bar{X} + zs_{\bar{x}}$ (upper confidence limit)
where $\bar{X}$ is the sample mean; z is the z score obtained from the normal curve table, such that it cuts off the appropriate area of the normal curve corresponding to the required probability of the confidence interval; and $s_{\bar{x}}$ is the sample standard error, which is equal to s (the sample standard deviation) divided by rn, that is, $s_{\bar{x}} = s/\sqrt{n}$.

Let us turn to the previous example to illustrate the use of the above equation. Here $\bar{X} = 148$, and $s_{\bar{x}} = 10\sqrt{100}$. Assume that we want to calculate a 95% confidence interval. We are looking for a pair of z scores which have 95% of the standard normal curve between them. In this case, 1.96 is the value for z which cuts off 95% of a normal distribution. That is, we looked up the value of z corresponding to an area (probability) of 0.4750, since the 0.05 has to be divided among the two *tails* of the distribution, given 0.025 at either end. Substituting into the equation above we have:

$$148 = (1.96)\,(10/\sqrt{100}) \leq \mu \leq 148 + (1.96)\,(10/\sqrt{100})$$
$$= 146.04 \leq \mu \leq 149.96$$

That is, the investigator is 95% confident that the true population mean, the true mean BP of smokers, lies between 146.04 and 149.96. There is only a 5% or 0.05 probability that it lies outside this range.

If we chose a 99% confidence interval, then using the formula as above, we have:

$$148 - (2.58)\,(10/\sqrt{100}) \leq \mu \leq 148 + (2.58)\,(10/\sqrt{100})$$
$$= 145.42 \leq \mu \leq 150.58$$

Here, the 2.58 is the value of z which cuts off 99% of a normal distribution (Fig. 17.6). That is, the investigator is 99% confident that the true population mean lies somewhere between 145.42 and 150.58. Clearly, the 99% interval is wider than the 95% interval; after all, here the probability of including the true mean is greater than for the 95% interval.

CONFIDENCE INTERVALS WHERE *n* IS SMALL: THE *t* DISTRIBUTION

It was previously stated that: 'as n becomes large, the distribution of sample means approaches a normal distribution' (central limit theorem). The questions left to explain are:

- How large must be the sample size, n, before the sampling distribution of the mean can be considered a normal curve?
- What are the implications for the sampling distribution if n is small?

It has been shown by mathematicians that the sample size, n, for which the sampling distribution of the mean can be considered an approximation of a normal distribution is $n \geq 30$. That is, if n is 30 or more, we can use the standard normal curve (Appendix A) to describe the sampling

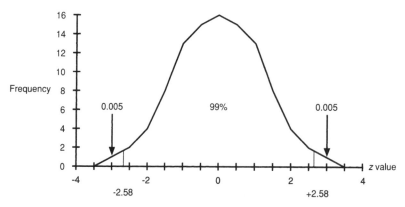

Fig. 17.6 *z* scores for 99% confidence interval.

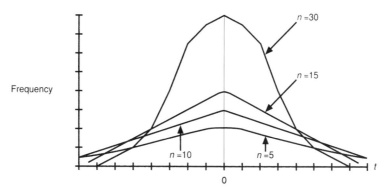

Fig. 17.7 *t* distributions.

distribution of the mean. However when $n < 30$, the sampling distribution of the mean is a rather rough approximation to the normal distribution. Instead of using the normal distribution, we use the **t distribution**, which takes into account the variability of the shape of the sampling distribution due to low n.

The *t* distributions (Fig. 17.7) are a family of curves, representing the sampling distributions of means drawn from a population when sample size, n, is small ($n < 30$). A 'family of curves' means that the shape of *t* distribution varies with sample size. It has been found that the distribution is determined by the **degrees of freedom** of the statistic.

The degrees of freedom (df) for a statistic represents the number of scores which are free to vary when calculating the statistic. Since the statistic we are calculating in this case is the mean, all but one of the scores could vary. That is, if you were inventing scores in a sample with a known mean, you would have a free hand until the very last score. For the *t* distribution, df is equal to $n - 1$ (the sample size, minus one). Each *row* of figures shown in Appendix B represents the critical values of *t* for a given distribution.

1. The *t* distribution is symmetrical about the mean.
2. The values of *t* along the *x* axis cut off specific areas under the curve, just as for *z*. These areas are given at the top of the page, under 'Directional' and 'Non-directional' probabilities.

3. The *t* distribution approaches a normal distribution as *n* becomes larger. As stated earlier, when $n \geq 30$, for all practical purposes the *t* and *z* distributions coincide.

The *t* distribution, just as the *z* distribution, can be used to approximate the probability of drawing sample means of a given magnitude from a population; *t* can also be used for calculating confidence intervals. Let us re-examine the example presented on page 215. Let us assume that $n = 25$, with the other statistics remaining the same: $\bar{X} = 148$ $s = 10$. The general formula for calculating the confidence intervals for small samples is:

$$\bar{X} - ts_{\bar{x}} \leq \mu \leq \bar{X} + ts_{\bar{x}}$$

You will note the similarity to the equation on page 216; here *t* replaces *z*. If we want to show the 95% confidence interval, then we use the same logic as for *z* distributions (Fig. 17.8).

To look up the *t* values from the tables (Appendix B) consider (i) direction, (ii) probabilities and (iii) degrees of freedom.

We are looking at a 'non-directional' or 'two-tail' probability in the sense that the *t* values cut off 95% of the area of the *t* curve between them, leaving 5% distributed at the two tails of the *t* distribution: $p = 0.05$ (see Fig. 17.8); df = 25 − 1 = 24. Therefore $t = 2.064$ (from tables in Appendix B). Substituting into the equation for calculating confidence intervals:

$$148 - (2.1)(10/\sqrt{25}) \leq \mu \leq 148 + (2.1)(10/\sqrt{25})$$
(Note $s_{\bar{X}} = s\sqrt{n}$)

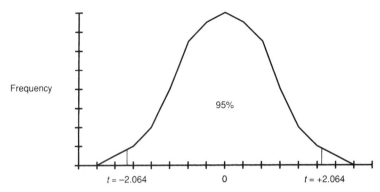

Fig. 17.8   The 95% confidence interval for sample size of 25.

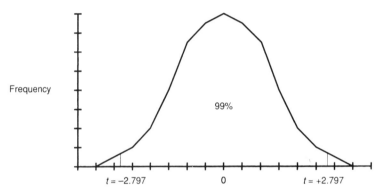

Fig. 17.9   The 99% confidence interval for sample size of 25.

$148 - 4.2 \le \mu \le 148 + 4.2$
$143.8 \le \mu \le 152.2$

Note that this is a wider interval than that which was obtained when n was 100. As sample size, n, becomes smaller, our confidence interval becomes wider, reflecting a greater probability of sampling error.

To calculate the 99% confidence interval (Fig. 17.9), we need to look up $p = 0.01$, non-directional, df = 24; in Appendix B to obtain the critical value of t, which is 2.797.

$148 - (2.8)(10/\sqrt{25}) \le \mu \le 148 + (2.8)(10\sqrt{25})$
$142.4 \le \mu \le 153.6$

As for the 95% confidence interval, and for the same reasons, we can see that when $n = 25$, the 99% confidence interval was wider than for $n = 100$. That is, the bigger our sample size, the narrower (more precise) becomes our estimate

of the range of values which includes the true population parameter.

SUMMARY

It was argued in this chapter that even with randomly selected samples, the possibility of sampling error must be taken into account when making inferences from sample statistics to population parameters. It was shown that probability theory can be applied to generating sampling distributions, which express the probability of obtaining a given sample from a population. With discontinuous, nominal data, the binomial theorem provides an adequate mathematical distribution for estimating the probability for obtaining possible samples. However, with continuous data, the central limit theorem is applied to generate the sampling distributions of the mean. The standard distribution of the mean enables the calculation of the probability-specified sample mean(s) by random selection. The sampling error of the mean ($s_{\bar{x}}$ or $\sigma_{\bar{x}}$), which expresses statistically the range of the sampling error, depends inversely on the sample size, such that the larger n the smaller $s_{\bar{x}}$ or $\sigma_{\bar{x}}$.

One of the applications of sampling distributions is for calculating confidence intervals for continuous data. Confidence intervals represent a range of scores which specify, from sample data, the probability of capturing the true population parameters. When sample sizes are small ($n < 30$), the t distribution is appropriate for representing the sampling distribution of the mean. With large sample sizes, the two distributions merge together. As the next chapter will demonstrate, sampling distributions are essential for testing hypotheses, a procedure which uses inferential statistics to calculate the level of probability at which sample statistics support the predictions of hypotheses.

SELF ASSESSMENT

Explain the meaning of the following terms:

> confidence interval
> sampling distribution
> sampling distribution of the mean
> standard error of the mean
> degrees of freedom
> sampling error
> population parameter
> probability
> t distribution
> central limit theorem

TRUE OR FALSE

1. If death and taxes are an absolute certainty, then the probability of their occurrence is infinite.
2. Probability values fall between 0 and 1.
3. When a score occurs at a relatively high level of frequency the probability of randomly selecting it from a distribution is $p = 1$.
4. The higher the corresponding z score, the lower the probability of randomly selecting the score from a distribution.
5. For a normal distribution, σ is the score which has the highest probability of random selection.
6. It is possible to have a negative z scores but not a negative probability.

7. For a continuous normal distribution, the probability of selecting a score up to and including the mode is $p = 0.5$.
8. The probability of randomly selecting a score 2 standard deviations above the mean is $p = 0.2$.
9. We can generate appropriate sampling distributions for statistics derived from nominal or ordinal data.
10. Statistical inference involves the estimation of population parameters from sample statistics.
11. Statistical inference depends on knowing the true population parameters before beginning research.
12. The sampling distribution of the mean is a frequency polygon of mean scores.
13. Using the sample mean as an estimate for the population mean is an example of statistical inference.
14. The sampling distribution of the mean is always normally distributed.
15. As n increases, the variability of the sampling distribution of the mean increases.
16. $\mu_{\bar{x}} = \mu$ regardless of the shape of the sampling distribution of the mean.
17. The characteristics of the sampling distribution of the mean vary with the size of the sample.

SELF ASSESSMENT

18. If a random selection method is used, sampling error will be zero.
19. The bigger the sampling error the smaller the confidence interval.
20. Generally speaking, the higher level of confidence we have that an interval contains the population mean, the larger is that interval.

MULTIPLE CHOICE

1. The mean age of the Canadian population is known to be 31 years. A small randomly selected sample of Canadians is found to have a mean age of 32. This discrepancy is an example of:

   a a sampling error
   b a measurement error
   c a problem in ecological validity
   d failure to control for the effects of maturation.

At a large maternity hospital the following hypothetical data are compiled concerning the birth weights and survival of neonates.

Weight of neonates (g)	Numbers (n)	Percentage of neonates surviving
0–499	25	40
500–999	50	60
1000–1499	75	80
1500–1999	150	90
2000–2499	250	95
2500 +	450	98

Questions 2–5 refer to this table.

2. What is the probability that a randomly selected neonate will weigh under 500 g?

   a 0.4000
   b 0.1700
   c 0.0250
   d 0.0025

3. What is the probability that a randomly selected neonate will have a birth weight of 2000 g or over?

   a 0.7000
   b 0.9638
   c 0.3000
   d 0.9500

4. What is the probability that a neonate weighing 499 g or under will survive?

   a 0.4000
   b 0.1700
   c 0.040
   d 0.025

5. What is the probability that a neonate weighing 2500 g or over will not survive?

   a 0.400
   b 0.300
   c 0.006
   d 0.020

A test of reaction times has a mean of 10 and a standard deviation of 4 in the normal adult population with a normal distribution. Questions 6–12 refer to this information.

6. A person scores 8. That person's z score is:

   a 2
   b −2
   c −0.5
   d −1

7. What percentage of the population would have scores up to and including 14 on this test?

   a 84.13
   b 15.87
   c 65.87
   d 34.13

8. What is the percentile rank of a score of 8 on this test?

   a 19.15

b 30.85
c 80.85
d 53.28

9. What score (to the nearest whole number) would cut off the highest 10% of scores?

a 1
b 14
c 15
d 18

10. What is the probability that a randomly selected individual will score greater than 6 on this test?

a 0.4987
b 0.3413
c 0.8413
d 0.6587

11. What is the probability that a randomly selected individual will score between 8 and 14 on this test?

a 0.1498
b 0.5328
c 0.6816
d 0.4671

12. What is the probability that a randomly selected individual will score either more than 14 or less than 10 on this test?

a 0.6587
b 0.6816
c 0.3184
d 0.8184

13. Sampling error of the mean:

a occurs because of poor sampling techniques
b decreases as sample size increases
c is independent of the standard deviation
d is always equal to 1.

14. Samples of 100 are drawn from a normally distributed population with a mean of 50 and a standard deviation of 10. The distribution of sample means will:

a have a mean of 50
b have a standard deviation of 1
c be normally distributed
d all of the above.

15. Increasing the sample size, in 'n':

a decreases sampling error
b increases sampling error
c has no effect on standard error of the mean
d requires increasing correction of sample estimates of population parameters
e none of these.

16. If the dispersion of the raw score population increases while n is held constant $\sigma_{\bar{x}}$:

a decreases
b increases
c remains the same
d need more information.

17. The sampling distribution of the mean:

a is always positively skewed for continuous data
b is normally distributed if the population raw scores are not normally distributed
c is approximately normally distributed if sample size is large
d all of the above.

18. As the degrees of freedom decrease, the similarity between the t and z distributions:

a increases
b decreases
c remains the same
d approaches infinity.

SELF ASSESSMENT

19. The theoretical sampling distributions of the *t* statistics depend on:

    a p
    b r
    c $s_{\bar{x}}$
    d df.

A normally distributed population has a mean of 80 and a standard deviation of 12. Questions 20–24 refer to this information.

20. For samples of $n = 36$, what is the standard error of the mean?

    a 12
    b 0.33
    c 2
    d 3

21. A sample of 64 cases is found to have a mean of 83. What is the *z* score of this mean?

    a 2
    b 0.25
    c 4
    d 1.5

22. A sample of $n = 144$ has a mean of 77. What is the probability that a mean this low would occur by chance?

    a 0.0300
    b 0.0013
    c 0.4989
    d 0.9987

23. A sample of 36 cases is selected. What is the probability that its mean falls outside the range of 79–81?

    a 0.6813
    b 0.8085
    c 0.3085
    d 0.6170

24. Which is more likely, that a randomly selected sample of $n = 36$ will have a mean greater than 82 or that it will have a mean less than 77?

    a Greater than 82
    b Less than 77
    c Both are equally probable
    d Impossible to tell.

25. The *t* distribution differs from the *z* distribution in which of these ways?

    a Its mean is not exactly equal to 0.
    b It is not quite symmetrical.
    c It is somewhat wider and flatter.
    d All of the above.

26. The 95% confidence interval arrived at from a particular experiment is 72–79. Therefore:

    a the probability is 0.05 that μ falls between 72–79
    b the probability is 0.95 that the interval 72–79 contains $\bar{X}$
    c the probability is 0.95 that the interval 72–79 contains μ
    d *a* and *c*.

27. Compared with a 99% confidence interval, a 95% confidence interval is:

    a larger
    b smaller
    c more likely to contain the population mean
    d less likely to contain the sample mean.

The following information should be used in answering questions 28–31: a random sample of 25 clients is selected, and their systolic blood pressures measured; the mean BP is 115 mmHg, with a standard deviation of 10.

28. This is an example of:

    a an experiment
    b a natural comparison study
    c a survey
    d field research.

29. What is the standard error of the mean for a sample of this size?

    a 10
    b 20
    c 2
    d 2.5

30. In order to calculate the 99% confidence interval of the mean, what t score will be used?

    a 2.492
    b 2.787
    c 2.797
    d 1.711

31. What is the 99% confidence interval of the mean in this example?

    a $110.0 \leq \mu \leq 120.0$
    b $109.4 \leq \mu \leq 120.6$
    c $111.6 \leq \mu \leq 118.4$
    d $113.0 \leq \mu \leq 117.0$

32. A random sample of 25 university students is found to have a mean IQ of 110, with a standard deviation of 10. Between what two possible scores can we be 99% confident that the true mean IQ for the students at the university lies?

    a 95.5–112.5
    b 85–135

    c 102.4–117.6
    d 104.1–115.9

In order to establish the mean weight of newborn babies at a large maternity hospital, a random sample of 64 babies is weighed. Their mean weight is 2500 g, with a standard deviation of 80 g.

Questions 33–35 require the information above.

33. What is the standard error of the mean?

    a 80
    b 10
    c 1.25
    d 0.1

34. In calculating the 95% confidence interval of the mean, what z value is used?

    a 1.96
    b 2.33
    c 2.58
    d 1.64

35. What is the 95% confidence interval of the mean in this example (to the nearest whole number)?

    a $2480 \leq \mu \leq 2520$
    b $2477 \leq \mu \leq 2523$
    c $2474 \leq \mu \leq 2526$
    d $2484 \leq \mu \leq 2516$

INTRODUCTION

In the previous chapter we introduced the use of inferential statistics for estimating population parameters from sample statistics. In the case of some non-experimental research projects such as descriptive surveys (see Section 3), parameter estimation is adequate for analyzing the data. After all, these investigations aim at describing the characteristics of specific populations. However, other research strategies involve data collection for the purpose of testing hypotheses such as whether two therapeutic techniques have different effectiveness. Here, the investigator has to establish if the data support or refute the hypotheses being investigated. The key issue here is that hypotheses are generalizations concerning differences in patterns and associations in *populations*. Inferential statistics enables us to calculate the probability (level of significance) for asserting that what we are seeing in our sample data is generalizable to the population.

The aim of this chapter is to introduce the logical steps involved in hypothesis testing in quantitative research. Given that hypothesis testing is probabilistic, special attention must be paid to the possibility of making erroneous decisions, and to the implications of making such errors.

The specific aims of the chapter are to:

1. Examine the logic of hypotheses testing for retaining or rejecting null hypotheses.
2. Outline how decisions are made with directional and non-directional alternative hypotheses.

3. Introduce the use of the single sample z and t test for analyzing the statistical significance of the data.
4. Outline the probability and implications of making Type 1 and Type II decision errors.

A SIMPLE ILLUSTRATION OF HYPOTHESIS TESTING

One of the simplest forms of gambling is betting on the fall of a coin. Let us play a little game. We, the authors, will toss a coin. If it comes out heads (H) you will give us £1; if tails (T) we will give you £1. To make things interesting, let us have 10 tosses. The results are:

Toss	1	2	3	4	5	6	7	8	9	10
Outcome	H	H	H	H	H	H	H	H	H	H

Oh dear, you seem to have lost. Never mind, we were just lucky, so send along your cheque for £10. What is that, you are a little hesitant? Are you saying that we 'fixed' the game? There is a systematic procedure for demonstrating the probable truth of your allegations:

1. We can state two competing hypotheses concerning the outcome of the game:
   (a) The authors fixed the game; that is, the outcome does not reflect the fair throwing of a coin. Let us call this statement the 'alternative hypotheses', H_A. In effect, the H_A claims that the sample of 10 heads came from a population other than P (probability of heads) = Q (probability of tails) = 0.5;
   (b) The authors did not fix the game; that is, the outcome is due to the tossing of a fair coin. Let us call this statement the 'null hypothesis', or H_0. H_0 suggests that the sample of 10 heads was a random sample from a population where $P = Q = 0.5$.
2. It can be shown that the probability of tossing 10 consecutive heads with a fair coin is $p = 0.001$, as discussed previously (see Ch. 15). That is, the probability of obtaining such a sample from a population where $P = Q = 0.5$ is extremely low.

3. Now we can decide between H_0 and H_A. It was shown that the probability of H_0 being true was $p = 0.001$ (1 in a 1000). Therefore, in the balance of probabilities, we can reject it as being true and accept H_A, which is the logical alternative. In other words, it is likely that the game was fixed and no £10 cheque needs to be posted.

The probability of calculating the truth of H_0 depended on the number of tosses (n = the sample size). For instance, the probabilities of obtaining all heads with up to five tosses, according to the binomial theorem (Ch. 17) are shown in Table 18.1. The table shows that as the sample size (n) becomes larger, the probability at which it is possible to reject H_0 becomes smaller. With only a few tosses we really cannot be sure if the game is fixed or not: without sufficient information it becomes hard to reject H_0 at a reasonable level of probability.

A question emerges: 'What is a reasonable level of probability for rejecting H_0?' As we shall see, there are conventions for specifying these probabilities. One way to proceed, however, is to set the appropriate probability for rejecting H_0 on the basis of the implications of erroneous decisions.

Obviously, any decision made on a probabilistic basis might be erroneous. Two types of elementary decision errors are identified in statistics as *Type I* and *Type II* errors. Type I error involves mistakenly rejecting H_0, while Type II error involves mistakenly retaining H_0.

In the above example, Type I error would involve deciding that the outcome was not due to chance, when in fact it was. The practical outcome of this would be to falsely accuse the authors of fixing the game. A Type II error would

Table 18.1 Probability of obtaining all heads in coin tosses

n (number of tosses)	p (all heads)
1	0.5000
2	0.2500
3	0.1250
4	0.0625
5	0.0313

represent the decision that the outcome was due to chance, when in fact it was due to a 'fix'. The practical outcome of this would be to send your hard-earned £10 to a couple of crooks. Clearly, in a situation like this, a Type II error would be more odious than a Type I error, and you would set a fairly high probability for rejecting H_0. However, if you were gambling with a villain, who had a loaded revolver handy, you would tend to set a very low probability for rejecting H_0. We will examine these ideas more formally in subsequent parts of this chapter.

THE LOGIC OF HYPOTHESIS TESTING

Hypothesis testing is the process of deciding statistically whether the findings of an investigation reflect chance or real effects at a given level of probability.

The mathematical procedures for hypothesis testing are based on the application of probability theory and sampling, as discussed previously. Because of the probabilistic nature of the process, decision errors in hypothesis testing cannot be entirely eliminated. However, the procedures outlined in this section enable us to specify the probability level at which we can claim that the data obtained in an investigation support experimental hypotheses. This procedure is fundamental for analyzing data, as well as being relevant to the logic of clinical decision making.

STEPS IN HYPOTHESIS TESTING

The following steps are conventionally followed in hypothesis testing:

1. State the *alternative hypothesis* (H_A), which is the prediction intended for evaluation. The H_A claims that the results are 'real' or 'significant': i.e. that the independent variable influenced the dependent variable, or that there is a real difference among groups.
2. State the *null hypothesis* (H_0), which is the logical opposite of the H_A. The H_0 claims that any differences in the data were just due to chance: that the independent variable had no

effect on the dependent variable, or that any difference among groups is due to random effects.
3. Set *decision level*, α (*alpha*). There are two mutually exclusive hypotheses (H_A and H_0) competing to explain the results of an investigation. Hypothesis testing, or statistical decision making, involves establishing the probability of H_0 being true. If this probability is very small, we are in a position to reject the H_0. You might ask 'how small should be the probability (α) for rejecting H_0?' By convention, we use the probability of $\alpha = 0.05$. That is, if the H_0 being true is less than 0.05 we can reject H_0. We can choose an α of < 0.05, but not more, That is, by convention among researchers results are *not significant* if $p > 0.05$.
4. Calculate the probability of H_0 being true. That is, we assume that H_0 is true and calculate the probability of the outcome of the investigation being due to chance alone, that is, due to random effects. We must use an appropriate sampling distribution for this calculation.
5. Make decision concerning H_0. The following *decision rule* is used. If the probability of H_0 being true is less than α, then we reject H_0, at the level of significance set by α. However, if the probability of H_0 is greater than α, then we must retain H_0. In other words, if:

$$p \, (H_0 \text{ is true}) \leq \alpha; \text{ reject } H_0$$
$$p \, (H_0 \text{ is true}) > \alpha; \text{ retain } H_0$$

It follows that if we reject H_0, we are in a position to accept H_A, its logical alternative. If we reject H_0, we conclude that the H_A is probably true.

Let us look at an example. A rehabilitation therapist devises an exercise programme which is expected to reduce the time taken for people to leave hospital following orthopaedic surgery. Previous records show that the recovery time for patients has been $\mu = 30$ days, with $\sigma = 8$ days. A sample of 64 patients are treated with the exercise programme, and their mean recovery time is found to be $\overline{X} = 24$ days. Do these results show that patients who had the treatment recovered significantly faster than previous patients? We can apply the steps for hypothesis testing to make our decision.

1. State H_A: 'The exercise programme reduces the time taken for patients to recover from orthopaedic surgery'. That is, the researcher claims that the independent variable (the treatment) had a 'real' or 'generalizable' effect on the dependent variable (time to recover).
2. State H_0: 'The exercise programme does not reduce the time taken for patients to recover from orthopaedic surgery'. That is, the statement claims that the independent variable had no effect on the dependent variable. The statement implies that the treated sample with $\bar{X} = 24$, and $n = 64$ is in fact a random sample from the population $\mu = 30$; $\sigma = 8$. Any difference between $\bar{X}$ and μ can be attributed to sampling error.
3. Decision level, α, is set before the results are analyzed. The probability of α depends on how certain the investigator wants to be that the results show real differences. If they set $\alpha = 0.01$, then the probability of falsely rejecting a true H_0 is less than or equal to 0.01 (1/100). If they set $\alpha = 0.05$, then the probability of falsely rejecting a true H_0 is less than or equal to 0.05 or (1/20). That is, the smaller α, the more confident the researcher is that the results support the alternative hypothesis. We

also call α the level of *significance*. The smaller α, the more significant the findings for a study, if we can reject H_0. In this case, say that the researcher sets $\alpha = 0.01$. (Note: by convention, α *should not* be greater than 0.05.)

4. Calculate the probability of H_0 being true. As stated above, the H_0 implies that the sample with $\bar{X} = 24$ is a random sample from the population with $\mu = 30$, $\sigma = 8$. How probable is it that this statement is true? To calculate this probability, we must generate an appropriate sampling distribution. As we have seen in Chapter 17, the sampling distribution of the mean will enable us to calculate the probability of obtaining a sample mean of $\bar{X} = 24$ or more extreme from a population with known parameters. As shown in Figure 18.1, we can calculate the probability of drawing a sample mean of $\bar{X} = 24$ or less. Using the table of normal curves (Appendix A) as outlined previously, we find that the probability of randomly selecting a sample mean of $\bar{X} = 24$ (or less) is extremely small. In terms of our table, which only shows the exact probability of up to $z = 4.00$, we can see that the present probability is less than 0.00003. Therefore, the probability that H_0 is true is less than 0.00003.
5. Make a decision. We have set $\alpha = 0.01$. The calculated probability was less than 0.0001. Clearly, the calculated probability is far less than α. Therefore, the investigator can reject

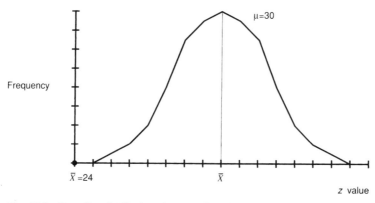

Fig. 18.1 Sampling distribution of means. Sample size = 64; population mean = 30; standard deviation = 8.

the statement that H_0 is true and accept H_A, that patients treated with the exercise programme recover earlier than the population of untreated patients.

DIRECTIONAL AND NON-DIRECTIONAL HYPOTHESES AND CORRESPONDING CRITICAL VALUES OF STATISTICS

In the previous example, H_A was *directional*, in that we asserted that the difference between the mean of the treated sample and the population mean was expected to be in a particular direction. If we state that there was some effect due to the dependent variable, but do not specify which way, then H_A is called *non-directional*. In the previous example, if the investigator stated the H_A as 'The exercise programme *changes* the time taken to recover following surgery' then H_A would have been non-directional.

In general, an alternative hypothesis is directional if it predicts a specific outcome concerning the direction of the findings by stating that one group mean will be higher or lower than the other(s). An alternative hypothesis is non-directional if it predicts a difference, without specifying which group mean is expected to be higher or lower than the others.

If we propose a directional H_A, it is understood that we have reasonable information on the basis of pilot studies or previously published research for predicting the direction of the outcome. The advantage of a directional H_A is that it increases the probability of rejecting H_0. However, the decision of the directionality of H_A must be decided *before* the data are collected and analyzed.

Let us now examine the concept of the 'critical' value of a statistic. The critical value of a statistic is the value of the statistic which bounds the proportion of the sampling distribution specified by α. The critical value of the statistic is influenced by whether H_A is directional or non-directional.

Figures 18.2 and 18.3 represent the sampling distributions of the mean where n is large; that is, the sampling distribution for the statistic $\bar{X}$.

As we have seen in Chapter 17, these are the sampling distributions for $\bar{X}$ we would expect by the random selection of samples, as specified by H_0. Therefore, we can estimate from the distributions the probability of selecting any sample mean, $\bar{X}$, by chance alone (Ch. 17). The α value (the level of significance) specifies the criterion for rejecting H_0. We can see that the critical value for the statistic (in this case z_{crit}) cuts off an area of the distribution corresponding to α ($p = 0.05$ or $p = 0.01$).

In Figure 18.2, we can see that $z_{crit} = 1.65$ (for $\alpha = 0.05$) and $z_{crit} = 2.33$ (for $\alpha = 0.01$). (These values are obtained from Appendix A.) Therefore, for any sample mean, $\bar{X}$, where the transformed (z) value is greater than or equal to z_{crit}, we will reject H_0 (that the sample mean was a random sample). However, if the absolute value of the transformed statistic is less than z_{crit}, then we must retain H_0. Note that when $\alpha = 0.01$, the z_{crit} is greater than when $\alpha = 0.05$. Clearly, the higher the level of significance set for rejecting H_0, the greater the absolute critical value of the statistic. Figure 18.2 shows statistical decision making with a directional H_A, where the probabilities associated with only one of the tails of the distribution are used.

Figure 18.3 shows the critical values for z with a non-directional H_A. Here, the probabilities associated α (0.05 or 0.01) are divided between the two tails of the distribution. That is, where $\alpha = 0.05$, half (0.025) goes into each tail and where $\alpha = 0.01$, half (0.005) also goes into each tail. This changes the values of z_{crit}, which becomes ± 1.96 or ± 2.58, respectively, as shown in Figure 18.3. Here, we reject H_0 if the calculated transformed z value of $\bar{X}$ falls beyond the values of z_{crit}. When we compare the values of z_{crit} for the one-tail and two-tailed decisions, we find that the critical values are greater for the two-tail decisions. This implies that it is more difficult to reject H_0 if we are making two-tail decisions on the basis of a non-directional H_A.

Decision rules

In general, Figures 18.2 and 18.3 illustrate the decision rules for statistical decision making for

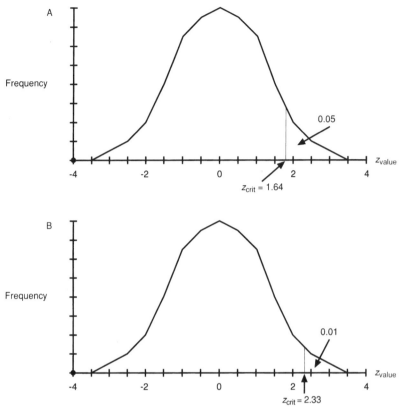

Fig. 18.2 Two examples of statistical decision-making with directional (one tail) hypothesis, H_A.

hypotheses concerning sample means. These rules are:

$$|z_{obt}| \geq |z_{crit}|; \text{reject } H_0$$
$$|z_{obt}| < |z_{crit}|; \text{retain } H_0$$

The same decision rules hold for the t distributions associated with the sampling distribution of the mean when n (the sample size) is small (see Ch. 16).

$$|t_{obt}| \geq |t_{crit}|; \text{reject } H_0$$
$$|t_{obt}| < |t_{crit}|; \text{retain } H_0$$

z_{obt} and t_{obt} refer to the calculated value of the statistic, based on the data:

$$z_{obt} = \frac{\bar{X} - \mu}{S_{\bar{x}}}$$

$$t_{obt} = \frac{\bar{X} - \mu}{S_{\bar{x}}}$$

z_{crit} and t_{crit} are the critical values of the statistic obtained from the tables in Appendices A and B. As we have seen, the values of these depend on α and the directionality of H_A. $|\ |$ is the symbol for modulus, implying that we should look at the absolute value of a statistic. Of course, the sign is important when considering if $\bar{X}$ was greater or smaller than μ. However we can ignore the sign (+ or −) when making statistical decisions. In effect, the greater z_{obt} or t_{obt}, the more deviant or improbable the particular sample mean, $\bar{X}$, is under the sampling distribution specified by H_0.

STATISTICAL DECISIONS WITH SINGLE SAMPLE MEANS

The following examples illustrate the use of statistical decision making concerning a single

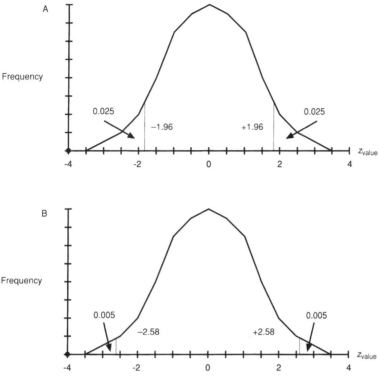

Fig. 18.3 Two examples of statistical decision-making with non-directional (two tail) hypothesis, H_A.

sample mean, $\bar{X}$. Such decisions are relevant when our data consists of a single sample and we are to decide if the $\bar{X}$ of the sample is significantly different to a given population, with a mean of μ.

A *statistical test* is a procedure appropriate for making decisions concerning the significance of the data. The z test and the t test are procedures appropriate for making decisions concerning the probability that sample means reflect population differences. (As shown in Chapter 19, there is a variety of statistical tests available for hypothesis testing.)

Example 1

A researcher hypothesizes that males now weigh more than in previous years. To investigate this hypothesis they randomly select 100 adult males and record their weights. The measurements for the sample have a mean of $\bar{X} = 70$ kg. In a census taken several years ago, the mean weight of males was $\mu = 68$ kg, with a standard deviation of 8 kg.

1. Directional H_A: males are heavier. That is, $\bar{X} = 70$ is not a random sample from population $\mu = 68$.
2. H_0: males are not heavier. That is, $\bar{X} = 70$ is a random sample from population with $\mu = 68$.
3. Decision level: $\alpha = 0.01$
4. Calculate probability of H_0 being true. Here, $\alpha = 0.01$, one-tail. We can find from the tables (Appendix A) z_{crit}, the z score which cuts off an area of 0.01 of the total curve. $z_{crit} = +2.33$ ($\alpha = 0.01$; one-tail)

Calculating the z score (z_{obt}) representing the probability of the sample being drawn from the population under H_0 ($\mu = 68$) we use the formula:

$$z_{obt} = \frac{\bar{X} - \mu}{S_{\bar{x}}}$$

$$\text{where } S_{\bar{x}} = \frac{S}{\sqrt{n}}$$

$$z_{obt} = \frac{70 - 68}{8 / \sqrt{100}}$$

$$= 2.5$$

Here, $z_{crit} = 2.33$

5. The decision rule is that if:

$$|z_{obt}| \geq |z_{crit}|; \text{ reject } H_0$$
$$|z_{obt}| < |z_{crit}|; \text{ retain } H_0$$

$2.5 > 2.33$, so the z_{obt} falls into the area of rejection, as shown in Figure 18.4. Therefore, the researcher can reject H_0, and accept H_A at a 0.01 level of significance. That is, the results of the investigation indicated that the mean weight of males has increased (consistently with the predictions of the research hypothesis).

Example 2

A researcher hypothesized that men today have different weights (either more or less) than in previous years (assume the same information as for Example 1).

1. Non-directional H_A: males are of different weight, that is, $\bar{X} = 70$ is not a random sample from population $\mu = 68$.
2. H_0: males are not different, that is $\bar{X}$ is a random sample from $\mu = 68$.
3. Decision level: $\alpha = 0.01$
4. Calculate the probability of H_0 being true. Here, $\alpha = 0.01$ (two-tail).
   The value of $z_{crit}| = 2.58$ (from Appendix A)
   The value of $|z_{obt}| = 2.5$ (as calculated in Example 1).

5. Decision: applying the decision rule as outlined in Example 1
   $|z_{obt}| < |z_{crit}|$; as $2.5 < 2.58$

z_{obt} falls into the area of acceptance, as shown in Figure 18.5. Therefore, the researcher must retain the H_0, and conclude that the study did not support H_A at a 0.01 level of significance. Therefore, the investigation has not provided evidence that the mean weight of males has increased.

Example 3

The previous two examples involved sample sizes of $n > 30$. However, as we saw in Chapter 17 if $n < 30$, the distribution of sample means is not a normal, but a t distribution. This point must be taken into account when we calculate the probability of H_0 being true. That is, for small samples, we use the t test to evaluate the significance of our data.

Assume exactly the same information as in Example 1, except that sample size is $n = 16$.

1. Directional H_A: as in Example 1.
2. H_0: as in Example 1.
3. $\alpha = 0.01$, one-tail.
4. We can find from the t table (Appendix B) the value for t_{crit}. To look up t_{crit} we must have the following information:
   (a) α, the level of significance (0.05 or 0.01);
   (b) direction of H_A (directional or non-directional);
   (c) the degrees of freedom, (df).

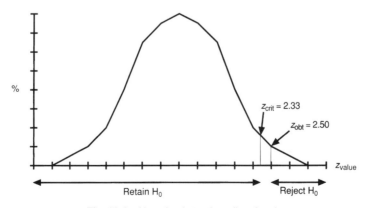

Fig. 18.4 Hypothesis testing: directional.

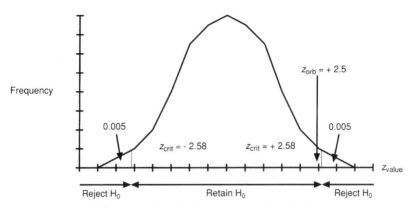

Fig. 18.5   Hypothesis testing: non-directional.

In this instance:

(a) $\alpha = 0.01$;

(b) H_A is directional, therefore we must look up a one-tail probability;

(c) $df = n - 1 = 16 - 1 = 15$

Looking up the appropriate value for t; $t_{crit} = 2.602$. Calculating the t score (t_{obt}) representing the probability of the sample being drawn from the population under H_0, we use the formula:

$$t_{obt} = \frac{\overline{X} - \mu}{S_{\overline{x}}}$$
$$= \frac{70 - 68}{8/\sqrt{16}}$$
$$= 1.0$$

5. As we stated earlier, the decision rule is identical to that of the z test:

$$|t_{obt}| \geq |t_{crit}|\ ;\ \text{reject}\ H_0$$
$$|t_{obt}| < |t_{crit}|\ ;\ \text{retain}\ H_0$$

Here, $1.0 < 2.602$, such that t_{obt} falls into the area of retention. Therefore, we must retain H_0 at a 0.01 level of significance. Clearly, when $n = 16$, the investigation did not show a significant weight increase for the males.

Summary

The above examples demonstrate the following points about statistical decision making:

- We are more likely to reject H_0 if we use a one-tail test (directional H_A) than a two-tail test (non-directional H_A). In effect, we are using the prediction of which way the differences will go to increase the probability of rejecting H_0, and therefore accepting H_A. Examples 1 and 2 demonstrate this point; in Example 1 we rejected H_0 with a directional H_A, while we retained H_0 in Example 2, with exactly the same data.

- The larger the sample size, n, the more likely we are to reject H_0 for a given set of data. Comparing Examples 1 and 3 demonstrates this; although μ, σ, and $\overline{X}$ were the same, where n was small, we had to retain H_0. Also, when n is small, ($n < 30$), we must use the t test to analyze the significance of our sample mean being different.

- The more demanding the decision level (that is, if α is small) the less likely we are to reject H_0. To illustrate this point, repeat Example 2, but set $\alpha = 0.05$. Here, $z_{crit} = 1.96$ so that z_{obt} is greater than z_{crit}. Therefore, we can reject H_0, and accept H_A at a 0.05 level of significance. That is, with exactly the same data, we have rejected or accepted H_0, depending on the level of significance, α.

ERRORS IN INFERENCE

When we say our results are *statistically significant* we are making the inference that the results for our sample are true for the population. It should be evident from the previous discussion that statistical decision making might result in

Table 18.2 Decision outcomes

Reality	Decision: reject H_0	Decision: retain H_0
H_0 correct (no difference or effect)	'False alarm' Type I error	Correct decision
H_0 incorrect (real difference or effect)	Correct decision	'Miss' Type II error

incorrect decisions. There are two main types of inferential error; *Type I* and *Type II*.

Type I error occurs when we mistakenly reject H_0; that is when we claim that our experimental hypothesis was supported when it is, in fact, false. The probability of a Type I error occurring is less than or equal to α. For instance, in Example 1 we set $\alpha = 0.01$. The probability of making a Type 1 error is less than or equal to 0.01; the chances are equal to or less than 1/100 that our decision in rejecting H_0 was mistaken. Therefore, the smaller α, the less the chance of making a Type I error.

Type II error occurs when we mistakenly retain H_0; that is, when we falsely conclude that the experimental hypothesis was not supported by our data. The probability of a Type II error occurring is denoted by β (beta). In Example 3 we retained H_0, perhaps falsely. If n were larger, we might well have rejected H_0, as in Example 1. Type 1 errors represent a 'false alarm' and Type II errors represent a 'miss'. Table 18.2 illustrates this.

Table 18.2 illustrates that if we reject H_0, we are making either a correct decision or a Type I error.

If we retain H_0, we are making either a correct decision or a Type II error. While we cannot, in principle, eliminate these from scientific decision making, we can take steps to minimize their occurrence.

We minimize the occurrence of Type I error by setting an acceptable level for α. In scientific research, editors of most scientific journals require that α should be set at 0.05 or less. This convention helps to reduce false alarms to a rate of less than 1/20. Replication of the findings by other independent investigators provides important evidence that the original decision to reject H_0 was correct.

How do we minimize Type II error rate?

1. Increase the sample size, n.
2. Reduce the variability of measurements ($S_{\bar{X}}$, either by increasing accuracy (Ch. 12) or by using samples that are not highly variable for the measurement producing the data).
3. Use of a directional H_A, on the basis of previous evidence about the nature of the effect.
4. Set a less demanding α, Type I error rate. There is a relationship between α and β, such that the smaller α, the greater β. This relationship is illustrated in Figure 18.7. Figure 18.7 shows that as α decreases, β increases. Inevitably, as we decrease Type I error rate, we increase the probability of Type II error. This is the reason why we do not normally set α at lower than $p = 0.01$.

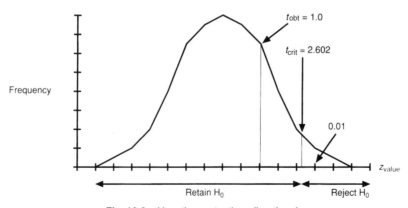

Fig. 18.6 Hypotheses testing: directional.

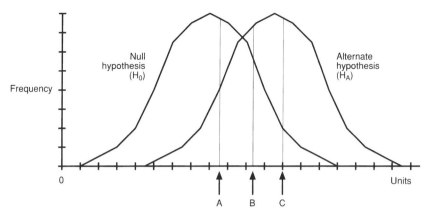

Fig. 18.7 Change of decision level to increase β and decrease α. As the decision criterion is moved from A to B to C, the relative frequency of Type I and Type II errors alters.

Although a significance level such as say α = 0.001 would reduce 'false alarms' it would also increase the probability of a 'miss'.

SUMMARY

It was argued in this chapter that once the data have been collected and summarized, the investigator must analyze the evidence to demonstrate its statistical significance. Significant results for an investigation mean that differences or changes demonstrated were real, rather than just the outcome of random sampling error.

The general steps in using tests of significance were explained, and several illustrative examples using the z and t tests for single sample designs were presented. A critical value is set for the statistic (in this case z_{crit}, t_{crit}) as specified by α. If the magnitude of the obtained value of the statistic (z_{obt}, t_{obt}) exceeds the critical value, H_0 is rejected. In this case, the investigator concludes that the data supported the differences predicted by the alternative hypothesis (at the level of significance specified by α). However, if the obtained value of the statistic is calculated to be less than the critical value, then the investigator must conclude

that the data did not support the hypothesis. It was noted that following these steps does not guarantee the absolute truth of decisions made about the rejection or acceptance of the alternative hypotheses, but rather specifies the probability of the decisions being correct.

Two types of erroneous decisions were specified, Type I and Type II errors. Type I error involves falsely concluding that differences or changes found in a study were real, that is concluding that the data supported a hypothesis (which is, in fact, false). Type II error involves falsely concluding that no differences or changes exist, that is concluding that the data did not support a hypothesis (which is, in fact, true). It was demonstrated that the probability of these errors depended on factors such as the size of n, the directionality of H_A and the variability of the data.

The procedures of hypothesis testing and error were related to the logic of clinical decision making. The probabilities (α and β) of making Type I and Type II errors are interrelated. In this way, both researchers and clinicians must take into account the implications of possible error when setting levels of significance for interpreting the data.

SELF ASSESSMENT

Explain the meaning of the following terms:

> alternative hypothesis
> critical value of a statistic
> decision rule
> directional or non-directional alternative hypothesis
> null hypothesis
> one tail or two tail test of significance
> region of acceptance
> region of rejection
> significance (level of)
> Type I and Type II error
> z test or t test

TRUE OR FALSE

1. The alternative hypothesis states that there is an effect or difference in the results.
2. If the probability of H_0 being true is greater than α, we can reject H_0.
3. Sampling distributions are used to enable the calculation of H_0 being true.
4. The critical value of a statistic is the value which cuts off the region for the rejection of H_0.
5. If the critical value of a statistic is less than the obtained or calculated value, we can reject H_0.
6. α is a probability, usually set at 0.01 or 0.05.
7. The t test requires that the sampling distribution of t should be normally distributed.
8. Hypothesis testing involves choosing between two mutually exclusive hypotheses, H_0 and H_A.
9. If α is set at 0.01 instead of 0.05, then the probability of making a Type I error decreases.
10. If we retain H_0, then we must conclude that the investigation did not produce significant results.
11. If n is greater than 30, the t test is more appropriate than the z test.
12. If results are statistically significant, the independent variable must have had a very large effect.
13. A directional H_A should be used when there is theoretical justification for the existence of a directional effect in the data.
14. When the results are statistically significant, they are unlikely to reflect sampling error.
15. It is impossible to prove the truth of H_A when using sample data as opposed to population data.
16. If we reject H_0 then we are in a position to accept H_A.
17. If alpha decreases (is made more stringent) then beta increases.
18. If H_0 is true and we reject it, we have made a Type I error.
19. If H_0 is false and we reject it, we have made a Type II error.
20. If H_0 is false, and we fail to reject it, we have made a Type II error.

MULTIPLE CHOICE

1. Hypothesis testing involves:

   a deciding between two mutually exclusive hypotheses H_0 and H_A
   b deciding if the investigation was internally and externally valid
   c deciding if the differences between groups was large or small
   d none of the above.

2. An α level of 0.01 indicates that:

   a the probability of falsely rejecting H_0 is limited to 0.05
   b the probability of Type II error is 0.01
   c the probability of a correct decision is 0.01
   d none of the above.

3. If α is changed from 0.01 to 0.001:

   a the probability of making a Type II error decreases

b the probability of a Type I error increases
c the error probabilities stay the same
d the probability of Type I error decreases.

4. If we reject the null hypothesis, we might be making:

a a Type II error
b a Type I error
c a correct decision
d a or c
e b or c.

5. Statistical tests are used:

a only when the investigation involves a true experimental design
b to increase the internal validity of experiments
c to establish the probability of the outcome of an investigation being due to chance alone
d a and b.

6. The outcome of a statistical analysis is found to be $p = 0.02$. This means that:

a the alternative hypothesis was directional
b we can reject H_0 at $\alpha = 0.05$
c we must conclude that H_A must be true
d a and c.

7. When the results of an experiment are non-significant, the proper conclusion is:

a the experiment fails to show a real effect for the independent variable
b chance alone is at work
c accept H_0
d accept H_A.

8. It is important to know the possible errors (Type I or Type II) we might make when rejecting or failing to reject H_0:

a to minimize these errors when designing the experiment

b to be aware of the fallacy of accepting H_0
c to maximize the probability of making a correct decision by proper design
d all of the above.

9. An α level of 0.05 indicates that:

a if H_0 is true, the probability of falsely rejecting it is limited to 0.05
b 95% of the time, chance is operating
c the probability of a Type II error is 0.05
d the probability of a correct decision is 0.05.

10. A directional alternative hypothesis asserts that:

a the independent variable has no effect on the dependent variable
b a random effect is responsible for the differences between conditions
c the independent variable does not have an effect
d there are differences in the data in a given direction.

11. If α is changed from 0.05 to 0.01:

a the probability of a Type II error decreases
b the probability of a Type I error increases
c the error probabilities stay the same
d the probability of Type II error increases.

12. If the null hypothesis is retained, you may be making:

a a correct decision about the data
b a Type I error
c a Type II error
d a or c
e a or b.

13. When the results are statistically significant, this means:

a the obtained probability is equal to or less than α.

SELF ASSESSMENT

b the independent variable has had a large effect

c we can reject H_0

d all of the above

e a and c.

14. β refers to:

a the probability of making a Type I error

b the probability of the $(1 - \alpha)$

c the inverse of the probability of sampling error

d the probability of making a Type II error.

15. Setting $\alpha = 0.0001$ would reduce the probability of Type I error. However, it would:

a increase Type II error probability

b increase the standard error of variance

c reduce external validity

d all of the above.

16. We retain H_0 if:

a $|t_{obt}| \leq |t_{crit}|$

b $|t_{obt}| > |t_{crit}|$

c $|t_{obt}| < |t_{crit}|$

d none of the above.

17. If α is changed from 0.01 to 0.001:

a the probability of a Type II error decreases

b the probability of a Type I error increases

c the error probabilities stay the same

d none of the above.

The researcher believes that the average age of unemployed persons has changed. To test this hypothesis, the ages of 150 randomly selected unemployed are determined. This mean age is 23.5 years. A complete census taken a few years before showed a mean age of 22.4 years, with a standard deviation of 7.6.

Questions 18–22 refer to this data.

18. The alternative hypothesis should be:

a $\bar{X}_A = \bar{X}_B$

b $\mu_A = \mu_B$

c $\mu_A \neq \mu_B$

d $\bar{X}_A \neq \bar{X}_B$

19. z_{crit} where $\alpha = 0.01$ is:

a +2.58

b +1.64

c +2.33

d −1.64

20. The obtained value of the appropriate statistic for testing H_0 is:

a 2.88

b 2.35

c 1.84

d 1.77

21. What do you decide, using $\alpha = 0.01$?

a retain H_0

b reject H_0

c it is not possible to decide

d a and b.

22. Therefore, the researcher should conclude that:

a unemployed persons are getting older on the average

b there is no evidence supporting the hypothesis that the average age of unemployed people has changed

c too many young people are unemployed

d b and c.

23. When the results are not statistically significant, this means that:

a the experimental hypothesis was not supported by the data at a given level of probability *b* the null hypothesis was retained at a given level of probability

c the alternative hypothesis must have been directional

d the investigation was internally valid

e *a* and *b*.

24. If $\alpha = 0.05$ and the probability of the statistic calculated from the data is $p = 0.02$, then:

a we should retain H_0

b we should reject H_A

c we should reject H_0 at $\alpha = 0.05$

d we should restate H_0 so that the findings will become significant at the 0.05 level.

19

Selection and use of statistical tests

INTRODUCTION

In the previous chapter, we examined the logic of hypothesis testing and the use of z and t tests for testing hypotheses about single sample means. There are numerous statistical tests available which are used in a conceptually similar fashion to analyze the statistical significance of the data. That is, all statistical tests involve setting up the relevant hypotheses H_0, H_A, and then on the basis of the appropriate inferential statistics, computing the probability of the sample statistics obtained occurring by chance alone. This probability is used to determine whether the experimental hypothesis has been supported by the data. We are not going to attempt to examine all of the various statistical tests in this introductory book. These are described in various statistics text books or in data analysis manuals. Rather, in this chapter we will examine the criteria used for selecting tests appropriate for the analysis of the data obtained in specific investigations. To illustrate the use of statistical tests we will examine the use of the chi-square test (χ^2). This is a statistical test commonly employed to analyze nominally scaled data.

The aims of this chapter are to:

1. Discuss the criteria by which a statistical test is selected for analyzing the data for a specific study.
2. Demonstrate the use of the χ^2 test for analyzing nominal scale data.

THE RELATIONSHIP BETWEEN DESCRIPTIVE AND INFERENTIAL STATISTICS

As we have seen in the previous chapters, statistics may be classified as descriptive or inferential. Descriptive statistics are concerned with issues such as 'What is the average length of hospitalization of a group of patients?' Inferential statistics are used to address issues such as whether the differences in average lengths of hospitalization of patients in two groups are statistically significantly different. Thus, descriptive statistics describe aspects of the data such as the frequencies of scores, the average, or the range of values for samples; whereas when using inferential statistics, one attempts to infer whether differences between groups or relationships between variables represent persistent and reproducible trends in the populations.

In Section 5 we saw that the selection of appropriate descriptive statistics depends on the characteristics of the data being described. For example, in a variable such as incomes of patients, the best statistics to represent the typical income would be the mean and/or the median. If you had a millionaire in the group of patients, the mean would give a distorted impression of the central tendency. In this situation the median would be most appropriate. The mode is most commonly used when the data being described are categorical. For example, if in a questionnaire respondents were asked to indicate their sex and 65 said they were male and 35 female then 'male' is the modal response. It is quite unusual to use the mode only with data that are not nominal. As a rule, the scale of measurement used to obtain the data and its distribution determine which descriptive statistics are selected.

In the same way, the appropriate inferential statistics are determined by the characteristics of the data being analyzed. For example, where the mean is the appropriate descriptive statistic, the inferential statistics will determine if the differences between the means are statistically significant. In the case of ordinal data, the appropriate inferential statistics will make it possible to decide if either the medians or the rank orders are significantly different. With nominal data, the appropriate inferential statistic will decide if proportions of cases falling into specific categories are significantly different.

Thus, when the data have been adequately described, the appropriate inferential statistic will follow logically. However, when selecting an appropriate statistical test, the design of the investigation must also be taken into account.

SELECTION OF THE APPROPRIATE INFERENTIAL TEST

Before addressing the issue of the selection of the appropriate inferential statistical test, it is useful to reiterate the reason why a statistical test should be employed.

In many studies, inferential statistical tests are not required. For example, if a health care needs-assessment survey is conducted in a particular community, using a full population, the investigator might not be overly concerned with generalizing the results to other communities, or with demonstrating that certain relationships between variables are reliable. It may be enough to be able to say, for example, that '35% of the respondents indicated that they were dissatisfied with the existing level of medical services'. In this instance, descriptive statistics are all that the investigator requires since the complete population was studied. If, however, the investigator wishes to argue that certain differences between groups or that certain *correlations* between variables for a *sample* are generalizable to the population, then inferential statistical tests are necessary.

The inferential statistic provides the investigator with a means of determining how reproducible the obtained results are, by enabling access to a probability. The probability associated with the value of an inferential statistic informs the investigator of the likelihood that the results obtained were due to chance factors, or if they are significant at a given level of probability.

Please note that we are not going to examine all of the numerous statistical tests available for decision making. Rather, the aim of this chapter is to examine the criteria used for selecting tests appropriate for the analysis of data obtained in

Table 19.1 Selection of tests of significance

Scale	Two groups Independent	Two groups Dependent	Three or more groups Independent	Three or more groups Dependent
Nominal	χ^2 test	McNemar test	test-χ^2	Cochran's Q test
Ordinal	Mann-Whitney U test	Sign test	Kruskal–Wallis H test	Friedman two-way analysis of variance
Interval or ratio	t test (independent groups)	t test (dependent groups)	ANOVA (F) (independent groups)	ANOVA (F) (dependent groups)

investigations. To illustrate the use of statistical tests we will look at the χ^2 test, commonly employed for analyzing nominal data. We examine the interpretation of findings which do not reach statistical significance and the relationship between statistical and clinical significance. In Chapter 20 we will consider some of the personal and social values implicit in making decisions concerning the actual adoption and use of treatments and diagnostic tests in clinical settings.

There is a variety of statistical tests, some of which are named in Table 19.1. The selection of the appropriate statistical test is determined by the following considerations:

1. The *scale* of measurement used to obtain the data (nominal, ordinal, interval, or ratio).
2. The *number of groups* used in an investigation (one or more).
3. Whether the measurements were obtained from *independent* subjects or from *related* samples, such as those involving repeated measurements of the same subjects.
4. The *assumptions* involved in using a statistical test, such as the distribution of the scores or the minimum required sample size.

Table 19.1 offers a sample of statistical tests in order to illustrate how statistical tests are selected for analyzing data. Several points are worth noting.

1. It can be seen that appropriate tests are selected on the basis of the four criteria outlined above. When we have determined these four criteria for a given investigation, the cell containing the appropriate test can be readily selected. We might need additional

criteria for deciding between two tests within a cell. For instance, we saw in the previous section that if n < 30, we use the t test rather than z test.

2. The tests appropriate for analyzing ordinal and nominal data are called *non-parametric* or *distribution free*. The tests for analyzing interval or ratio data are called *parametric* tests. The parametric tests (for example, z, t, or F) require that certain assumptions (such as normality and equal variance) be valid for the populations from which the samples were drawn. The non-parametric tests (e.g. χ^2, Mann Whitney U) require few, if any, assumptions about the underlying population distributions.

3. Even before the data are collected, an investigator should have a good idea of which statistical test is appropriate for analyzing the data. Sometimes, however, the distribution of the data is such that the test that was initially selected is found to be inappropriate.

Let us look at some examples to illustrate how statistical tests are selected.

An investigator wishes to evaluate the effectiveness of a new treatment in contrast to a conventionally used treatment. Assume that the outcome (dependent variable) is measured on a five-point ordinal scale. Each subject is assigned to one of the two treatment groups. Which test would the investigator use to analyze the significance of sample data when:

1. The measurement was ordinal.
2. There were two groups (new treatment, conventional treatment).
3. Subjects were independently assigned to a specific group.

By inspection of Table 19.1 the investigator would select the Mann–Whitney U test to analyze the significance of the data.

If we change the above example by stating that the dependent variable was measured on an interval scale, the appropriate test would now be a t test (for independent groups).

Let us say that three groups were used (by the inclusion of a placebo group) by the investigator. Now, if the outcome measurement remained ordinal, the appropriate test for analyzing the data is the Kruskal–Wallis H test. If, however, the outcome measures were interval, it follows from Table 19.1 that the appropriate test for analyzing the results would be ANOVA (analysis of variance).

Finally, say that in the original example *each* of the subjects was treated with both the new and old treatments. Now, the data would have been obtained from the repeated measurement of the same subjects, and the appropriate statistical test would be the Sign test (ordinal, two groups, dependent).

Table 19.1 does not include all the available statistical tests and their uses. In fact, mathematical statisticians can generate inferential tests appropriate for a whole variety of designs. The basic idea is to use probability theory to generate appropriate sampling distributions in terms of which the probability of H_0 being true can be calculated, and the *statistical significance* of the findings evaluated.

Rather than examining all the tests and their underlying assumptions, we will look at the use of the χ^2 test in some detail. As well as being a very useful test for analyzing nominal data, it (along with the z and t) illustrates how statistical tests are carried out to test hypotheses.

THE χ^2 TEST

As shown in Table 19.1, χ^2 (chi-square) is appropriate for statistical analysis when:

1. Variables were measured on a nominal scale.
2. Measurements were of independent subjects.

The χ^2 test is appropriate for deciding if proportions of cases falling into categories are different at a given level of significance.

Table 19.2 Treatments offered

Psychotherapy	Drugs	Electroconvulsive therapy
$n = 45$	$n = 40$	$n = 65$

The statistic, χ^2, is given by the formula:

$$\chi^2 = \Sigma \frac{(f_o - f_e)^2}{f_e}$$

where f_o = observed frequency for a given category and f_e = expected frequency for a given category, assuming H_0 was true.

The sampling distribution for χ^2 is a family of curves, which, like t, vary with degrees of freedom. The use of this inferential statistic is best illustrated by an example.

Suppose that an investigator is interested in finding out whether there is a difference in the relative frequency of different kinds of treatments currently offered to extremely depressed patients. A random sample of 150 patients is selected from a population of patients in Australia, and the type of treatment offered to them is determined from their medical records, as shown in Table 19.2.

The entries in each cell represent the frequency with which patients were given the various treatments. Thus, 45 patients were offered psychotherapy, 40 drugs and 65 electroconvulsive therapy. The χ^2 is the appropriate test for analyzing these data. Let us follow the steps involved in hypothesis testing, as outlined in Chapter 18.

1. H_A: there is a difference in the population proportions for the three treatments. H_A is non-directional when we use χ^2.
2. H_0: there is no difference in the population proportions of the three treatments. The frequencies shown in each cell in the table occurred through random sampling from a population where there is an equal frequency of the three treatments.
3. Decision level, α: say the investigator sets a significance level of 0.05 for rejecting H_A ($\alpha = 0.05$).
4. Calculation of the statistic: χ^2_{obt} is the value of χ^2 calculated from the data obtained. To

Table 19.3 Treatments; *fe* is shown in parentheses

Psychotherapy	Drugs	Electroconvulsive therapy
45	40	65
(50)	(50)	(50)

calculate χ^2_{obt}, we must determine f_e for each cell (f_o is, of course, determined by the data). If the null hypothesis is true, then our expectation is that the frequencies in each cell should be the same. In this case, $n = 150$, so that f_e should be $150/3 = 50$, given that there are three cells. Let us show this in tabular form (Table 19.3).

We can now calculate χ^2_{obt}, by calculating $(f_o - f_e)^2/f_e$ for each cell, and then summing the values.

$$\chi^2_{obt} = \Sigma \frac{(f_o - f_e)^2}{f_e}$$

$$= \frac{(45 - 50)^2}{50} + \frac{(45 - 50)^2}{50} + \frac{(65 - 50)^2}{50}$$

$$= 0.5 + 2.0 + 4.5$$

$$= 7.0$$

The greater the discrepancy between f_e and f_o the greater the calculated value of the chi-square statistic (χ^2_{obt}). The direction of the difference is of no account as the difference between f_e and f_o is squared.

5. Making decisions concerning H_0: The decision rule for χ^2 is similar to that of the z and t test, as shown in the previous section:

$$\chi^2_{obt} \geq \chi^2_{crit}, \text{ reject } H_0$$
$$\chi^2_{obt} < \chi^2_{crit}, \text{ retain } H_0$$

Here, χ^2_{crit} is the critical value of the statistic χ^2, which cuts off a proportion of the sampling distribution equal to α. The value of χ^2_{crit} is obtained from the tables in Appendix C. To look up this statistic, we need to know:
(a) α, which was set at 0.05 for this example
(b) the degrees of freedom, df.
Note that with χ^2 the degrees of freedom with one variable is $k - 1$, where k stands for the number of categories or groups. In this instance, we have $k = 3$ (three treatments) so

that df $= 3 - 1 = 2$. Now we can look up the tables in Appendix C. In this case, $\alpha = 0.05$ and df $= 2$, therefore $\chi^2_{crit} = 5.99$.

Here, since $\chi^2_{obt} > \chi^2_{crit}$ we can reject H_0 at a 0.05 level of significance. The investigator is in a position to accept H_A (that the three treatments are offered at *different* frequencies to depressed patients). Clearly, electroconvulsive therapy is given most frequently for the condition (in this hypothetical example).

χ^2 AND CONTINGENCY TABLES

In the previous example of χ^2 we had clear expectations of the expected frequencies (f_e), and were dealing with only one variable. The χ^2 test is also relevant for analyzing nominal data where f_e is not known, and where we are interested in the effects of more than one variable. Thus, χ^2 is a statistical test appropriate for deciding whether two variables are significantly related.

For example an investigator compares the effectiveness of drug therapy with coronary artery surgery in males 55–60 years old, suffering from coronary heart disease. A sample of 40 patients consenting to the investigation is selected from this population, and randomly divided into the two treatment groups (drugs only or coronary artery surgery). The treatment outcome is measured in terms of survival over 5 years. The outcome of this hypothetical study is shown in Table 19.4.

Table 19.4 is called a contingency table. A *contingency table* is a two-way table showing the relationship between two or more variables. Note that the levels of the variables have been classified into mutually exclusive categories ('drug or surgery' for the independent variable,

Table 19.4 Contingency table showing obtained frequencies for a hypothetical study comparing survival after treatments

	Drugs	Surgery	Row marginal
Dead	11	8	19
Alive	9	12	21
Column marginal	20	20	$n = 40$

and 'dead or alive' for the dependent variable, in this instance). The cells in the contingency table show the frequency of cases falling into each joint category (for example, 11 people who had 'drugs only' died during the 5 years). The row and column marginal scores are the sums of the frequencies. The row and column marginals necessarily add up to n, the sample size ($n = 40$ for this example).

Table 19.4 is called a two-by-two (2×2) contingency table. Depending on the number of categories (or levels) in each of the two variables, we might have 3×2 tables, 3×3 tables, etc. Let us now turn to analyzing the data.

1. H_A: there is a difference in the proportion of patients surviving for 5 years following the two types of treatment.
2. H_0: there is no difference in the frequency of survival rates; any difference between observed and expected frequencies in the sample is due to chance.
3. Decision level: $\alpha = 0.05$.
4. Calculation of the statistic χ^2_{obt}

$$\chi^2_{obt} = \Sigma \frac{(f_o - f_e)^2}{f_e}$$

To make our explanation of the calculation easier, let us label the cells and the marginal values, as shown in Table 19.5. We calculate χ^2_{obt} by calculating f_e for each of the cells and then substituting this value into the equation for χ^2_{obt}. In order to calculate the expected frequencies, f_e for each of the cells, we use the formula:

$$\frac{\text{row total} \times \text{column total}}{n}$$

Substituting into the above formula for each of the cells:

$$A: f_e = \frac{j \times l}{n}, \ B: f_e = \frac{j \times m}{n}, \ C: f_e = \frac{k \times l}{n}, \ D: f_e = \frac{k \times m}{n}$$

Table 19.5 General format for 2×2 contingency table

A	B	j
C	D	k
l	m	n

Now f_o are the observed frequencies as in the data, summarized in contingency Table 19.5. Substituting the values for f_e and f_o for each cell is shown in Table 19.6.

5. Making decisions concerning H_0: the degrees of freedom for a contingency table are calculated by the following formula:

$$df = (r - 1)(c - 1)$$

where r = the number of rows and and c = the number of columns. In this instance, given a 2×2 contingency table:

$$df = (2 - 1)(2 - 1) = 1$$

Now we can look up χ^2_{crit}, for $\alpha = 0.05$ and $df = 1$. From Appendix C, $\chi^2_{crit} = 3.84$ Therefore, since $\chi^2_{obt} < \chi^2_{crit}$ we must retain H_0: there is no difference in the frequencies of survival over 5 years following the two kinds of treatments. Our data shows that either there is no difference in the outcomes of the two treatments or we made a Type II error.

The χ^2 test can be used to analyze the statistical significance of nominal data arising from experimental or non-experimental investigations. This non-parametric test can be used provided that two simple assumptions are met:

1. Each subject has provided only one entry into the χ^2 table; that is, each of the entries are independent.
2. The expected frequency (f_e) in each cell is at least five. Therefore, if the sample size is too small, χ^2 may not be used.

If either of these assumptions is violated, the use of χ^2 is inappropriate for statistical decision making. Assumption 2 is particularly important when the degrees of freedom is one (df = 1) for a contingency table.

Table 19.6 Sample calculation of Chi squared

	f_o	f_e	$(f_o - f_e)^2$	$(f_o - f_e)^2/f_e$
A	11	9.5	2.25	0.236
B	8	9.5	2.25	0.236
C	9	10.5	2.25	0.214
D	12	10.5	2.25	0.214
n	40			$\chi^2 = 0.90$

χ^2: SAMPLE SIZE AND STATISTICAL SIGNIFICANCE

We demonstrated earlier that the larger the sample size selected for a study the more likely it is that we will decide that the findings are statistically significant. The reason for this principle is quite straight-forward. Data collection with a large sample yields more information on the basis of which we can test our hypotheses more accurately than with smaller samples. This is the case when we use χ^2 to analyze the significance of nominal scale data.

As an illustration, consider the following hypothetical example: you are working to retrain people recovering from severe brain injury as safe drivers. This is a rather arduous task which has a rather low success rate of around 40%. A new but rather expensive computerized driving simulation system has become available and you have been assigned the task of evaluating the effectiveness of the computerized system. A representative sample of 20 patients with brain damage are selected and are randomly assigned to one of two independent groups. The control group (C) are given standard treatment while the experimental group (E) are trained with the new computerized system. An independent instructor is used to assess if the patients were safe to drive following treatment. The obtained data are shown in Table 19.7.

The sample data indicates that 60% of the patients were assessed as safe drivers following the experimental treatment while only 40% were safe following standard treatment. This is true for the sample; the question is whether we can generalize these results to the population at large. In other words, we need to demonstrate the statistical significance of the results.

Given nominal scale data and independent groups, χ^2 is the appropriate test for analyzing the data. Following the procedure outlined in (Table 19.4), we have Table 19.8.

1. H_A: There is a difference in the proportion of patients who can be trained as safe drivers.
2. H_0: There is no difference in the population proportions for the two treatments.
3. Decision level : $\propto$ = .05
4. Calculation of χ^2_{obt}

$$\chi^2_{obt} = \Sigma \frac{(f_o - f_e)^2}{f_e}$$
$$= 0.8$$

5. For df = 1, $\propto$ = .05, χ^2_{crit} = 3.84 (Appendix C)

Therefore, since $\chi^2_{obt} < \chi^2_{crit}$, we must retain H_0 at a 0.05 level of significance.

Our data can be interpreted as showing that either the new equipment does not in general improve safe driving in patients with brain injury; or that we have made a Type II error in our inference (see also in Chs 18 and 20). Our decision hinges on the probability (B) of having made a Type II error.

As discussed in Chapter 18 one of the ways of reducing Type II error probability is to increase the sample size, n. Say that we had a sample size of n = 100 for the previously described study and we obtained the same proportions as described before, the data would now look as shown in Table 19.9.

The expected values f_e = 25 for each cell.

$$\frac{(20-25)^2}{25} \quad \frac{(30-25)^2}{25} \quad \frac{(30-25)^2}{25} \quad \frac{(20-25)^2}{25}$$

Therefore χ^2_{obt} = 4.0

As before, χ^2_{crit} = 3.84 ($\propto$ = 0.05, df = 1)

Decision: As $\chi^2_{obt} > \chi^2_{crit}$

Table 19.7 Hypothetical data for driving safety following control and experimental treatment

	Treatment	
Driving Outcome	Control	Experimental
Safe	4	6
Not safe	6	4

Table 19.8 Contingency table showing obtained frequencies for a hypothetical study comparing control and experimental treatments

	C	E	Total
Safe	4	6	10
Not safe	6	4	10
Total	10	10	20

C = Control   E = Experimental

Table 19.9 Contingency table showing obtained frequencies for a hypothetical study comparing control and experimental treatments with increased sample size

	Treatment	
Driving Outcome	C	E
Safe	20	30
Not safe	30	20

C = Control   E = Experimental

With an increased sample size, the results are significant at a 0.05 level and we can draw the inference that the new equipment does, in fact increase the proportion of patients who benefit from driver instruction.

Another influence on decision making is effect size. If you are looking for a needle in a haystack it helps if it is a very big one. Say that for the previous example there was a 90% recovery rate for the experimental group as opposed to 40% in the control group; with a sample size of $n = 20$ the data would look as shown in Table 19.10.

Table 19.10 Contingency table showing obtained frequencies for a hypothetical study comparing control and experimental treatments with changed recovery rates

	Treatment		
Driving Outcome	C	E	Total
Safe	4	9	13
Not safe	6	1	7
Total	10	10	20

C = Control   E = Experimental

Using the formula $f_e = \dfrac{\text{Row} \times \text{column}}{n}$

Table 19.5 shows that f_e for each of the four cells:

$$\text{Cell A:} f_e = \frac{10 \times 13}{20} = 6.5 \quad \text{Cell B:} f_e \frac{10 \times 13}{20} = 6.5$$

$$\text{Cell C:} f_e = \frac{10 \times 7}{20} = 3.5 \quad \text{Cell D;} f_e = \frac{10 \times 7}{20} = 3.5$$

$$\text{Therefore } \chi^2_{obt} = \frac{(4 - 6.5)^2}{6.5} + \frac{(9 - 6.5)^2}{6.5} + \frac{(6 - 3.5)^2}{3.5} + \frac{(1 - 3.5)^2}{3.5}$$

$$= \frac{(-2.5)^2}{6.5} + \frac{(2.5)^2}{6.5} + \frac{(2.5)^2}{3.5} + \frac{(-2.5)^2}{3.5}$$

$$= 5.49$$

$$\chi^2_{crit}, (df = 1, \propto = 0.05) = 3.84$$

Therefore, with a 90% recovery rate as $\chi^2_{obt} > \chi^2_{crit}$, we can conclude that there is a significant difference in the proportions, even when we only had a small sample size.

The above example demonstrates, with nominal scale data, two of the principles which were discussed in Chapter 18.

1. Increasing n, the sample size, increases the probability for obtaining significant findings.
2. When the effect size, as indicated by the differences between the groups is large, the results are more likely to be significant.

We will revisit these issues again when we look at the concept of 'power' in Chapter 20.

SUMMARY

There is a variety of statistical tests available for analyzing the significance of the obtained data. The statistical test appropriate for analyzing a given set of data is selected on the basis of:

1. The scaling of the data.
2. The dependence/independence of the measurements.
3. The number of groups being studied.
4. Specific requirements for using a statistical test.

Generally, parametric and non-parametric statistical tests were distinguished on the grounds of the scaling of the data and the assumptions underlying the sampling distributions.

None of the individual statistical tests was discussed in detail, except the χ^2 test which was presented as an example. Together with the discussion on the z and t tests in Chapter 18, the χ^2 test illustrates the principle that theoretical sampling distributions can be generated, and the probability of obtaining specific obtained outcomes can be calculated. If the obtained value of the inferential statistic is greater than or equal to the critical value, the null hypothesis can be rejected at the level of significance specified by the Type 1 error rate (α). This is the case regardless of which particular statistical test is being used.

The retention of H_0 might reflect a correct decision, or a Type II error. Sample size is a factor which contributes to Type II error rate, as shown in both Chapters 18 and 20.

SELF ASSESSMENT

Explain the meanings of the following terms:

> chi-square
> contingency table
> expected frequency
> non-parametric test
> observed frequency
> parametric test

TRUE OR FALSE

1. Inferential statistics are used to decide if differences obtained in sample data are persistent, 'real' trends.
2. The selection of descriptive and inferential statistics is independent of the scaling of the data.
3. Inferential statistics must be used, regardless of the nature and aims of an investigation.
4. Parametric tests are used to analyze the significance of interval or ratio data.
5. The use of non-parametric tests depends on the normal distribution of the underlying population.
6. Each statistical test entails the use of sampling distributions for calculating the probability of the obtained sample outcomes.
7. It is impossible to select an appropriate statistical test before the data is collected.
8. The number of groups being compared in an investigation influences the selection of the appropriate statistical test.
9. A basic assumption for using t is that the samples were drawn from a normally distributed population. A basic assumption of χ^2 is that the scores in each cell are independent.
10. When using χ^2, the closer the observed

frequency for each cell is to the expected frequency, the higher the probability of rejecting H_0.
11. In order to reject the null hypothesis, $\chi^2_{obt} > \chi^2_{crit}$.
12. The χ^2 sampling distribution is a family of curves, the distribution of which varies with the degrees of freedom.
13. The χ^2 test is appropriate for testing hypotheses about proportions.
14. Each entry in a χ^2 table is a frequency.
15. The value of f_e is looked up in the appropriate χ^2 table.
16. If the f_e and f_o values are the same for each cell, χ^2_{obt} will not be statistically significant.
17. The decision level, α is generally set at 0.05 or 0.01 with χ^2.
18. If we use sample data to calculate the values of f_e, then we use contingency tables for calculating χ^2_{obt}.
19. A 2×2 contingency table shows the relationship between two variables.
20. 'rc' stands for the degrees of freedom for a 2×2 contingency table.

MULTIPLE CHOICE

1. In a study, three independent samples are compared and the dependent variable is measured on a ratio scale. A statistical test appropriate for analyzing these findings is:

   a χ^2
   b Mann–Whitney U
   c t
   d ANOVA (analysis of variance).

2. In a study two independent samples are compared and the dependent variable is

SELF ASSESSMENT

measured on an ordinal scale. A statistical test appropriate for analyzing these findings is:

a χ^2
b Mann–Whitney U
c t
d Wilcoxon.

3. Which of the following is a 'non-parametric' test?

a ANOVA (analysis of variance)
b t
c z
d Kruskal–Wallis H.

4. Which of the following is a 'parametric test'?

a Median test
b McNemar's test
c z
d Cochran's Q.

5. Which of the following tests is appropriate for analyzing data where three or more groups were used?

a z
b t
c χ^2
d sign test.

6. The larger the discrepancy between f_o and f_e for each cell in a contingency table:

a the more likely it is that the results will not be significant
b the more likely it is that H_0 will be rejected
c the more likely it is that the population proportions are the same
d the more likely it is that the population proportions are different
e a and c
f b and d.

7. For any given level of significance, χ^2_{crit}:

a increases with increases in sample size
b decreases with increases in degrees of freedom
c increases with increases in degrees of freedom
d decreases with increases in sample size.

8. A contingency table:

a always involves two degrees of freedom
b always involves two dependent frequencies
c always involves two variables
d all of the above
e a and b.

9. Entries into the cells of a contingency table should be:

a frequencies
b means
c percentages
d degrees of freedom.

10. The degrees of freedom for a contingency table:

a equal $n - 1$
b equal rc $- 1$
c cannot be determined if r = c
d equal $(r - 1)(c - 1)$.

11. χ^2 should not be used with a 2×2 contingency table if:

a df > 1
b f_e is below 5 in any cell
c f_o is below 5 in any cell
d $f_e = f_o$
e b and c.

An investigator is interested in determining whether there is a relationship between gender and susceptibility to a substance known to trigger an allergic response. 'Susceptibility' is measured as yes or no.

Questions 12–15 refer to this example. The raw data are presented in the contingency table below.

	Not susceptible	Susceptible	Total
Female	90	110	200
Male	60	140	200
Total	150	250	400

12. The value of χ^2_{obt} is:

 a 2.50
 b 8.09
 c 9.60
 d 11.05

13. The value of df is:

 a 2
 b 1
 c 3
 d need more information.

14. Using $\alpha = 0.05$, χ^2_{crit} is:

 a 3.841
 b 5.412
 c 2.706
 d –3.841

15. Using $\alpha = 0.05$, what is your conclusion?

 a Accept H_0: there is no relationship between gender and susceptibility
 b Reject H_0: there is a significant relationship between gender and susceptibility
 c Fail to reject H_0: the study does not show a significant relationship between gender and susceptibility
 d Fail to reject H_0: this study shows a significant relationship between gender and susceptibility.

16. In selecting an appropriate statistical test:

 a z should be used as it is most powerful
 b t should be used as it takes the sample size into account
 c the choice depends on the design of the study
 d χ^2 should be avoided.

17. The χ^2 test requires that:

 a data be measured on a nominal scale
 b data conform to a normal distribution
 c expected frequencies are equal in all cells
 d all of the above occur.

The following information should be used in answering questions 18–25: aerobics classes are conducted by the student union of a tertiary institution; although there are equal numbers of male and female students enrolled at the institution, it is observed that far more female than male students attend. A test is performed to see whether the proportions of the two sexes at the class is representative of the proportions of the two sexes enrolled at the institution as a whole. Of the 50 students who attend the classes, 10 are male. A χ^2 is conducted on these data.

18. What type of χ^2 will be conducted?

 a one-way
 b two-way
 c contingency analysis
 d parametric.

19. How many cells will there be in the χ^2 table?

 a 1
 b 2
 c 3
 d 4

20. What is the expected frequency of male students at the aerobic classes?

 a 10
 b 40

SELF ASSESSMENT

c 25

d 8

21. What is the obtained value of χ^2?

    a 4.5
    b 2.5
    c 18.0
    d 9.0

22. What are the degrees of freedom?

    a 1
    b 2
    c 49
    d 48

23. If α is set at 0.01, what is the critical value of χ^2?

    a 0.0201
    b 4.605
    c 9.210
    d 6.635

24. What statistical decision should be made on the basis of these data?

    a Reject null hypothesis
    b Retain null hypothesis
    c Increase α
    d Increase size of sample.

25. What conclusion can be drawn on the basis of these data?

    a Overall, the tendency for more females than males to attend the classes is not statistically significant.
    b There is a statistically significant tendency for more females than males to attend the classes ($\alpha = 0.01$)
    c The aerobics classes should have their format changed to attract more male students.
    d There is a statistically significant trend ($\alpha = 0.01$) for differential attendance by

the two sexes, but it is impossible to state the direction of this trend.

The following information should be used in answering questions 26–31: in a test of the effectiveness of phenothiazine in treating schizophrenia, 60 patients are randomly assigned to receive either the drug or a placebo; after 2 weeks of daily treatment, each patient is assessed by the chief psychiatrist as 'improved' or 'not improved'. A 2 × 2 table is constructed to indicate improved number of patients falling into each category:

Assessment	Treatment	
	Phenothiazine	Placebo
Improved	20	10
Not improved	10	20

26. The degrees of freedom in this table are:

    a 1
    b 2
    c 3
    d 4

27. The obtained χ^2 is:

    a 1.33
    b 13.5
    c 8.71
    d 6.67

28. With α set at 0.05, the critical value of χ^2 is:

    a 3.841
    b 5.991
    c 6.635
    d 0.013

29. The correct statistical decision in this case is to:

    a reject H_0
    b retain H_0

c decrease α

d decrease α.

30. The appropriate conclusion to be drawn from these data is:

    a Patients receiving the active drug are not significantly more likely to get an 'improved' rating than those receiving the placebo.
    b Those receiving the active drug are significantly more likely to be rated as 'improved' (α = 0.05).
    c The drug cures schizophrenia.
    d The improvements cannot be due to the drug, as some people received the drug and did not improve.

31. Following the publication of this study, it is revealed that the psychiatrist who did the ratings of improvement was also the person who had assigned the patients to phenothiazine or placebo groups. What type of problem could have invalidated these findings?

    a Rosenthal effects
    b Placebo effects
    c Instrumentation effects
    d All of the above.

20

The interpretation of the evidence

INTRODUCTION

At the outset, it is important to recognize the distinction between establishing the statistical significance of an outcome in a study and the process of interpreting the importance and implications of the results.

As discussed earlier, in the process of data analysis, the investigator assembles the data, chooses an appropriate statistic, calculates the value of the statistic and then consults a table relating the values of the statistics to probabilities to find whether the results are *statistically significant*. Statistical significance is agreed to be reached when the probability value is lower than a predefined value (1 in 20 or 0.05 is a commonly used value). If the results are statistically significant the researcher is justified in generalizing the sample findings to the population from which the sample was selected. Of course, we assume that the sample was *representative* (Chapter 3). Unfortunately, many researchers stop at this point, believing that if they have established statistical significance, no further analysis or interpretation is required. Nothing could be further from the truth.

It is necessary to consider, in addition to statistical significance of the results, a set of further issues, including:

1. Effect size, that is, how large are the relationships or differences observed in the data.
2. The social and clinical significance of factors such as cost effectiveness and quality of life issues.

255

EFFECT SIZE

The effect size in a study refers to the actual size of the differences observed between groups or the strength of relationships between variables, as opposed to the statistical significance of these effects.

It is important to recognize that although statistical significance may be reached, the effect size in a study may not be clinically significant, or may be of such minimal size as to be theoretically uninteresting. Many students new to the research process believe that the reaching of statistical significance implies that the results in question necessarily illustrate important or 'significant' trends. This is not the case.

This situation can be illustrated by results from two student research projects supervised by the authors.

Study 1: Test–retest reliability of a force measurement machine

In the first study, the student was concerned with demonstrating the test–retest reliability of a device designed to measure maximum voluntary forces being produced by patients' leg muscles under two conditions (flexion and extension).

21 patients took part and the reliability of the measurement process was tested by calculating the Pearson correlation between the readings obtained from the machine in question during two trials separated by an hour for each patient. The results were as shown in Table 20.1.

Both results reach the 0.01 level of significance.

The student was ecstatic when the computer data analysis programme informed them that the correlations were statistically significant at the 0.01 level (indicating that there was less than a 1 in 100 chance that the correlations were illusory or actually zero.) We were somewhat less ecstatic because, in fact, the results indicated

that approximately 69% $(1-0.56^2)$ and 71% $(1-0.54^2)$ of the variation was not shared between the measurements of the first and second trial. In other words, the measures were 'all over the place', despite statistical significance being reached. Thus, far from being an endorsement of the measurement process, these results were somewhat of a condemnation. This is a classic example of the need for careful interpretation of effect size in conjunction with statistical significance.

Study 2: A comparative study of improvement in two treatment groups

The second project was a comparative study of two groups; one group suffering from suspected repetition strain injuries (RSI) induced by computer keyboard input and a group of 'normals'. An Activities of Daily Living (ADLs) assessment scale was used and yielded a 'disability' index of between 0 and 50. There were 60 people in each group. The results were as shown in Table 20.2.

The appropriate statistic for analyzing these data happens to be the independent groups t test, although this is not important to the understanding of this example. The t value for these data was significant at the 0.05 level. Does this finding indicate that the difference is clinically meaningful or significant? There are two steps in interpreting the clinical significance of the results.

First, we calculate the *effect size*. For interval or ratio scaled data the effect size 'd' is defined as:

$$\propto = \frac{\mu_1 - \mu_2}{\sigma}$$

Where $\mu_1 - \mu_2$ refers to the difference between the population means and σ the population standard deviation.

Table 20.1 Pearson correlations between trials 1 and 2

Flexion	Extension
0.56	0.54

Table 20.2 Mean ADL disability scores

	RSI group	Normals
Mean	33.2	30.4
Standard deviation	1.6	1.2

Since we rarely have access to population data we use sample statistics for estimating population differences. The formula becomes:

$$d = \frac{\bar{X}_1 - \bar{X}_2}{S_1}$$

where $\bar{X}_1 - \bar{X}_2$ indicates the difference between the sample means and S_1 refers to the standard deviation of the 'normal' or 'control' group. Therefore, for the above example, substituting into the equation yields:

$$d = \frac{30.4 - 33.2}{1.2}$$

$$= -2.33$$

In other words, the average ADL score of the people with suspected RSI was 2.33 standard deviations under the mean of the distribution of 'normal' scores. The meaning of d can be interpreted in accordance with using z scores as described in Chapter 15.

Second, we need to consider the clinical implications of the evidence. It might be that the difference of 2.8 units of ADL scores is important and clinically meaningful. However, if one inspects the means, the differences are slight, notwithstanding the statistical significance of the results. This example further illustrates the problems of interpretation that may arise from focusing on the level of statistical significance and not on the effect sizes shown by the data.

When we say that the findings are *clinically significant* we mean that the effect is sufficiently large to influence clinical practices.

HOW TO INTERPRET NULL (NON-SIGNIFICANT) RESULTS

As we discussed in previous chapters (18 and 19), the researcher will analyze data that show no relationships or effects according to the chosen statistical test and criteria. In other words, the researcher cannot reject the null hypothesis. There are several reasons why the researcher may obtain a null result.

1. There really is not the trend or difference that the researcher believes exists.

2. The sample of cases and observations included in the analysis is biased.
3. There are insufficient cases in the sample to detect the trend; this is especially a problem if the trends are subtle (ie. Type II error).
4. The measurements chosen have very high or inherent random variability.

Therefore, if the researcher obtains a null result, it is difficult, if not impossible, to determine which one or more of the above explanations is appropriate. There are, however, measures that can be taken to minimize the chance of missing real effects. In order to understand these measures, it is necessary to again invoke the table illustrating the possible outcomes of a statistical decision (Table 20.3 similar to Table 18.2).

There are four possible outcomes. On the basis of the statistical evidence you may (i) correctly conclude there is an effect when there is indeed an effect; (ii) you may decide that there is an effect when there is not (false alarm); (iii) you may decide statistically that there is not an effect when there really is (miss); or (iv) correctly decide there is not an effect when indeed there is not. The probability that researchers consult in their statistical tables is in fact the probability of a false alarm or Type I error. Thus, if I decide that any time my obtained statistical probability value is below 0.05 I will assume that there is an effect, only one time out of 20 will I be wrong in the sense of making a false alarm error. How many times, however, will I miss an effect? The probability of making this type of error is affected by the size of the effect and number of cases, among other things. In other words, if you have large effects and large samples the number of misses will be small. If the effect is small, larger samples are needed to detect it.

Table 20.3 Statistical decision outcomes

Reality	Decision: Effect	Decision: no effect
Effect	Correct	'Miss' Type II error
No effect	'False alarm' Type I error	Correct

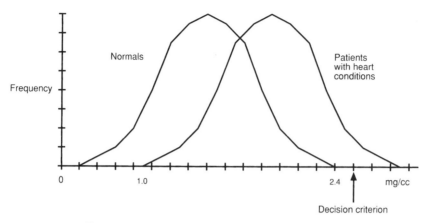

Fig. 20.1 Decision criterion: risk of Type II error (miss).

STATISTICAL POWER ANALYSIS

For any analysis, it is often useful to know how likely a miss is to occur. We can do this by calculating the *statistical power* of a design. The statistical power for a given effect size is defined as 1 − probability of a miss (Type II error or β). Thus, if the power of a particular analysis is 0.95, for a given effect size we will correctly detect the existence of the effect 95 times out of 100. Power is an important concept in the interpretation of null results. For example, if a researcher compared the improvements of two groups of only five patients under different treatment circumstances, the power of the analysis would almost certainly be low, say 0.1. Thus 9 times out of 10, even with an effect really present, the researcher would be unable to detect it.

It is well to be careful in the interpretation of null results where they are used to demonstrate a lack of superiority of one treatment method over another, especially when there is a low number of cases. This may be purely a function of low statistical power rather than lack of superiority. Unfortunately the calculation of statistical power is complicated and beyond the scope of this text. However, there are books of tables available to look up the power of various analyses; there are also statistical programmes which ensure that we are collecting sufficient information for detecting the phenomena in which we are studying. The best defence against low power is a good-sized sample.

CLINICAL DECISION MAKING

It should be noted that decision procedures confronting a clinician making a diagnosis on the basis of uncertain information is exactly analogous to the scientist's hypothesis testing procedure.

As a hypothetical example, assume that a clinician wishes to decide whether a patient has heart disease on the basis of the cholesterol concentration in a sample of the patient's blood. Previous research of patients with heart disease and 'normals' has shown that, indeed, heart patients tend to have a higher level of cholesterol than normals.

When the frequency distributions of cholesterol concentrations of a large group of heart patients and a group of normals are graphed, they appear as shown in Figure 20.1. You will note that if a patient presents with a cholesterol concentration between 1.0 and 2.4 mg/cc, it is not possible to determine with complete certainty whether they are normal or have a heart disease, due to the overlap of the normal and heart disease groups in the cholesterol distribution.

Therefore, the clinician, like the scientist, has to make a decision under uncertainty: to diagnose pathology (that is, reject the null hypothesis) or normality (that is retain the null hypothesis). The clinician risks the same errors as the scientist, as shown in Table 20.4.

The relative frequency of the type of errors made by the clinician can be altered by moving the point above which the clinician will decide

Table 20.4   Clinical decision outcomes

Reality	Decision Pathology	Decision No pathology
No pathology	'False alarm' Type 1 error	Correct decision
Pathology	Correct decision	'Miss' Type II error

that pathology is indicated (that is the decision criterion). For example, if the clinician did not bother their colleagues or patients with false alarms (Type I errors), they might shift the decision criterion to 2.5 mg/cc (Fig. 20.2). Any patient presenting with a cholesterol level below 2.5 mg/cc would be considered normal. In this particular case with a decision point of 2.5 mg/cc no 'false alarms' would occur. However, a huge number of people with real pathology would be missed (Type II errors).

If the clinician values the sanctity of human life (and their bank balance after a successful malpractice suit) they will probably adjust the decision criterion to the points shown in Figure 20.1. In this case, there would be no misses but lots of false alarms.

Thus, most clinicians are rewarded for adopting a conservative decision rule, where misses are minimized, by receiving lots of false alarms. Unfortunately, this generates a lot of useless, expensive and sometimes even dangerous clinical interventions.

The scientist considers it more acceptable to make a Type II error (a miss) rather than a Type I error (a false alarm). This is even more so the case since the integrity of some medical researchers has been questioned because of 'irregularities' in their data. That is, claims of breakthroughs or novel findings have been made but other researchers have been unable to replicate the results.

SUMMARY

In the interpretation of a statistical test, the researcher calculates the statistical value and then compares this value against the appropriate table to determine the probability level. If the probability is below a certain value (0.05 is a commonly chosen value), the researcher has established the statistical significance of the analysis in question.

The researcher must then interpret the implications of the results by determining the actual size of the effects observed. If these are small, the results may be statistically significant but clinically unimportant. Statistical significance does not imply clinical importance.

A null result (indicating no effects) must be carefully interpreted. It is possible that the researcher has missed an effect because of its small size and/or insufficient cases in the analysis. The statistical analysis measures the chance of correctly detecting a real effect of given size.

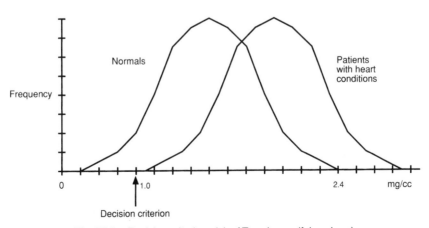

Fig. 20.2   Decision criterion: risk of Type I error (false alarm).

Thus, a null result may be a function of low statistical power, rather than there being no real effect.

There are several criteria, beyond statistical significance, which need to be considered before making decisions concerning the clinical applications of investigations. These criteria are to a large extent influenced by values and economic limitations concerning the administration of health care in a given community.

SELF ASSESSMENT

Explain the meanings of the terms:

      effect size
      clinical significance
      null result
      power analysis
      social significance
      statistical significance

TRUE OR FALSE

1. If the effect size is small, clinical significance will be large.
2. In order to establish statistical significance, clinical significance must first be established.
3. In order to establish clinical significance, statistical significance must first be established.
4. The effect size in an analysis is directly measured by the size of the p value associated with the statistic.
5. High inherent variability in measures will promote the detection of effects within data.
6. If a statistical analysis has high power, this means that β will be low.
7. A 'miss' is a correct rejection of the null hypothesis.
8. If a statistical analysis has low power, the null hypothesis will be accepted more frequently.
9. Power = $1 - \beta$ (Type II error).
10. It is more difficult to detect small effects in data where the statistical power is high.

MULTIPLE CHOICE

1. If $\beta = 0.80$ and $\alpha = 0.1$, the power of an analysis equals:

   a 0.9
   b 0.7
   c 0.2
   d 0.65

2. In a study there was a 1% difference in improvement of systolic blood pressure for two groups of patients receiving different treatments. This was statistically significant at $p = 0.05$. The results probably demonstrate:

   a clinical and statistical significance for the difference
   b clinical significance only
   c statistical significance only
   d neither clinical nor statistical significance.

3. A study of the relationship between family income and probability of occurrence of nutritionally related disorders demonstrated a correlation of 0.8 with $p < 0.001$. The results probably demonstrate:

   a clinical and statistical significance of the relationship
   b clinical significance only
   c statistical significance only
   d neither clinical nor statistical significance.

4. If the effect size in a study is large, the results are likely to have:

   a clinical and statistical significance for the difference
   b clinical significance only
   c statistical significance only

d neither clinical nor statistical significance.

5. If the power of the statistical analysis of a study is high there will be:

   a fewer misses
   b fewer correct rejections
   c fewer correct acceptances
   d more misses.

6. The effect of large sample sizes in a study upon statistical power is generally to:

   a increase it
   b decrease it
   c not affect it.

7. In a study, the effect of larger sample sizes upon clinical significance is generally to:

   a increase it
   b decrease it
   c not affect it.

8. In a study, the effect of a larger sample size upon obtained statistical significance as measured by *p* is generally to:

   a increase it
   b decrease it
   c not affect it.

9. If a null result is obtained in an experimental clinical study, the clinical significance of any observed differences between treatment groups:

   a cannot be supported
   b can be supported if it is big
   c can be supported if it is small
   d should be determined by power analysis.

10. If a power analysis is not performed, is it sensible to accept a null result from a study at face value?

   a Yes
   b No.

SECTION 6

Discussion, Questions and Answers

Inferential statistical tests arise from the desire of the clinical researcher to generalize from the data they have collected in a sample to the population from which the sample has been drawn. 'Is what I have found in my sample a true representation of the population (and hence other samples)?' is the basic question to be answered through the use of inferential statistical tests.

Inferential statistical tests all have the same basic format. The data are processed using the appropriate calculation procedure (often with the support of a computer programme) and the value of the statistic is calculated. This value obtained is then compared with a table of known values in order to interpret the outcome of the statistical test. This is very much like the application of clinical tests where, in order to interpret the value of the test result, it is compared with a known standard. As with the clinician, the clinical researcher needs to know which test to choose in which circumstance. It would not be appropriate to try to measure the weight of a patient by giving them an X-ray. Similarly, it is not appropriate to use a χ^2 test when the t test is required. It is beyond the scope of an introductory text to have an extended discussion of the various types of statistical tests and when they might be used (although it should be noted that there are many fewer statistical than clinical tests). However, it is essential that the student understands the basic use of inferential tests.

Consider the following analysis using χ^2. This statistic is designed to test the relationship between variables with nominal or categorical scales (i.e. the values are categories).

The clinical researcher is using the χ^2 test to examine the relationship between length of stay in hospital and the rate of unplanned readmissions. These data are described more fully in Section 5. The goal is to determine whether there is a statistically significant association between the two variables. The raw data appear in Table D20.1.

As demonstrated in Section 5, we could use the Pearson correlation to analyze these data. However, to illustrate the use of χ^2 we will recode the data to categorical data and use this technique. The data will be recoded using the averages for each variable to convert the data from ratio data to categorical data. For example, all those cases (hospitals) with a mean length of stay of 13.6 days or greater will

Table D20.1 Average lengths of stay and readmission rates per 100 patients for patients with fractured neck of femur at 30 hospitals

Hospital	Average length of stay (days)	Unplanned readmission rates per 100 patients
1	11.100	7.800
2	11.200	6.500
3	11.200	4.300
4	11.200	5.500
5	11.700	5.100
6	12.100	5.200
7	12.100	5.000
8	12.100	4.900
9	12.300	4.800
10	12.400	3.400
11	12.400	5.000
12	12.500	4.300
13	13.100	3.900
14	13.100	3.300
15	13.200	4.700
16	13.200	4.500
17	13.200	5.500
18	13.300	4.100
19	13.700	3.200
20	13.900	3.400
21	14.100	3.500
22	14.200	3.400
23	14.200	6.000
24	14.900	4.400
25	15.300	3.300
26	15.400	4.200
27	15.400	4.300
28	15.500	4.100
29	16.300	3.200
30	22.400	3.300

Discussion, Questions and Answers

considered as having an 'above average' length of stay. Those cases (hospitals) with a stay below 13.6 days will be considered as having a 'below average' length of stay. The same procedure will be followed for readmissions rates of 4.47 or greater. These are the respective means for the two variables shown in the table above. The recoded data appear as Table D20.2.

From these data we can construct a contingency table which shows the relationship between the two newly coded variables. We do this by counting the number of times the 30 cases fall into the appropriate categories.

Table D20.2 Recoded average lengths of stay and readmission rates per 100 patients for patients with fractured neck of femur at 30 hospitals

Hospital	Average length of stay (days)	Unplanned readmission rates per 100 patients
1	Below average	Above average
2	Below average	Above average
3	Below average	Below average
4	Below average	Above average
5	Below average	Above average
6	Below average	Above average
7	Below average	Above average
8	Below average	Above average
9	Below average	Above average
10	Below average	Below average
11	Below average	Above average
12	Below average	Below average
13	Below average	Below average
14	Below average	Below average
15	Below average	Above average
16	Below average	Above average
17	Below average	Above average
18	Below average	Below average
19	Above average	Below average
20	Above average	Below average
21	Above average	Below average
22	Above average	Below average
23	Above average	Above average
24	Above average	Below average
25	Above average	Below average
26	Above average	Below average
27	Above average	Below average
28	Above average	Below average
29	Above average	Below average
30	Above average	Below average

As can be seen from Table D20.3, only one hospital with an above average length of stay had an above average readmission rate, while 11 hospitals with above average lengths of stay had below average readmission rates.

These data can be subjected to χ^2 analysis. If these calculations are performed, we obtain a χ^2 value of 9.98, df = 1, $p < 0.01$. In other words there is a statistically significant association between length of stay and readmission rates for the 30 hospitals. This confirms the analysis conducted in Section 5.

Questions

1. From Table D20.1, how many hospitals have a below average length of stay, if the average length of stay is 13.6 days? How many have an above average length of stay? Why is it not 15 above and below?
2. From Table D20.3, why is there one degree of freedom in this analysis?
3. On the basis of this analysis, what would you conclude about the relationship between average length of stay in hospital and unplanned readmission rate for patients with fractured neck of femur at the 30 hospitals?
4. To what other groups of patients could these findings be generalized?

Answers

1. In this sample, 18 hospitals have a below-

Table D20.3 Contingency table of relationship between average length of stay and readmission rates at 30 hospitals for patients with fractured neck of femur

	Unplanned readmission rate	
	Above average	**Below average**
Length of stay		
Above average	1	11
Below average	12	6

Discussion, Questions and Answers

average length of stay. 12 hospitals have an above-average length of stay. Although that is how the median is defined, i.e. the score above which and below which half of the cases fall, the mean does not always fall at the exact half-way point of the sample.

2. The number of degrees of freedom in a contingency table is calculated by the formula (rows − 1) multiplied by (columns − 1) = (2 − 1) × (2 − 1) = 1.

3. There is a moderately sized statistical association between average length of stay in hospital and unplanned readmission rate. That is, those hospitals with shorter lengths of stay for patients with a fractured neck of femur tend to have higher unplanned readmission rates.

4. It is difficult to say. The current data include patients with one condition only, i.e. fractured neck of femur. These patients may be atypical of other acute/surgical patients; they are likely to be older and perhaps more debilitated. These analyses would need to be extended to other types of patients before the results could be generalized. The country in which the study has been performed also needs to be considered, as procedures and incentives may vary considerably from one country to the next.

Dissemination and critical evaluation of research

Having completed the analysis and interpretation of our data, we are now ready to communicate our results to the community of health scientists and professionals. Depending on the context in which our research was carried out, this entails the writing up of a report, a thesis or a 'paper' for a health sciences journal. The most common way of communicating research findings by established researchers is to first report the results at a professional conference and then to write a more formal paper for a relevant journal.

Each journal has its particular set of rules and requirements for how research projects should be written up for publication. In general, at least for quantitative research, the format for presenting our research follows the sequential stages of the research process outlined in the present book. This general format is outlined in Chapter 21, which includes a detailed discussion of the specific sections of a research paper and outlines some 'stylistic' considerations required by journal editors.

It is an ethical requirement that we report our results in an accurate and honest fashion. Before a paper is published in a reputable journal, it is critically evaluated by experts in the area (called referees) for errors or problems. However, sometimes problems remain unidentified. Ultimately, it is our task, as health professionals, to read important publications in a critical fashion. We owe it to our patients and clients to be cautious and critical concerning recent developments in theories and practices. However, being critical does not imply the adoption of a cynical or derogatory approach towards the work of other health researchers. We are aware that ethical and economic constraints, and the complex nature of the subject matter, as discussed in Section 2, make it difficult to ensure the external and internal validity of research projects.

The critical evaluation of a paper is not like

judging a dog show; we do not simply award or subtract points for the strengths and weaknesses of a research project. Rather, if the information is relevant to advancing the effectiveness of our practices, we have a stake in the project (even as readers). In this way, we take an active role in trying to 'repair' the problems which might cloud or invalidate the evidence.

In Chapter 22, we outline some of the criteria which we generally apply to evaluate specific sections of a research paper. We also discuss the implications of finding serious problems with the design, data collection, and analysis and interpretations of a research project.

In effect, a single research project is rarely sufficient either to verify or falsify a theory, or to convincingly demonstrate the effectiveness of a treatment programme. Rather, we need to evaluate and summarize the literature as a whole, that is, produce a literature review. Conflicting findings or gaps in the knowledge for a given area of health care identified in our literature review provide the impetus for further research, as outlined in Section 2. In this way research is a circular process.

21

Presentation of health science research

INTRODUCTION

Knowledge in the health sciences is the sum of the individual efforts of investigators working all over the world. Professional journals in science and health care provide the dominant medium for disseminating information about the outcome of specific investigations. Investigators must report their procedures and results in an accurate and complete fashion. In this chapter, we outline the format and style generally followed for presenting the results of empirical investigations.

The specific aims of this chapter are to:

1. Describe the conventional way in which quantitative research is presented for publication
2. Discuss the style or language used to describe research
3. Outline briefly the way in which research papers are selected for publication.

THE STRUCTURE OF RESEARCH PUBLICATIONS

The format of a professional publication reporting empirical research reflects the stages of the research process discussed in this book. Table 21.1 represents the relationship between the stages of research and the commonly used publication format. This format is generally used to report quantitative empirical research, although you will find that some variations on this theme are adopted by some professional journals. This format is not necessarily followed for certain types of scholarly communications, such as for

Table 21.1 Format of research publications and the research process

Publication format	Research process
Title	
Abstract	
Introduction	Research planning
Method:	Design
Subjects	
Apparatus	Measurement
Procedure	
Results	Descriptive statistics
	Inferential statistics
Discussion	Interpretation of the data
References	
Appendices	

qualitative research, theoretical papers or literature reviews. In the subsections following, we examine in detail each of the components of a research report shown in Table 21.1.

Title and abstract

The *title* is a descriptive sentence stating the exact topic of the report. Many titles of research reports take one of the following two forms:

- y as a function of x
- The effect of x upon y

In casual research, such as experiments, y refers to the dependent variable being measured and x refers to the independent variable being manipulated. For example:

- The incidence of alcoholism in health professionals as a function of work-related stress.
- The effect of major tranquilizers on the cognitive functioning of persons with schizophrenia.

For descriptive or qualitative research the title should inform the reader about the groups being studied and the characteristics being reported. For example, 'The Attitudes of Physicians to the Professional Functions of Podiatrists'.

In general, titles should be concise and informative, enabling a prospective reader to identify the nature of the investigation. Immediately below the title should appear the name(s) of the investigator(s) and their affiliation.

The *abstract*, is a short (not more than 250 words) description of the entire report. The purpose of this section is to provide the reader with a general overview of the communication. It should provide enough details to enable the reader to decide whether or not the article is of interest. This section can be difficult to write because of its precise nature. When writing an abstract you should include:

1. A brief statement about previous findings which led you to conduct your own research.
2. The hypothesis and/or aim of your research.
3. Methods, including subjects, apparatus and procedure.
4. A short description of what you found and how you interpreted your results.
5. What you concluded.

In some journals, this section may appear at the end of the manuscript in the form of a *summary*. For our purposes, however, we will treat this section as an abstract.

The title and the abstract together are important and should contain key words that enable the efficient retrieval of the information.

Introduction

The *introduction* is equivalent to the planning stages of research discussed in Section 2. A good introduction will set the stage for the hypotheses being tested. It should do this by discussing the theoretical background of the problem under consideration and evaluating the relevant research done previously. The introduction thus serves as a link between the past and the present.

Generally, all aspects of the literature cannot be covered in a relatively brief research paper, therefore, the review of past research is done with a bias towards only those aspects of the problem which are of direct relevance to your report. In this way the hypotheses being tested can be derived in a logical manner. For this reason, a good introduction starts out by making a few general statements about the field of research, leading logically to a narrow and specific set of statements which represent the aims or hypotheses. The final paragraph of the introduction should state the precise aims or the hypotheses being investigated.

Method

The purpose of the *method* section is to inform the reader of how the investigation was carried out. It is important to remember that the method section should contain enough detail to enable another researcher to replicate your investigation. (Of course, replications may not be feasible for a unique event, such as a case study of a specific individual). Conventionally, three subsections are used: *Subjects*, *Apparatus* and *Procedure*.

- *Subjects*. Three questions must be answered concerning the subjects: who were they, how many were there and how were they selected. Specific information must be given concerning the subjects, as results may vary from one sample to another.
- *Apparatus*. A description of all equipment, including questionnaires, etc., used in the research must be provided. If it is commercially available, provide the reader with the manufacturer's name and the commercial identification of the equipment. Alternatively, if the equipment was privately made, provide the reader with enough information to allow replication. Measurements and perhaps a diagram will be necessary.
- *Procedure*. Once again, this section should provide enough information for other researchers to replicate the investigation. Details of how research was carried out should include how subjects were assigned to groups, how many subjects per group, the experimental procedure and a description of how the data were collected.

In a sense, the method section should read like a cookbook. The subjects subsection describes the ingredients. The apparatus subsection describes the equipment necessary for baking (note we did *not* say 'cooking' the experiment) and, finally, the procedure subsection describes

how the ingredients were mixed to produce the final outcome: the results section.

Results

The *results* section presents the findings of the investigation and draws attention to points of interest. Raw data and statistical calculations are not presented in this section. Rather, we use the principles of descriptive and inferential statistics to present the summarized and analyzed data: graphs, tables and the outcomes of statistical tests are presented in this section. It is essential that all the findings are presented and that the graphs and tables are correctly identified.

Discussion

The *discussion* section restates the aim(s) of the investigation and discusses your results with reference to the aims or experimental hypothesis stated in the introduction. Did you find what you expected? How do the present results relate to previous research?

It is important to remember that one experiment in isolation cannot make or break a theory or establish the effectiveness of a practice. Thus, the discussion should connect the findings with similar studies and especially with the theory underlying such studies. If unexpected results were obtained, possible reasons for the outcome (such as faulty design and controls) should be discussed. By this, the discussion will point the way to further problems which remain to be solved. Unconstructive, negative or unimportant criticism should be avoided, so that the report does not end with long discussions of possible reasons for the outcome. Brief, concise discussion is more appropriate.

In the *conclusion*, which is usually the last paragraph of the discussion section, the main findings are summarized and suggestions made for further research. For example, you may have demonstrated certain phenomena which may have implications for explaining broader concepts which can be empirically tested. You are therefore taking your findings and generalizing them to phenomena not directly tested in the present research.

References and appendices

It is expected that all the literature discussed in the paper is listed in the *references* section. This enables your reader to evaluate your sources. You should refer to appropriate style manuals for information on how references should be listed. Sufficient information must be provided for an interested reader to be able to identify and retrieve the sources. In addition, a report may include labelled *appendices*. These might include a full description of questionnaires or other measuring instruments, raw data, or statistical calculations if required.

THE STYLE OF RESEARCH PUBLICATIONS

It is essential that you read research publications in your professional area to gain a 'feel' for the appropriate style of writing. In general, the following points should be kept in mind when writing reports:

1. Avoid long phrases or complicated sentences. Short, simple sentences are far more easily understood by your reader. In other words, try not to posture but to communicate.
2. Use quotations sparingly; put ideas in your own words. Quotations are used only when it is necessary to convey precisely the ideas of another researcher, for instance, while conducting a critique of a paper.
3. Use past tense when writing your research report.
4. Use an objective style, avoiding personal pronouns wherever possible.
5. Make sure you are writing to your audience; if the material is specialized or difficult, explain it clearly.
6. Make sure that you are concise and clear; do not introduce issues and concepts which are not strictly relevant to reporting your investigation. Raising interesting but superfluous issues might distract and confuse your reader.

In general, you should aim to improve your report writing and your ability to communicate your finding and ideas by seeking constructive criticism from your colleagues and supervisors.

THE PUBLICATION PROCESS

The formal knowledge representing the empirical and professional basis for your professional practice is in a large part stored in journals, books and conference reports, Journals are published by appropriate professional associations, government departments or private companies. Having completed a research project, how does one publish it in a professional journal? After all, the value of research is negligible if it is not made public.

In general, the prospective author will:

1. Select a professional or scientific journal appropriate for the material.
2. Present the research report in a format required by the journal.
3. Send the completed manuscript to the journal's editor.

The editor is generally a person of high standing in a given scientific or professional area. If the article is judged as being appropriate for the journal, the editor will send the article to two or more referees and, on the basis of the referees' report, publish or reject the manuscript. Sometimes the referees recommend certain additions or changes which have to be made by the author before the manuscript is judged to be publishable.

Therefore, when you read research publications in refereed journals, you can be confident that the articles have been scrutinized by experts. However, as shown in the next subsection, this does not necessarily guarantee the truth of either the evidence or the conclusions.

ETHICS OF PRESENTING RESEARCH

The health science researcher has an obligation to publish honest and accurate results that would not harm those people who participated in the research.

Most ethics committees in health care institutions and universities have the twin objectives of not only advancing knowledge for the common good but also preventing harm to those participating in the research. This is particularly so in the situation where the participants may have a diminished capacity to freely consent to their involvement (e.g. children or people who are unconscious or seriously ill). It is crucial to maintain the dignity and confidentiality of participants in health research.

Therefore, in the process of ethical evaluation of health science research, the researcher can expect to be closely questioned on these issues. If they cannot convince the ethics committee that the research will deliver knowledge for the common good and that it will not harm the participants, then the research will not usually proceed.

In research performed for a higher degree, many universities will not accept a thesis without an accompanying ethical clearance from the relevant ethics committee. Most hospitals and universities have strict ethical procedures that must be followed before any research work is commenced by their staff. Most, if not all, health research grant bodies require an ethical clearance before they will release the funds to successful applicants. Many journals also require certification from the researcher that the work complies with ethical principles. It is likely that this trend towards tightening of procedures will continue.

The ultimate unethical act is to manufacture data. Broad & Wade (1982), in their book *Betrayers of the Truth* describe this problem. It would seem to be a growing problem that may be associated with the 'publish or perish' requirements placed upon health science researchers by granting bodies and employers.

In the health sciences, it is not only the participants in research who may be harmed or assisted by the research. If an erroneous research finding is widely applied, it may harm many thousands of people. Ethics are therefore not simply concerned with whether the researcher has good intentions and treats the research participants well, there is also the issue of competence. Poorly designed research is unethical in that it may bring great harm to others. Thus, the ethical researcher must also be a competent researcher.

SUMMARY

In this chapter we outlined the general format followed by researchers for publishing their results. The format is related to the logical steps of planning, conducting and interpreting research. The style involves clarity, accuracy and sufficient completeness for colleagues to understand or replicate the research project. Research is published in journals, which are generally edited by persons of high standing in the field. Every effort is made by editors to ensure the validity of the research published in their journals. The individual researcher is also ethically bound to report findings in an unbiased and truthful fashion.

Although the format and style outlined in this chapter might seem rather arduous, poor presentation may destroy the intrinsic value of a research project.

SELF ASSESSMENT

Explain the meaning of the following terms:

abstract
apparatus
discussion

method
plagiarism
procedure
refereed journal
subjects

SELF ASSESSMENT

TRUE OR FALSE

1. As a rule, the title of a research investigation should not contain more than seven words.
2. Generally, the research hypothesis should be presented in the introduction.
3. A research report should contain sufficient information so that the investigation can be replicated.
4. The results section should contain all computational details for each statistic.
5. The abstract should normally contain the key tables of the results.
6. The design of an investigation influences the content of the method section.
7. All the names and addresses of your subjects must be published to enable replication of your investigation.
8. Quotations should be used sparingly in a research report.
9. A research report should be written in the past tense.
10. The outcomes of statistical analyses are reported in the results section.
11. Scientists do not normally report the results of their investigations, in case their work is stolen or misrepresented.
12. Calculations are best presented in appendices.
13. The 'referees' are hired by the investigator in order to convince the editor that an investigation should be published.
14. The role of an editor for a scientific journal is to censor research publications for pornographic, blasphemous or politically undesirable material.
15. Good research is unique and cannot be replicated.
16. A researcher should report data even if it is inconsistent with the researcher's original preconceptions.
17. Scientific and professional journals are important for disseminating and storing knowledge.
18. Fortunately, there have been no major scandals concerning scientists publishing fabricated data.
19. Provided that the results are statistically significant, there is no need to present descriptive statistics.

MULTIPLE CHOICE

1. Scientific journals:

   a only publish empirical evidence
   b depend on the services of referees to comment on the validity of the research project
   c publish only true knowledge
   d b and c

2. The literature review is normally found in which section of a research report?

   a Abstract
   b Introduction
   c Discussion
   d References

3. A literature review for a research report should:

   a contain a detailed review of all previously published reports
   b contain a selective review of evidence pertinent to the current research project
   c be at least 5000 words
   d a and c.
   e b and c.

4. Which of the following is most inadequate as a title for a research report?

   a The effects of the twentieth century culture on being human: an empirical evaluation of personal functioning in declining cultures
   b Electrical stimulation of the limbic system: effects on emotion and memory

   c A survey of the incidence of mental illness in the London metropolitan area

   d Popularity, friendship selection and specific peer interaction among children.

5. The methods section of a research report:

   a informs the reader of the purpose of an investigation

   b informs the reader about the state of methodological advances in the subject area

   c informs the reader as to how the investigation was carried out

   d informs the reader as to how the hypothesis or aim of the investigation was formulated.

6. When writing a scientific report one should:

   a make sure the Introduction contains 250 words or less

   b use personal pronouns as much as possible

   c try to impress the readers by one's level of general knowledge

   d use the past tense.

7. In which part of a research report are the descriptive and inferential statistics normally reported?

   a Abstract

   b Results

   c Discussion

   d Appendices.

8. In writing a Discussion, one should:

   a relate the results to findings reported in previous publications

   b establish if the results of the investigation supported the hypothesis

   c neither *a* nor *b*

   d both *a* and *b*.

9. Which of the following statements is true?

   a The discussion section should relate present findings to previous research.

   b The literature review should be conducted in a special appendix labelled references.

   c The results section should contain only tables and graphs, but not any verbal descriptions of the data.

   d All the above statements are true.

   e None of the above statements is true.

10. Which of the following statements is false?

   a The abstract should be a brief summary of the research.

   b It is unethical to fabricate data.

   c A refereed journal is one in which experts independently evaluate a research report before it is published.

   d A well-designed research project need not have a procedure section.

22

Critical evaluation of published research

INTRODUCTION

By the time a research report is published in a reputable journal, it has been critically scrutinized by several experts. Nevertheless, even this detailed evaluation procedure does not necessarily guarantee the validity of the design or the conclusions. Ultimately, as a health professional, you must be responsible for judging the validity and relevance of published material.

The proper attitude to published material is hard-nosed scepticism. This attitude is based on our understanding of the probabilistic and provisional nature of scientific and professional knowledge. In addition, health researchers deal with the investigation of complex phenomena, where it is often impossible for ethical reasons to exercise desired levels of control. The aim of critical evaluation is to identify the strengths and weaknesses of a research publication, to ensure that patients receive assessment and treatment based on the best available evidence.

This is essentially a revision chapter. Its general aim is to demonstrate how select concepts in design, measurement and statistics can be applied to the critical evaluation of published research. The chapter is organized around the evaluation of specific sections of research publications.

The specific aims of this chapter are to:

1. Examine the criteria used for the critical evaluation of a quantitative research paper
2. Discuss the implications of identifying problems in design, measurement and analysis in a given publication

3. Outline briefly strategies for summarizing and analyzing evidence from a set of papers
4. Discuss the implications of critical evaluation of research for health care practices.

CRITICAL EVALUATION OF THE INTRODUCTION

The introduction of a paper essentially reflects the planning of the research. Inadequacies in this section might signal that the research project was erroneously conceived or poorly planned. The following issues are essential for evaluating this section.

Adequacy of the literature review

The literature review must be sufficiently complete so as to reflect the current state of knowledge in the area. Key papers should not be omitted, particularly when their results could have direct consequences for the research hypotheses or aims. Researchers must be unbiased in presenting evidence which is unfavourable to their points of view. A particular 'howler' occurs when a research project is undertaken in ignorance of the fact that the same research has been already conducted and published.

Clearly defined aims or hypotheses

As stated in Chapter 2, the aims or hypotheses of an investigation should be clearly and operationally stated. If this is lacking, how the evidence obtained in the investigation is to be used for conceptual advances in the area will be ambiguous.

Selection of an appropriate research strategy

In formulating the aims of the investigation, the researcher must have taken into account the appropriate research strategy. For example, if the demonstration of causal effects is required, a survey may be inappropriate for satisfying the aims of the research.

Selection of appropriate variables

The operational definition of the variables being investigated calls for selection of appropriate measurement strategies. If the selection of the variables is inappropriate to the construct being investigated, then the investigation will not produce useful results.

CRITICAL EVALUATION OF THE METHODS SECTION

A well-documented methods section is a necessary condition for understanding, evaluating and perhaps replicating a research project. In general, critical evaluation of this section will reveal the overall internal and external validity of the investigation.

Subjects

This section shows if the sample was representative of the target population and the adequacy of the sampling model used.

Sampling model used. In Chapter 3, we outlined a number of sampling models which can be employed to optimize the representativeness of a sample. If the sampling model is inappropriate, then the sample might be biased, raising questions concerning the external validity of the research findings.

Sample size. Use of a small sample is not necessarily a fatal flaw of an investigation, if the sample is representative. However, given a highly variable, heterogenous population, a small sample will not be adequate to ensure representativeness (Ch. 3). A small sample size could also decrease the power of the statistical analysis (Ch. 20).

Description of the sample. A clear description of key sample variables (for example, age, sex, type and severity of condition) should be provided. When necessary and possible, demographic information concerning the population should be provided. If not, the reader cannot judge the representativeness of the sample. Also, the reader might not be able to decide if the findings are applicable to the specific groups of patients being treated.

Instruments/apparatus

The validity and reliability of observations and measurements are fundamental characteristics of good research. In this section, the investigator must demonstrate the adequacy of the equipment used for data collection.

Validity and reliability. The investigator should use standardized apparatus, or establish the validity and reliability of new apparatus used. The lack of proven validity and reliability will raise questions about the adequacy of the empirical findings.

Description of instrumentation. A full description of the structure and use of novel instrumentation should be presented so that the instrument can be replicated by independent parties.

Procedure

A full description of how the investigation was carried out is necessary for both replication and for the evaluation of its internal and external validity.

Adequacy of the design. It was stated previously that a good design should control for alternative interpretations of the data. A poor design will result in uncontrolled influences by extraneous variables, negating the unequivocal evaluation of causal effects. In Section 3, we looked at a variety of threats to internal validity which must be considered when critically evaluating an investigation.

Control groups. A specific way of controlling for extraneous effects is the use of control groups (such as placebo, no treatment or conventional treatment). If control groups are not employed, then the internal validity of the investigation might be questioned. Also, if placebo or untreated groups are not present, the size of the effect due to the treatments might be difficult to estimate.

Subject assignment. When using an experimental design, care must be taken in the assignment of subjects to avoid significant initial differences between treatment groups (see Ch. 4). Even when quasi-experimental or natural comparison strategies are used, care must be

taken to establish the equivalence of the groups (see Chs 5 and 6).

Treatment parameters. It is important to describe all the treatments given to the different groups. If the treatments differ in intensity or in the equality of the administering personnel, the internal validity of the project is threatened.

Rosenthal and Hawthorne effects. Whenever possible, studies should be double or single blind. If the subjects, experimentors or observers are aware of the aims and predicted outcomes of the investigation, then the validity of the investigation will be threatened through bias and expectancy effects (see Ch. 4).

Settings. The setting in which a study is carried out has implications for external (ecological) validity. An adequate description of the setting is necessary for evaluating the generalizability of the findings (see Ch. 3).

Times of treatments and observations. The sequence of treatments and observations must be clearly indicated, so that issues such as series and confounding effects can be detected. Identification of variability in treatment and observation times can influence the internal validity of experimental, quasi-experimental or $n = 1$ designs, resulting in, for example, internal validity problems.

CRITICAL EVALUATION OF THE RESULTS

The results should represent a statistically correct summary and analysis of the data (see Sections 5 and 6). Inadequacies in this section could indicate that inferences drawn by the investigator were erroneous.

Tables and graphs. Data should be correctly tabulated or drawn and adequately labelled for interpretation. Complete summaries of all the relevant findings should be presented.

Selection of statistics. Both descriptive and inferential statistics must be selected according to specific rules outlined in Sections 5 and 6. The selection of inappropriate statistics could distort the findings and lead to inappropriate inferences.

Calculation of statistics. Clearly, both descriptive

and inferential statistics must be correctly calculated. The use of computers generally ensures this, although some attention must be paid to gross errors when evaluating the data.

CRITICAL EVALUATION OF THE DISCUSSION

In the discussion, the investigator draws inferences from the data in relation to the initial aims or hypotheses of the investigation. Unless the inferences are correctly made, the conclusions drawn might lead to useless and dangerous treatments being offered to clients.

Drawing correct inferences from the data. The inferences from the data must take account of the limitations of descriptive and inferential statistics. We have seen, for instance in Chapter 16, that correlations do not necessarily imply causation, or that a lack of significance in the analysis could imply a Type II error (see Ch. 20).

Logically correct interpretations of the findings. Interpretations of the findings must follow from the statistical inferences, without extraneous evidence being introduced. For example, if the investigation used a $n = 1$ design, the conclusions should not claim that a procedure is generally useful.

Protocol deviations. In interpreting the data, the investigator must indicate, and take into account, unexpected deviations from the intended design. For example, a placebo/active treatment code might be broken, or 'contamination' between control and experimental groups might be discovered. If such deviations are discovered by investigators, they are obliged to report these, so that the implications for the results might be taken into account.

Generalization from the findings. Strictly speaking, the data obtained from a given sample are generalizable only to the population from which the sample was drawn. This point is sometimes ignored by investigators and the findings are generalized to subjects or situations that were not considered in the original sampling (see Ch. 3).

Statistical and clinical significance. As was explained in Chapter 20, statistical significance does not necessarily imply that the results of an investigation are clinically applicable. In deciding on clinical significance factors such as the size of the effect, side-effects and cost effectiveness, as well as value judgements concerning outcome, must be considered.

Theoretical significance. It is necessary to relate the results of an investigation to previous relevant findings which have been identified in the literature review. Unless, the results are logically related to the literature, the theoretical significance of the investigation remains unclear. The processes involved in comparing the findings of a set of related papers are introduced in the next subsection.

Table 22.1 summarizes some of the potential problems and their implications, which might emerge in the context-critical evaluation of an investigation. A point which must be kept in mind is that even where an investigation is flawed, useful knowledge might be drawn from it. The aim of critical analysis is not to discredit or tear down published work, but to ensure that the reader understands its implications and limitations with respect to theory and practice.

CRITICAL EVALUATION OF THE LITERATURE: META-ANALYSIS

By 'literature' we mean publications relevant to a specific area of science or clinical practice. Given the complexity of health care problems, it is unusual when the results of a single research publication are adequate for making clinical decisions.

As stated before, in preparing literature reviews and evaluating research findings, a multiplicity of papers must be considered, according to the following steps:

1. Identify relevant literature (see Section 2).
2. Evaluate critically the key papers, as discussed in this section. You might decide to discard some papers if irreparable problems are discovered.
3. Identify general patterns of findings in the literature. Tabulate findings.

Table 22.1 Checklist for evaluating published research

Problems which might be identified	Possible implications in a research article
1 Inadequate literature review	Misrepresentation of the conceptual basis for the research
2 Vague aims or hypothesis	Research might lack direction; interpretation of evidence might be ambiguous
3 Inappropriate research strategy	Findings might not be relevant to the problem being investigated
4 Inappropriate variables selected	Measurements might not be related to concepts being investigated
5 Inadequate sampling method	Sample might be biased, investigation could lack external validity
6 Inadequate sample size	Sample might be biased; statistical analysis might lack power
7 Inadequate description of sample	Application of findings to specific groups or individuals might be difficult
8 Instruments lack validity or reliability	Findings might represent measurement errors
9 Inadequate design	Investigation might lack internal validity; i.e. outcomes might be due to uncontrolled extraneous variables
10 Lack of adequate control groups	Investigation might lack internal validity; size of the effect difficult to estimate
11 Biased subject assignment	Investigation might lack internal validity
12 Variations or lack of control of treatment parameters	Investigation might lack internal validity
13 Observer bias not controlled (Rosenthal effects)	Investigation might lack internal and external validity
14 Subject expectations not controlled (Hawthorne effects)	Investigation might lack internal and external validity
15 Research carried out in inappropriate setting	Investigation might lack ecological validity
16 Confounding of times at which observations and treatments are carried out	Possible series effects; investigation might lack internal validity
17 Inadequate presentation of descriptive statistics	The nature of the empirical findings might not be comprehensible
18 Inappropriate statistics used to describe and/or analyze data	Distortion of decision process, false inferences might be drawn
19 Erroneous calculation of statistics	False inferences might be drawn
20 Drawing incorrect inferences from the data analysis (e.g. Type II error)	False conclusions might be made concerning the outcome of an investigation
21 Protocol deviations	Investigation might lack external or internal validity
22 Overgeneralisation of findings	External validity might be threatened
23 Confusing statistical and clinical significance	Treatments lacking clinical usefulness might be encouraged
24 Findings not logically related to previous research findings	Theoretical significance of the investigation remains doubtful

4. Identify crucial disagreements and controversies.
5. Propose valid explanations for the disagreements. Such explanations provide a theoretical framework for resolving controversies and proposing future research.

Dooley (1984) discussed the availability of two general types of strategies for summarizing research findings from multiple papers:

1. *Qualitative*. A qualitative review involves the selection of key features of related publications, such as designs, subject characteristics or measures used in the studies. These features are presented in a table form, such that differences in the features of the research can be related to outcomes.

2. *Quantitative*. A quantitative review calls for the condensation of the results from several papers into a single statistic. This statistic represents an average effect size.

These procedures are also related to meta-analyses, which are systematic procedures for summarizing the overall implications of a set of research papers.

There are advantages and disadvantages in these two review approaches, but discussion of the quantitative approach is beyond the scope of the present text. To illustrate the qualitative method, consider a set of four hypothetical studies reporting on levels of compliance by diabetics to insulin administration. The results and key

Table 22.2 Compliance with insulin use by diabetics (hypothetical reports)

Publication	Sample size	Average age of patients (years)	Method of measuring compliance	Percentage of patients compliant
Smith (1980)	50	55	Self-report	85
Jones (1981)	60	58	Self-report	82
Brown (1980)	50	59	Blood sugar level	40
Miller (1981)	55	56	Blood sugar level	35

features of these hypothetical studies are tabulated in Table 22.2.

Table 22.2 represents how findings from several publications might be tabulated. Key information about each study, as well as the outcomes, is presented in the table, enabling the emergence and demonstration of an overall pattern.

Unfortunately, in some reviews no clear pattern will emerge from the tabulated findings. Even when controlling for the quality of the individual publications, a conflict might emerge concerning the nature and causes of the findings. In the rather simple, hypothetical example above, the percentage of compliance reported by Smith (1980) and Jones (1981) is over twice that reported by Brown (1980) and Miller (1981). A possible explanation for this discrepancy might emerge by the inspection of Table 22.1. Clearly, neither differences in sample size nor the average ages of the patients suggest an explanation of the difference. However, the method by which compliance was measured emerges as a plausible explanation. The investigators, Smith and Jones, who relied on the patients' self-reports might have overestimated compliance levels, in contrast to Brown and Miller who used a more objective method. Of course, this explanation is not necessarily true, but is simply a hypothesis to guide future investigations of the problem.

One should not underestimate the difficulty of writing adequate literature reviews on the basis of the above simple illustrative example. Writing an adequate literature review should bring into play your knowledge of research design, measurement and statistics as well as your understanding of health science issues.

SUMMARY

The critical evaluation of published material at a level of detail suggested by this chapter is a time-consuming, even pedantic task. One undertakes such detailed analysis only when professional communications are of key importance, for example, when writing a formal literature review or when evaluating current evidence for adopting a new treatment. Nevertheless, it is a necessary process for an in-depth understanding of the empirical and theoretical basis of your clinical practice.

Even when problems are identified with a given research report, it is likely that the report will provide some useful empirical knowledge. Given the problems of generalization, an individual research project is usually insufficient for deciding on the truth of a hypothesis or the usefulness of a clinical intervention. Rather, the reader needs to scrutinize the range of relevant research and summarize the evidence using qualitative and quantitative review methods. In this way, individual research results can be evaluated in the context of the research area. Disagreements or controversies are ultimately useful for generating hypotheses for guiding new research and for advancing theory and practice.

SELF ASSESSMENT

Explain the meaning of the following terms:

> critical evaluation
> meta-analysis
> protocol deviation
> qualitative review
> quantitative review

TRUE OR FALSE

1. Critical analysis of a publication aims to identify the internal and external validity of the investigation.
2. If an investigation is published in a reputable journal by established investigators then the validity of the investigation can be taken for granted.
3. Random assignment of subjects to treatment groups ensures that the investigation uncovers casual effects.
4. The outcome of an investigation can be useful even with a small sample size.
5. If an investigation produces statistically significant results, its design must have been adequate.
6. Obtaining statistical significance in an investigation is a condition for the demonstration of the clinical significance of a quantitative study.
7. The replication of an investigation demonstrates the internal validity of the original investigation.
8. Without adequate controls the size of an effect might be difficult to estimate.
9. If a study is internally valid, the investigator is justified in generalizing the results to any other population.
10. Provided that the outcomes are statistically significant, it does not matter which statistical tests were chosen to analyze the data.
11. If the design of an investigation is inadequate, none of the empirical findings are of scientific or clinical use.
12. Controversies in an area of science usually reflect the presence of fraudulently published evidence.
13. One of the problems with using human subjects for research is the expectations of the subjects concerning the purpose of the investigation.
14. Even poorly planned research can provide some useful results.
15. The application of the scientific method ensures the validity of a researcher's conclusions.
16. Disagreements among researchers in an area are useful for generating new hypotheses.
17. A qualitative research review is useful for generating hypotheses concerning trends in the literature.
18. A quantitative research review is useful for estimating effect sizes.
19. To understand a clinical phenomenon we should review the range of relevant research findings.

MULTIPLE CHOICE

1. The aim of the critical analysis of a publication is to:

   a identify the relevance of the results for clinical practice
   b identify the internal and external validity of the investigation
   c identify and attack incompetent researchers in one's area of interest
   d a and b.

2. If the internal validity of a study is adequate, then:

   a the results will be statistically significant
   b the results will be clinically useful
   c the investigation may demonstrate casual effects
   d a and b.

3. Say that an investigation has generated some interesting findings. However, you

SELF ASSESSMENT

find that the investigators selected an inappropriate statistical test to analyze their findings. You should:

a regretfully discard the study as useless
b re-analyze the data from the descriptive statistics provided
c write to the investigators for their raw data, and re-analyze it yourself
d b or c.

4. The reason one should evaluate the 'literature' as a whole is to:

a identify general patterns of findings in the area
b condense results from related papers into a single statistic
c identify and attempt to explain controversies in the area
d all of the above.

5. In judging the clinical significance of a well-designed investigation one should consider:

a the cost effectiveness of the interventions
b the size of the therapeutic effects
c the possible undesirable side effects of the treatment
d a, b and c.

An investigation was carried out in order to show that 'prepared childbirth' was an effective method for reducing pain during delivery. A total of 90 women attending a large hospital constituted the sample. 60 of the women chose to participate in childbirth preparation, based on the Lamaze method, provided by trained instructors working at the hospital. This method encourages 'natural' (drug free) childbirth through teaching physical and mental strategies for coping with pain or discomfort occurring during childbirth. The other 30 women chose not to attend the childbirth preparation programme. The level of

pain experienced was assessed on the McGill pain questionnaire, which has been shown to be a valid and reliable interval scale for pain. It was administered following the childbirth. In addition the number of women seeking analgesia during childbirth was recorded as a measure of levels of discomfort experienced. The results for the investigation are as follows:

Groups	Mean pain scores
Women with no training ($n = 30$)	38
Women with childbirth preparation ($n = 60$) (The difference was statistically significant at $\alpha = 0.05$)	32

	Number given medication
Women with no training ($n = 30$)	24
Women with childbirth preparation ($n = 60$) The difference was not statistically significant at $\alpha = 0.05$	49

Questions 6–14 refer to the above investigation.

6. The strategy for the investigation is best described as:

a an experiment
b a quasi-experiment
c a correlational study
d an $n = 90$ design.

7. One of the problems with the above investigation was that:

a the subjects could not be randomly assigned to treatment groups *b* the dependent variable was irrelevant to the aims

c basic ethical issues were not considered

d the instructors teaching the Lamaze method were incompetent.

8. From the information given above, it is clear that the investigators controlled for:

a Hawthorne effect

b Rosenthal effects

c subject assignment

d none of the above.

9. If you wanted to calculate the proportion of women with no training who had greater McGill pain scores than women with childbirth preparation, then the required statistics are:

a the distribution of t for $n = 98$

b the normal distribution

c the indicies for reliability and validity

d the standard deviations for the two groups.

10. Which of the following statistical tests is most appropriate for analyzing the significance of the data for the McGill pain scores?

a Mann–Whitney U

b sign test

c z test for two means

d χ^2 test.

11. Which of the following statistical tests is most appropriate for analyzing the significance of the data for women requiring medication?

a Mann–Whitney U

b sign test

c t test for two means

d χ^2 test.

12. The lack of statistical significance for the data on medication implies that:

a the power for the test may have been too low

b equal sample sizes should have been used

c training has no effect

d both *a* and *c*.

13. The outcome of this investigation can be generalized to:

a women having children and undergoing Lamaze training

b women having children without Lamaze training

c women who chose the type of childbirth they undergo

d none of the above groups.

14. Considering the evidence provided, one concludes that:

a prepared childbirth is a waste of time

b there is evidence that Lamaze preparation at this hospital results in statistically significant reductions in pain during delivery

c that women undergoing childbirth find Lamaze preparation useless at this hospital

d *a* and *c*.

A decision is to be made concerning whether Treatment x or Treatment y is to be used to treat seriously ill cancer patients in a hospital. There are three published studies in the area, comparing the proportion of clients surviving up to 5 years with the treatments.

The results for the three hypothetical studies are:

SELF ASSESSMENT

		Number surviving	Number not surviving	Outcome
Study A				
Treatment *x*	$n = 10$	5	5	Not significant $a = 0.01$
Treatment *y*	$n = 15$	5	10	
Study B				
Placebo control	$n = 100$	20	80	Significant at $a = 0.01$
Treatment *y*	$n = 100$	40	60	
Study C				
Treatment *x*	$n = 50$	40	10	Significant at $a = 0.01$
Treatment *y*	$n = 60$	30	30	

Questions 15–18 refer to the above information.

15. Which of the following statements is true on the basis of the above?

    a Study C must be fraudulent
    b Study A is more powerful than Study B
    c In Study A, subjects must have been assigned on the basis of matching
    d χ^2 test was appropriate for analyzing the results.

16. Which of the above statements is false?

    a Treatment *y* appears more effective than placebo treatment
    b The scale of measurements used for the dependent variables was nominal in the three studies
    c None of the three studies controlled for the effects of 'history'
    d In Study A, 33.3% of patients followed Treatment *y*.

17. In Study A, 50% of patients survived for 5 years, following Treatment *x*, while in Study C, 80% of patients survived

following the same treatment. Which of the following is a possible explanation?

    a The therapists in Study C were more effective in carrying out the treatment
    b There is a random sampling error
    c Either *a* or *b* is a possible explanation
    d Neither *a* nor *b* is a possible explanation.

18. On the basis of the combined results of the three studies what is the approximate probability that a client will survive for over 5 years following Treatment *y*?

    a less than 0.33
    b between 0.3 and 0.4
    c between 0.33 and 0.5
    d 0.5 or more.

19. On the basis of the evidence provided by the above three studies, one should adopt for the treatment of patients:

    a Treatment *x*
    b Treatment *y*
    c Neither Treatment *x* nor Treatment *y*
    d the least expensive treatment.

SECTION 7

Discussion, Questions and Answers

This question is based on a survey which was published in an Australian newspaper. Of course, such surveys do not represent research published in scientific journals, but they are important sources for public knowledge or/and attitudes towards health sciences issues. The survey questioned a sample of adults concerning their smoking habits. Only one of the questions asked is discussed here and the results are hypothetical.

Survey characteristics

Sample:	1000 voters
Coverage:	Australia wide
Method:	Telephone
Question:	Do you smoke? (Yes or No)

Results

Percentage of replies to the question in two major cities:

	Melbourne	Sydney
Yes	24	18
No	76	82

Questions

The following questions involve the critical analysis of the above survey.

1. If we assume that cigarette smoking is now a 'stigmatized' behaviour, do you think the telephone survey produced valid answers?
2. A total of 180 people were interviewed in Melbourne and 220 in Sydney. If the population of Australia is 17 million and the populations of Melbourne and Sydney are 2.5 and 3.2 million respectively, do the samples appear to be quota samples?

3. Which categories of smokers may not have been reached by this survey? What implications might this have for the external validity of the survey?
4. A journalist commented on the results, saying: 'This difference is ironic, given that anti-smoking lobbyists have applauded Melbourne as a pacesetter for smoking law reform, such as tobacco tax-funded health promotion'.
   (a) Explain why this comment is inappropriate given the design of the survey?
   (b) What research design would be appropriate to show a causal effect on smoking due to health promotion on smoking? (Hint: see Ch. 6).
5. Explain why the comment quoted in question 4 is inappropriate, given that the statistical significance of the results was not calculated.
6. Which statistical test should be used to analyze the significance of the results concerning differences in smoking between the two cities? Justify your selection.
7. Setting $\alpha = 0.05$, calculate the statistic and decide if the results were significant (note that we gave the results in percentages).
8. Do you think the sample size ($n = 1000$) was adequate? Explain.

Answers

1. Although telephone interviews and mailed out questionnaires are a relatively cost-efficient strategy for collecting data, we have problems validating the responses. This is particularly true for conditions and behaviours which are socially stigmatized; why should the respondent disclose such information about themselves? In face-to-face interviews, we can explore issues; for example, if the respondents have nicotine-

Discussion, Questions and Answers

stained fingers or smell of cigarettes, we may pursue the issue further to establish the accuracy of the replies.

2. Given that $n = 1000$, 18% of the respondents were from Melbourne and 22% from Sydney. For a quota sample, the expected samples would be:

$$\text{Melbourne:} \frac{2.5}{17} \times 100 = 14.7\%$$

and

$$\text{Sydney:} \frac{3.2}{17} \times 100 = 18.8\%$$

Assuming that the information used to calculate the above figures is correct, it seems that the sample included more respondents from Melbourne. This may reflect the different proportion of 'voters' in the two cities, or a rather poor quota sample.

3. People who are not on the electoral roll, such as persons under 18 years of age, and people who do not have, or do not answer their telephones, would not have been contacted. In this way, the sample may not be representative of all the smokers in the city (e.g. young people, poor or itinerant people, people with unlisted telephone numbers). In this way, the survey may not be externally valid if we generalize to all persons in Australia who smoke.

4. The present surveys did not tell us how rates of smoking have changed over a period of time. We may use a quasi-experimental design and introduce the programme in one city (A) but not in the other equivalent city (B). If the reduction is greater over time in A than in B, we may argue that this difference could reflect the causal effect of health promotion.

5. Although results for the samples show a difference between the two cities, this may simply reflect sampling error. We must establish the significance of the results before we can draw inferences ('ironic' or

otherwise) about populations.

6. χ^2; nominal data and independent measurements or samples.

7. Convert the data into frequencies (see Ch. 19) before entering obtained values into a 2 × 2 contingency table (values rounded to closest whole number).

	Melbourne	Sydney	Total
Smokers	43	40	83
	Cell 1	Cell 2	
Non-smokers	137	180	317
	Cell 3	Cell 4	
Total	180	220	400

Expected values: (for calculation procedure, see Ch. 19)

$$f_e \text{ (cell 1)} = \frac{83 \times 180}{400} = 37.4$$

$$f_e \text{ (cell 2)} = \frac{83 \times 220}{400} = 45.7$$

$$f_e \text{ (cell 3)} = \frac{317 \times 180}{400} = 142.6$$

$$f_e \text{ (cell 4)} = \frac{317 \times 220}{400} = 174.3$$

Calculation of χ^2

Cell	f_o	f_e	$(f_o - f_e)^2$	$\dfrac{(f_o - f_e)^2}{f_e}$
1	43	37.4	31.36	0.84
2	40	45.7	32.49	0.71
3	137	142.6	31.36	0.22
4	180	174.3	32.49	0.19

$$\chi^2{}_{obt} = \Sigma \frac{(f_o - f_e)^2}{f_e} = 1.96$$

Critical value of χ^2; $\alpha = 0.05$ where (degrees of freedom) = 1 (Appendix C)

$$\chi^2{}_{crit} = 3.84$$

Discussion, Questions and Answers

In this case we would retain H_0: there is no association between the variables 'city' (M or S) and smoking (Yes or No). (For details of decision making process, refer to Chapter 19).

It is apparent that the results are not significant, therefore we are not justified in drawing any inferences concerning the different proportions of smokers in Melbourne and Sydney.

8. Although a sample size of $n = 1000$ appears quite large, this was an Australia wide sample which was divided up to represent regions.

It is possible that the null results obtained in question 7 are because there are no differences in smoking rates between the two cities, but there are other possibilities (see Ch. 20). Perhaps the sample size was inadequate and we made a Type II error in our decision. Replicating the study with larger sample sizes might enable us to show significant differences in smoking rates.

SECTION 8

Glossary of research terms

AB design   A type of experimental design in which the participant is monitored during a baseline phase followed by an intervention phase.

ABAB design   A type of experimental design in which the participant is monitored during a baseline phase followed by an intervention phase which, in turn, is followed by further baseline and intervention phases.

Abstract   An abbreviated summary of a research report, generally found at the beginning of the report.

Acquiescent response mode   A style of answering questions which results in the respondent choosing the middle category in a response scale.

Alternative hypothesis   Sometimes also known as the experimental hypothesis. This is the hypothesis for which the researcher is trying to gain support in a statistical analysis, by rejecting the null hypothesis. The alternative hypothesis is represented by the symbol H_A or H_1.

Apparatus   Any equipment or special facilities used in a research project.

Area sample   A type of sampling procedure in which the units of the sample are where people live or work, rather than who they are. The researcher divides the target area into sections and then samples the sections.

Assignment   The process in an experiment where the researcher allocates subjects to the various groups. Matching and random assignment are the two most common methods. The goal of assignment is to achieve identical groups.

Assignment errors   A situation that arises in an experiment where the assignment or allocation of people to groups results in groups with different characteristics.

Authority   An appeal to authority argument is based on the proposition that someone of high status knows best, not whether the argument is soundly based.

Bar graph   A method of displaying data where the frequency of a particular category is reflected in the height of the bar in the graph.

Baseline   A phase in an intervention study where the participant is receiving no intervention.

Bell shaped curve   This is the characteristic shape of the normal distribution.

Bias   In a questionnaire, bias is introduced by inappropriately framed questions, such as leading questions.

Biased sample   A biased sample is one that is not representative. It does not reflect the composition of the population to which the researcher is attempting to generalize.

Causal explanation   An attempt to explain the occurrence of a particular phenomenon or event by identifying the cause(s).

Causality   An event or factor (A) is generally argued to have caused another one (B) if the following conditions are met: (i) if (A) occurs then (B) occurs; (ii) if (A) does not occur then (B) does not occur; (iii) if (A) precedes (B) in time.

Central tendency   The central tendency of a frequency distribution is the average, middle or most common score. Measures of central tendency include the mean, the median and the mode.

Chi-square (χ^2)   A statistical test often used with categorical data. It is based on a comparison of the frequencies observed and the frequencies expected in the various categories.

Clinical significance   The clinical significance of a research finding is the extent to which that finding is clinically meaningful.

Closed response format   A method of eliciting answers from people in a questionnaire in which the researcher provides fixed response categories, e.g. yes or no.

Coding   A qualitative method of analysis of materials such as interviews where categories are formed and their interrelationships examined.

Complete observer   A type of research strategy in which the researcher observes social interactions with no direct personal input; for example, observation via a one-way mirror or through the analysis of a video tape.

Complete participant   A research strategy in which the researcher completely participates in the research setting in order to experience its characteristics.

Confidence interval   The confidence interval of a sample statistic is the expected range in which the actual population value will be found, at a given level of confidence or probability.

Content validity   The extent to which a test or assessment matches the real requirements of the situation e.g. a living skills assessment would have high content validity if it measured cooking, self care, etc.

Contingency table   A method of presenting the relationship between two categorical variables in the form of a table.

Continuous data   Data with values that do not fall into discrete categories. For example, measures of temperature and mass.

Control   In an experiment, the researcher attempts to control or eliminate the influence of extraneous variables so that any changes or differences may be attributed solely to the intervention.

Control group   In an experiment, a control group is generally a non-treatment group which is compared with the experimental group to study the effects of the intervention.

Correlation coefficient   A statistic designed to measure the size and direction of the association between two variables. The values vary between 0 and ± 1.

Correlational studies   Studies that are concerned with investigating the associations between variables.

Critical theory   In qualitative research, critical theory explains how personal meanings and actions are influenced by the person's social environment.

Critical value of a statistic   The value of the statistic (obtained from appropriate tables) that the calculated value for a given result must exceed, in order to attain statistical significance.

Curvilinear correlation coefficient   A measure of association between variables designed to investigate curved rather than straight-line relationships.

Data   The information collected by a researcher.

Deduction   A process where a general principle is applied to a particular case to explain it, e.g. all humans die; this is a human, therefore they will die.

Descriptive statistics   Statistics designed to describe characteristics of a sample. For example, the most common or typical value or the extent of variation among such values.

Determinism   The view that all events are caused by other events.

Directional hypothesis   A directional hypothesis is one that asserts that differences between groups in the data will occur in a particular direction. For example, the hypothesis 'smokers die younger than non-smokers' is a directional hypothesis.

Discontinuous data   Sometimes termed discrete data; variables that have discrete categories, for example male versus female.

Discussion   A section of a research report in which the research findings are discussed.

Dispersion   Sometimes known as variability; the extent to which scores in a group of scores vary. This may be measured by statistics such as the standard deviation, variance, range and semi-interquartile range.

Ecological validity   The extent to which the results of a study may be generalized to the real world.

Effect size   The amount of change created by an intervention, especially in an experimental study.

Empathy   In qualitative research, the ability to understand the perspectives of others.

Epidemiology   The study of the distribution and determinants of disease within a community.

Ethics   A project is ethical to the extent that its design and execution conforms to a set of standards or conventions guiding research.

Ethnography   A descriptive qualitative study, often of an individual or situation, usually written from the perspective of the participant(s) in the first person.

Ethnomethodology   A qualitative approach to research which involves the study of social processes associated with the ways in which people perceive, describe and explain the world.

Expected frequency   In the analysis of categorical data, the expected frequency is the one that would be expected in a particular category, under certain theoretical conditions. The expected frequency of women in a sample of 100 people would be 50, if equal proportions of sexes were assumed.

Experiment   A research design involving the random allocation of subjects to groups and the application of different interventions to these groups. A non-intervention control group is often employed in an experimental design. The aim of an experiment is to be able to conclude validly that differences in outcomes for the groups were caused by the different interventions.

External validity   The extent to which the results of the study may be generalized to the population.

Extreme response mode   A method of responding to questions in which the respondent chooses the most extreme available response categories.

Factorial design   A type of research design in which combinations of several independent variables are manipulated concurrently. A 2×2 factorial design involves the manipulation of two independent variables each with two levels.

False negative   The situation that occurs when a diagnostic test indicates that the person being assessed does not have a disease when they actually do.

False positive   The situation that occurs when a diagnostic test indicates the person being assessed has a disease when they do not.

Forced response format   A method of eliciting responses to a questionnaire in which there is no middle response category. This is sometimes done to avoid acquiescent response mode.

Frequency distribution   The way in which scores within a given sample or population are distributed.

Frequency polygon   A method of graphing frequency distributions.

Grounded theory   A qualitative research approach that advocates the development of theories to explain social phenomena grounded in data, following a process of induction, deduction and verification.

Hawthorne effect   An effect which results in the improvement of subjects performances through being observed and/or social contact. An example of a placebo effect.

Histogram   A method of graphing frequency distributions.

History   A threat to the validity of studies in which unforeseen and uncontrolled events occur to the participants during the study that are outside the control of the researcher and which may be responsible for changes in the participants.

Hypothesis   A proposition advanced by the researcher which is evaluated using the data collected.

Incidence rate   The occurrence of new cases of a disease or condition within a specified time frame. See also *prevalence*.

Incidental sample   A method of sampling in which the researcher takes the most conveniently available cases.

Independent variable   In an experiment an independent variable is the variable or condition manipulated by the researcher.

Induction   The process in which a set of observations is made and a general principle formed to explain them. For example, 'every human I have read about eventually dies; this is a human; therefore I expect them to die'.

Informed consent   The situation where a competent person, in possession of all the relevant facts, has agreed to participate in a research study.

Instrumentation   In a study, instrumentation may be a threat to internal validity. It refers to the situation when the instrumentation changes over the period of the study, thus invalidating comparison of measured results.

Internal validity   In a study, internal validity refers to the ability of the researcher to attribute differences in the groups or participants to the independent variable.

Interobserver reliability   The extent to which observers rating a particular phenomenon agree with each other.

Interrupted time series   A type of research design in which a case is repeatedly measured over time to produce a series of measurements. The series is interrupted by an intervention or event, the effects of which may then be monitored by continuing the measurement series.

Interval scale   A type of measurement scale with the following properties: (i) the values are distinguishable, (ii) they are ordered, (iii) the intervals between the points on the scale are equal, (iv) the zero point is not absolute, i.e. does not represent the absence of the quantity.

Interview   A conversation between one or more interviewers and interviewees with the purpose of eliciting certain information.

Intraobserver reliability   The extent to which an observer rating a particular phenomenon agrees with their own rating when presented with the same task on two different occasions.

Likert scale   A five-point response scale used in questionnaires, e.g. strongly agree, agree, undecided, disagree, strongly disagree.

Literature review   This is a section of a research report in which the previous research that has been done in the area is reviewed and related to the present problem being studied.

Matching   In a study, subjects may be assigned to their groups using matching or random assignment. In matching in a two-group study, pairs of similar 'matched' subjects are formed and then one member of the pair is randomly assigned to one group and the other member to the other group. This ensures that the two groups have similar characteristics.

Maturation   The phenomenon where participants in a study change spontaneously over time due to natural maturational changes. For example, children may grow older or an infection may spontaneously clear up.

Mean   The average of a group of scores. For example, the mean of the scores 7, 8 and 9 is $(7 + 8 + 9) \div 3 = 8$. In statistical notation the mean of a sample is represented by the symbol $\bar{X}$. The mean of a population is represented by the symbol μ.

Measurement   A procedure where qualities or quantities are attributed to characteristics of objects, persons or events. Weighing a patient involves a measurement process, as does a clinical judgment about whether a symptom is present or not.

Median   The 'middle' score of a group of scores. For example, the median of the scores, 7, 8 and 9 is 8. The median is the 50 percentile. The median is often used in preference to the mean when a group of scores contains a small number of extremely small or large scores because it is less sensitive to extreme values.

Mode   The mode is the most frequently occurring score in a group of scores. For example, the mode of the scores 7, 8, 8, 9, 10 is 8.

Mortality   Used to describe a situation where some participants in a study are unable to continue in a study. This might be because they died or because they refuse to continue. If there is high mortality in a group in a study this can jeopardize the internal validity of the study, because differences between the groups may be caused by differential mortality.

Multiple group time series   A type of research design where two groups or cases are repeatedly measured over time to produce a series of measurements. One group or case receives an intervention and the other does not. The effects of intervention may then be studied by comparing the two series.

n   The symbol used to represent the number of cases in a sample.

N   The symbol used to represent the number of cases in a population.

n **= 1 design**   A research design in which one subject rather than a group of subjects is studied.

Natural comparison study   A type of study in which naturally occurring groups are compared with one another. For example, the health status of smokers versus non-smokers may be studied in a natural comparison study. The researcher does not assign the participants to the groups. These are naturally occurring. Studies of gender differences are natural comparisons.

Natural setting   The normal setting of the phenomenon or people under study. Studies performed under laboratory conditions may sometimes have diminished external validity.

Negative correlation   A correlation is a measure of the strength and direction of the association between two variables. A negative correlation between two variables implies that as one variable gets bigger the value of the other variable becomes smaller.

Negative skew   A frequency distribution where there is a long tail towards the negative end of the *x*-axis. The figure below represents both positively and negatively skewed samples.

The position of 'tail' of the distribution determines whether the skew is positive or negative.

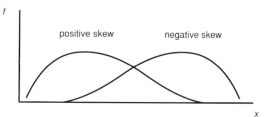

Nominal scale   Measurement scales may be either nominal, ordinal, interval or ratio. A nominal scale (often called a categorical scale) is one in which the values are distinct categories, e.g. male or female, Catholic or Protestant or Jewish or Muslim. It has the property of distinctiveness of values, but not ordering, equidistant intervals or an absolute zero.

Non-directional hypothesis   This asserts that there are differences between groups in the data but with no direction specified. For example, the hypothesis 'smokers and non-smokers have different life expectancies' is a non-directional hypothesis.

Non-experimental study   A study in which the researcher observes a situation but does not systematically manipulate or experiment with it. This may also be called a descriptive design.

Non-parametric test   Statistical tests are chosen on the basis of the type of scales that are being analyzed. Tests that are suitable for the analysis of ordinal or nominal data are termed non-parametric.

Normal curve   A bell-shaped curve as shown in the figure below.

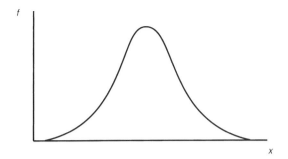

The normal curve is symmetrical and unimodal (has one peak).

Null hypothesis   The hypothesis in a study that asserts there is no difference between groups or relationship between variables. The statistician normally poses the null hypothesis and then tests it statistically. If it is rejected, the alternative hypothesis (that there is a difference between two groups or a relationship between variables) is accepted. The null hypothesis is represented by the symbol H_0.

Objective measures   Measures derived from a mechanical measuring process involving a minimum amount of human interpretation, e.g. weight measurements.

Observation   A situation where the researcher studies the phenomenon without deliberate intervention.

Observed frequency   The actual number of occurrences of an event observed by a researcher. For example, the observed frequency of females who passed the exam in a group of students might be 37 students. See also *expected frequency*.

Observer as participant   Where the researcher studies the behaviour of a group by actively participating in the group's activities and situation.

One-tailed test   A statistical test where a difference between two groups is expected to occur in a particular direction. For example, it may be hypothesized that smokers will have more health problems than non-smokers. This would be tested by applying a one-tailed test of significance.

Open-ended question   If a question is asked without a pre-defined set of responses it is an open-ended question. For example, the question, 'What did you think about the program?' is an open-ended question.

Operational definition   The specific way in which a concept or variable has been measured in a study. For example, the operational definition of anxiety in a study might be scores from the Spielberger State–Trait Anxiety Inventory scores or a self rating on a 1 to 10 scale.

Ordinal scale   Measurement scales may be either nominal, ordinal, interval or ratio. An ordinal scale has the following properties: (i) the values are distinguishable, (ii) they are ordered but the intervals between the points are not equidistant nor is there a meaningful zero point scale. The values of an ordinal scale are often ranked, e.g. 1st, 3rd.

Parametric test   Statistical tests are chosen on the basis of the type of data being analyzed. Statistical tests that are suitable for the analysis of interval or ratio data are termed parametric.

Participation   A situation where the researcher studies the phenomenon by actively participating.

Percentile   The position of a score on a frequency distribution expressed in standard score units such that the 50 percentile is the median and all scores fall below the 100 percentile.

Phenomenology   In qualitative research, the study and understanding of human conscious experience.

Pie diagram   A graphical method of representing the frequency distribution of a set of categorical data in the shape of a pie.

Pilot study   A preliminary study where the procedures and protocols are tested or 'piloted'.

Placebo effect   The phenomenon where an otherwise worthless intervention in a study nevertheless induces an improvement in the patient's condition or perception of their condition, perhaps due to the expectations of the participants in the study.

Population   A group of people, institutions, cases or objects defined as that under study by the researcher. Samples are drawn from populations. Examples of populations are all coronary heart disease cases in the UK, all Australian men, all 'not for profit' hospitals in Canada.

Population parameter   A value derived from a population. For example, the average age of all the patients in a population defined by the researcher is a population parameter. In statistical notation, population parameters are represented by Greek letters.

Population validity   The extent to which a sample reflects the characteristics of a population from which it is drawn.

Positive correlation   A correlation is a measure of the strength and direction of the association between two variables. A positive correlation between two variables implies that as the values of one variable get bigger, so do the values of the other variable.

Positive skew   A frequency distribution where there is a long tail towards the positive end of the x-axis.

Post-test only design   A type of experimental study in which measurements of the groups are taken only after an intervention has occurred. This is generally done to avoid the effects of measurement upon people's response to the interventions.

Power   The probability of rejecting the null hypothesis when the alternative hypothesis is true, i.e. correctly identifying an effect when it is there.

Pre-test/post-test design   A type of experimental study in which measurements of the groups are taken both prior to and following an intervention. This allows the direct comparison of pre-intervention and post-intervention results for individual subjects and groups of subjects.

Predictive validity   The extent to which a test or measure can validly predict a future event. For example, a clinical test may have high predictive validity with respect to 5-year mortality of people with cancer. It is often expressed in the form of a correlation coefficient.

Prevalence   The overall occurrence of a particular disease in a specific population at a specific point in time.

Probability   The chance or likelihood of an event. The probability of flipping a 'heads' with a fair coin is 0.5 or 1/2. Probabilities may vary in value from 0 ('no chance') to 1 (certain).

Procedure   A section in a research report that describes the protocol or procedure followed for the collection of data.

Proportion   The ratio of one value to another expressed as a fraction of one. For example, the proportion of women in the adult population is about 0.5.

Protocol deviation   A deviation from the ideal procedure described as having been followed in a study by the researcher.

Qualitative methods   An approach to research that emphasizes the non-numerical and interpretive analysis of social phenomena.

Quantitative methods   An approach to research that emphasizes the collection of numerical data and the statistical analysis of hypotheses proposed by the researcher.

Quasi experimental design   A structured research design that is experiment-like but does not involve its full characteristics such as a control group and random assignment of subjects to treatment groups.

Questionnaire   A means of collecting data from people where they provide written responses to a set of questions, either in their own words, or by selecting pre-defined answers.

Quota sample   The result of a sampling procedure in which the researcher sets quotas for the number of cases in particular categories to be included in the sample. For example, a sample of 100 might have quotas of 50 men and 50 women. The cases, however, are still selected on the basis of convenience rather than randomly. See also *stratified random sample*.

Random assignment   In an experiment, subjects are assigned to their groups by using a random assignment method. In random assignment, subjects are assigned to their groups using a random procedure. For example, in a two-group study the tossing of a coin to assign subjects to groups would be a random assignment procedure.

Random sample   A group of cases drawn from a population such that each member of the population has had an equal chance of selection.

Random sampling   The process of selecting cases from a population such that each member of the population has had an equal chance of selection.

Range   In a group of scores the range is the difference between the maximum and minimum scores.

Ratio scale   Measurement scales may be either nominal, ordinal, interval or ratio. A ratio scale has the following properties: the values are distinctive, ordered, equidistant and the zero point represents an absence of the quantity rather than being an arbitrary zero. Metres and kilograms are examples of ratio scales.

Refereed journal   A journal in which the articles are vetted by independent referees for quality and interest. Refereed journals generally carry more highly regarded articles.

Regression to the mean   The phenomenon where an individual who is measured on a test and obtains an extreme (very high or low) score and then upon remeasurement tends to move towards (regress) the average score (mean). Regression to the mean may be misinterpreted as representing a real change in score.

Relationships   Associations between variables.

Reliability   The extent to which a test or measurement result is reproducible.

Repeated measures   The situation where a group of cases are measured on more than one occasion, for example prior to and following an intervention.

Representative sample   A sample that accurately reflects the characteristics of the population from which it is drawn. Sometimes termed an 'unbiased' sample.

Reversal   Reversal of the order of interventions is often used in experimental studies to control for the effects of order of administration. For example, intervention B, preceded by intervention A may have a different effect than B followed by A.

Risk factors   In epidemiology, a risk factor is an agent that is believed to increase the probability of a certain outcome or illness. For example, smoking may be a risk factor for the onset of coronary heart disease.

Rosenthal effect   The phenomenon where the expectations of the researchers in a study influence the outcome. For example, if an observer believes that a particular intervention is effective they may under-report or discount symptoms inconsistent with this belief.

Sample   A group of cases selected from a population.

Sampling error   Because a sample is smaller than the population from which it is drawn, there is often a discrepancy between the values obtained for the sample and those that apply to the population. For example, the average age of a sample might be 22 years and the average age of the population might be 28 years. This discrepancy is termed the sampling error.

Sampling method   The method by which a sample is drawn from a population. Broadly, there are two approaches: random, in which every case in the population has an equal chance of selection and non-random in which cases have different chances of selection.

Scattergram   A graph displaying the relationship between two variables as shown in the following figure:

Semi interquartile range   A measure of the spread of a frequency distribution, being the distance between the first and third quartiles.

Sensitivity   The proportion of people who test as positive to a disease who really do have the disease. See also *true positive*.

Shared variance   In the examination of relationships between variables, researchers are concerned about the extent to which when one variable changes the other also changes. Shared variance refers to the extent to which this occurs.

Skewness   A characteristic of the shape of a frequency distribution. See also *negative skew*.

Specificity   The proportion of people who test negative to a disease who really do not have the disease. See also *true negative*.

Standard deviation   A measure of the dispersion or variability of a group of scores. The standard deviation of a sample is represented by the symbol s and by the symbol σ for a population.

Standard error of the mean   If a number of samples were taken from the same population and the mean calculated for each sample, the standard deviation of this distribution of means is known as the standard error of the mean. The standard error of the mean is used in statistical inferences about population means.

Standard normal curve   An idealized normal or bell-shaped frequency distribution with a mean of 0 and a standard deviation of 1 unit.

Standardized test   A standardized test is one that has known characteristics, especially known levels of reliability and validity. Researchers use standardized tests, wherever possible, in preference to unstandardized tests.

Statistic   A statistic is a number with known properties derived from sample data. There are two types of statistics: inferential statistics which are used to apply statistical tests, and descriptive statistics which are used to describe characteristics of the sample.

Statistical significance   When a researcher has demonstrated statistical significance through the application of a statistical test, they have demonstrated that the result obtained is probably not due to chance but is 'real'. This does not mean the result is important or interesting. See also *clinical significance*.

Stratified random sample   A type of sample in which the researcher wishes to ensure that important subgroups and their representation are preserved in the sample. For example, if a researcher randomly selected a subsample of 50 men and then 50 women, the sample has been stratified with respect to gender. See also *quota sample*.

Structured interview   An interview in which the questions are generally predefined, i.e. asked in a fixed order with the answers recorded by the researcher on a response sheet.

Subjective measures   Measures derived from a measurement process involving a substantial degree of human interpretation, e.g. subjective ratings of pain, clinical ratings of social skills.

Subjects   Participants in a study.

Surveys   A type of research design in which characteristics of the cases under study are systematically recorded without the researcher attempting to actively change the situation. A non-experimental type of study.

Systematic sample   A method of drawing a sample from a population where, for example, every 10th case is selected from a population list.

Test–retest reliability   When a test or assessment procedure is administered twice to the same group of people, the correlation between the first score and the second score is termed the test–retest reliability. This is a measure of the reproducibility of an assessment procedure.

Time series   A series of measurements taken repeatedly from the same person or group of people, over time.

Transcript   A verbatim written version of an interview.

Transformed score   A score that has been altered by an arithmetic manipulation, such as a z score.

True negative   The situation that occurs when a diagnostic test indicates the person being assessed does have a disease when in fact they do not.

True positive   The situation that occurs when a diagnostic test indicates the person being assessed does have a disease when they do.

Two tailed test   A statistical test where a difference between two groups is tested without reference to the expected direction of the difference.

Type I error   When a researcher, on the basis of a statistical test applied to a sample of data, wrongly concludes that there is evidence of an association between variables or difference between groups in the population, they have committed a Type I error. The probability of a Type I error is represented by the symbol α.

Type II error   A 'miss'. When a researcher, on the basis of a statistical test applied to a sample of data, wrongly concludes that there is no evidence of an association between variables or difference between groups in the population, they have committed a Type II error. The probability of a Type II error is represented by the symbol β.

Unstructured interview An interview in which there may be no preplanned questions or fixed agenda. The dialogue is usually recorded in a transcript or field notes which are subsequently analyzed.

Validity The extent to which a test measures what it is intended to measure.

Variability The extent to which a group of scores varies or is spread out. This is usually measured by a descriptive statistic such as the standard deviation range or semi-interquartile range.

Variable A property or attribute that varies. For example, gender, age, weight are all variables.

Variance A measure of the dispersion or variability of a group of scores. The variance of a sample is represented by the symbol s^2 and the symbol σ^2 for a population. See also *standard deviation*.

z scores Transformed scores which express how many standard deviations a specific score is above or below the mean. For instance, a corresponding z score of -2 implies that a given score is two standard deviations below the mean.

Zero correlation Correlation is used to measure the strength and direction of an association between two variables. A zero correlation implies that two variables are unrelated to one another.

References and further reading

REFERENCES

Anastasi A 1976 Psychological testing, 4th edn. Macmillan, New York

Bailey K D 1987 Methods of social research. Free Press, New York

Beecher H K 1959 Measurement of subjective responses. Oxford University Press, Oxford

Bloch R 1987 Methodology in clinical pain trials. Spine 12: 430–432

Bogdan R, Taylor S 1976 The judged, not the judges: an insider's view of mental retardation. American Psychologist 31(1):47–52

Broad W, Wade N 1982 Betrayers of the truth. Simon & Schuster, New York

Chalmers A F 1976 What is this thing called science? Queensland University Press, St Lucia

Coakes S J, Steed L G 1999 SPSS for Windows. Jacaranda Wiley, Brisbane

Cohen L, Manion L 1985 Research methods in education. Croom Helm, London

Cook T D, Campbell D T 1979 Quasi-experimentation: design and analysis issues for field settings. Rand McNally, Chicago

Coppleson L, Factor R, Strums S, Graff P, Rappaport H 1970 Observer disagreement in the classification and histology of Hodgkin's disease. Journal of the National Cancer Institute 45: 731–740

Denzin N K 1978 The research act: a theoretical introduction to sociological methods, 2nd edn. Aldine, Chicago

Dooley D 1984 Social research methods. Prentice Hall, New Jersey

Engel G 1977 The need for a new medical model: a challenge for biomedicine. Science 196: 129–136

Feyerabend P 1975 Against method. Verso, London

Field P A, Morse J M 1985 Nursing research: the application of qualitative approaches. Rockville, Aspen

Flaherty G, Fitzpatrick J 1978 Relaxation technique to increase comfort level of postoperative patients: a preliminary study. Nursing Research 27(6): 352–355

Gardner H (ed.) 1989 The politics of health: the Australian experience. Churchill Livingstone, Melbourne

Glaser B G, Strauss A 1967 The discovery of grounded theory: strategies for qualitative research. Aldine, New York

Grundy S 1987 Curriculum: product or praxis. Falmer Press, East Sussex

Guba E G, Lincoln Y S 1983 Epistemological and methodological bases of naturalistic enquiry. In: Madaus G F, Scriven M, Stufflebeam D L (eds) Evaluation models. Kluwer Nishoff, Boston, pp. 311–339

Hay D, Oken D 1977 The psychological stress of intensive care unit nursing. In: Monat A, Lazarus R S (eds) Stress and coping. Columbia University Press, New York, pp. 118–131

Hersen M, Barlow D H 1976 Single case experimental designs: strategies for studying behaviour change. Pergamon, New York

Huck S W, Cormier W H, Bounds W G 1974 Reading statistics and research. Harper & Row, New York

Krzyzwoski J 1989 The historical development of electroconvulsive therapy. European Journal of Psychiatry 3(1): 49–54

Kuhn T S 1970 The structure of scientific revolutions. Chicago University Press, Chicago

Laing R D, Esterson A 1970 Sanity, madness and the family. Penguin, London

Lakatos I 1970 Falsification and the methodology of scientific research programmes. In: Lakatos I, Musgrave A (eds) Criticism and the growth of knowledge. Cambridge University Press, Cambridge pp. 91–196

Lofland J 1971 Analyzing social settings. Wadsworth, Belmont California

McGartland M, Polgar S 1994 Paradigm collapse in psychology: the necessity for a 'two methods' approach. Australian Psychologist 29(1): 21–28

Melzack R F, Wall P D 1965 Pain mechanisms: a new theory. Science 1250: 971

Merton R K 1946 The focused interview. American Journal of Sociology 51: 541–557

Minichiello V, Aroni R, Timewell E, Alexander L 1991 In depth interviewing. Longman Cheshire, Melbourne

Mogan J, Wells N, Robertson E 1985 Effects of preoperative teaching and postoperative pain: a replication and expansion. International Journal of Nursing Studies 22(3): 267–280

Rosenhan D L 1975 On being sane in insane places. In: Krupat E (ed) Psychology is social. Scott Foresman, Glenview, Illinois, pp. 189–200

Rosenthal R 1976 Experimenter effects in behavioural research. Irvington, New York

Schatzman L, Strauss A L 1973 Field research: strategies for a natural sociology. Prentice Hall, Englewood Cliffs, New Jersey

Strauss A L 1987 Qualitative analysis for social scientists. Cambridge University Press, New York

Taylor R 1979 Medicine out of control. Sun Books, Melbourne

Taylor S J, Bogdan R C 1984 Introduction to qualitative research methods: the search for personal meanings, 2nd edn. Wiley, New York

Teltscher B, Polgar S 1981 Objective knowledge about

Huntington's disease and attitudes towards predictive tests of persons at risk. Journal of Medical Genetics 18(1): 31–39

Thomas S A, Henry P, McCoy A, Smith J 1989 Why do parents stay overnight with children in hospitals? Australian Health Review 12(2): 39–49

Thomas S A, Wearing A, Bennett M 1991 Clinical decision making for nurses and health professionals. Harcourt Brace Jovanovich, Sydney

Thomas S A, Steven I, Browning C, Dickens E, Eckermann E, Carey L, Pollard S 1992 Focus groups in health research: a methodological review. Annual Review of Health Social Sciences 2: 7–20

Thomas S A, Steven I, Browning C, Dickens E, Eckermann E, Carey L, Pollard S 1993 Patient knowledge, opinions, satisfaction and choices in primary health care provision: a progress report. In: Doessel D P (ed.) The general practice evaluation program: the 1992 work-in progress conference. Australian Government Publishing Service, Canberra

Walker Q, Langlands A 1986 The nurse of mammography in the management of breast cancer. Medical Journal of Australia 1435: 185–187

FURTHER READING

Babbie E 1979 The practice of social research, 2nd edn. Wadsworth, Belmont California. *This book offers a lucid theoretical account of social research methods.*

Bailey K D 1978 Methods of social research. Free Press, New York. *This is an excellent book with a very good set of chapters on survey design and execution.*

Castle W M 1976 Statistics in small doses, 2nd edn. Churchill Livingstone, Edinburgh. *This is a good little book for extra computational examples in statistics.*

Cook T D, Campbell D T 1979 Quasi-experimentation: design and analysis issues for field settings. Rand McNally, Chicago. *Following on from Campbell's earlier book with Stanley, this text offers an excellent account of design and control issues in quasi-experimental research, with an excellent chapter on philosophy of science issues.*

Hersen M, Barlow D H 1976 Single case experimental designs: strategies for studying behaviour change. Pergamon, New York *This is a useful book for additional reading in the area of single case experimental approaches. It is, however, rather lengthy in its descriptions of the theory rather than the practicalities of carrying out such research.*

Minichiello V. Aroni R, Timewell E, Alexander L 1991 In depth interviewing. Churchill Livingstone, Melbourne. *An excellent text for qualitative researchers who use interviews in their research.*

Moser C, Kalton G 1971 Survey methods in social investigation, 2nd edn. Heinemann, London. *An excellent book on survey methods.*

Answers to questions

Chapter 1

True or false

1. T
2. F
3. T
4. T
5. T
6. T
7. F
8. F
9. F
10. F
11. F
12. T
13. T
14. T
15. F
16. T
17. T
18. F
19. T
20. F

Multiple choice

1. d
2. b
3. b
4. a
5. c
6. a
7. c
8. d
9. b
10. c
11. a
12. d
13. c
14. d
15. c
16. a

Chapter 2

True or false

1. F
2. F
3. F
4. F
5. T
6. F
7. T
8. F
9. T
10. F
11. F
12. T
13. F
14. T
15. F
16. T
17. T
18. F
19. F
20. T
21. T
22. F
23. T

24. F
25. F
26. F
27. F
28. T

Multiple choice

1. e
2. d
3. b
4. a
5. b
6. b
7. c
8. d
9. d
10. d
11. c

Chapter 3

True or false

1. T
2. F
3. T
4. T
5. T
6. F
7. F
8. F
9. F
10. F
11. F
12. F
13. F
14. T
15. F
16. F
17. T
18. T
19. T
20. F
21. F
22. T
23. F

Multiple choice

1. a
2. d
3. a
4. c
5. d
6. a
7. d
8. b
9. a
10. c
11. b
12. c
13. c

Chapter 4

True or false

1. F
2. F
3. T
4. F
5. F
6. T
7. F
8. F
9. T
10. T

Multiple choice

1. a
2. b
3. c
4. d
5. c
6. a
7. a
8. d

Chapter 5

True or false

1. T
2. T
3. F

4. F
5. F
6. F
7. T
8. F

Multiple choice

1. d
2. c
3. b
4. c
5. d
6. c
7. e
8. a
9. d
10. a
11. d
12. c
13. a
14. c
15. a
16. d
17. b
18. a
19. d
20. d

Chapter 6

True or false

1. T
2. F
3. T
4. T
5. T
6. F
7. T
8. T
9. T
10. T
11. F
12. T
13. F
14. F
15. F

16. T
17. T
18. F
19. T
20. F
21. F
22. T

Multiple choice

1. d
2. b
3. d
4. a
5. d
6. d
7. a
8. b
9. d
10. b
11. d
12. a
13. c
14. d

Chapter 7

True or false

1. F
2. T
3. F
4. F
5. F
6. T
7. F
8. T
9. F
10. T
11. F
12. F
13. T
14. T
15. F
16. T

Multiple choice

1. c

2. b
3. c
4. a
5. b
6. c
7. c
8. c
9. c
10. c

Chapter 8

True or false

1. T
2. F
3. T
4. F
5. F
6. F
7. F
8. T
9. T
10. T
11. F
12. T

Multiple choice

1. b
2. d
3. d
4. b
5. a
6. a
7. c

Chapter 9

True or false

1. F
2. T
3. F
4. F
5. F
6. F
7. F
8. T

9. F
10. T

Multiple choice

1. a
2. a
3. d
4. c
5. c
6. d
7. b
8. b
9. c

Chapter 10

True or false

1. F
2. F
3. F
4. T
5. T
6. F
7. F
8. T

Multiple choice

1. a
2. b
3. d
4. c
5. c
6. d
7. c
8. a

Chapter 11

True or false

1. T
2. F
3. T
4. T
5. F
6. F

7. T
8. F
9. F
10. T

Multiple choice

1. b
2. a
3. c
4. c
5. d
6. c
7. a
8. c

Chapter 12

True or false

1. T
2. T
3. T
4. F
5. F
6. T
7. T
8. F
9. T
10. T
11. F
12. F
13. F
14. F
15. T
16. F
17. F
18. T
19. T
20. T
21. T
22. F
23. F
24. T
25. F
26. F
27. T
28. T

29. F
30. T

Multiple choice

1. a
2. e
3. b
4. e
5. c
6. d
7. b
8. a
9. b
10. b
11. a
12. c
13. a
14. a
15. d
16. a
17. c
18. d
19. c
20. a

Chapter 13

True or false

1. T
2. F
3. T
4. T
5. F
6. T
7. F
8. F
9. F
10. F
11. T
12. T
13. T
14. F
15. T
16. T
17. F
18. T

19. F
20. F
21. F
22. F

Multiple choice

1. b
2. e
3. c
4. e
5. d
6. d
7. c
8. b
9. d
10. c
11. d
12. c
13. a
14. a
15. a
16. a
17. c
18. c
19. b
20. a
21. a
22. c
23. c
24. b
25. a
26. d
27. d
28. b
29. d

Chapter 14

True or false

1. F
2. F
3. T
4. F
5. T
6. F
7. T
8. T

9. T
10. T
11. F
12. F
13. T
14. T
15. T
16. T
17. T
18. T
19. T
20. T
21. T
22. F
23. T
24. F
25. F

Multiple choice

1. b
2. d
3. a
4. d
5. c
6. b
7. a
8. d
9. b
10. c
11. a
12. d
13. d
14. c
15. d
16. a
17. c
18. b
19. a
20. b
21. c
22. b
23. d
24. b
25. a
26. d
27. a
28. c

Chapter 15

True or false

1. T
2. F
3. F
4. F
5. T
6. T
7. F
8. F
9. T
10. F
11. F
12. F
13. T
14. F
15. T
16. F
17. T
18. T
19. F
20. T

Multiple choice

1. d
2. c
3. c
4. d
5. a
6. b
7. d
8. e
9. a
10. c
11. b
12. c
13. d
14. d
15. b
16. d
17. c
18. a
19. b
20. c
21. d
22. c

23. b
24. a
25. d

Chapter 16

True or false

1. F
2. T
3. T
4. T
5. F
6. T
7. T
8. F
9. F
10. T
11. F
12. T
13. F
14. T
15. F
16. T
17. T
18. F
19. T
20. T
21. F
22. F
23. F
24. T
25. F
26. F
27. F
28. F
29. T

Multiple choice

1. a
2. d
3. e
4. b
5. c
6. d
7. a
8. b

9. c
10. b
11. c
12. c
13. d
14. c
15. b
16. e
17. a
18. b
19. d
20. e
21. c
22. b
23. a

Chapter 17

True or false

1. F
2. T
3. F
4. T
5. F
6. T
7. T
8. F
9. T
10. T
11. F
12. T
13. T
14. F
15. F
16. T
17. T
18. F
19. F
20. T

Multiple choice

1. a
2. c
3. a
4. a
5. d
6. c

7. a
8. b
9. c
10. c
11. b
12. a
13. b
14. d
15. a
16. b
17. c
18. b
19. d
20. c
21. a
22. b
23. d
24. a
25. c
26. c
27. b
28. c
29. c
30. c
31. b
32. d
33. b
34. a
35. a

Chapter 18

True or false

1. T
2. F
3. T
4. T
5. T
6. T
7. F
8. T
9. T
10. T
11. F
12. F
13. T
14. T
15. T

16. T
17. T
18. T
19. F
20. T

Multiple choice

1. a
2. d
3. a
4. e
5. c
6. b
7. a
8. d
9. a
10. d
11. d
12. d
13. e
14. d
15. a
16. a
17. d
18. c
19. a
20. d
21. a
22. b
23. e
24. c

Chapter 19

True or false

1. T
2. F
3. F
4. T
5. F
6. T
7. F
8. T
9. T
10. F
11. T
12. T

13. T
14. T
15. F
16. T
17. T
18. T
19. T
20. F

Multiple choice

1. d
2. b
3. d
4. c
5. c
6. f
7. c
8. c
9. a
10. d
11. b
12. c
13. b
14. a
15. b
16. c
17. a
18. a
19. b
20. c
21. c
22. a
23. d
24. a
25. b
26. a
27. d
28. a
29. a
30. b
31. a

Chapter 20

True or false

1. F

2. F
3. T
4. F
5. F
6. T
7. F
8. T
9. T
10. F

Multiple choice

1. c
2. c
3. a
4. a
5. a
6. a
7. c
8. a
9. a
10. b

Chapter 21

True or false

1. F

2. T
3. T
4. F
5. F
6. T
7. F
8. T
9. T
10. T
11. F
12. T
13. F
14. F
15. F
16. T
17. T
18. F
19. F

Multiple choice

1. b
2. b
3. b
4. a
5. c
6. d

7. b
8. d
9. a
10. d

Chapter 22

True or false

1. T
2. F
3. F
4. T
5. F
6. T
7. F
8. T
9. F
10. F
11. d
12. F
13. T
14. T
15. F
16. T
17. T
18. T
19. T

Multiple choice

1. d
2. c
3. d
4. d
5. d
6. b
7. a
8. d
9. b
10. c
11. d
12. d
13. d
14. b
15. d
16. d
17. c
18. c
19. a

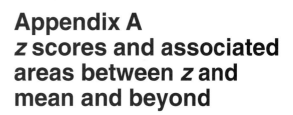

Appendix A
z scores and associated areas between *z* and mean and beyond

z	area between mean and z	area beyond z	z	area between mean and z	area beyond z	z	area between mean and z	area beyond z	z	area between mean and z	area beyond z	z	area between mean and z	area beyond z	z	area between mean and z	area beyond z
0.00	0.0000	0.5000	0.55	0.2088	0.2912	1.10	0.3643	0.1357	1.65	0.4505	0.0495	2.22	0.4868	0.0132	2.79	0.4974	0.0026
0.01	0.0040	0.4960	0.56	0.2123	0.2877	1.11	0.3665	0.1335	1.66	0.4515	0.0485	2.23	0.4871	0.0129	2.80	0.4974	0.0026
0.02	0.0080	0.4920	0.57	0.2157	0.2843	1.12	0.3686	0.1314	1.67	0.4525	0.0475	2.24	0.4875	0.0125	2.81	0.4975	0.0025
0.03	0.0120	0.4880	0.58	0.2190	0.2810	1.13	0.3708	0.1292	1.68	0.4535	0.0465	2.25	0.4878	0.0122	2.82	0.4976	0.0024
0.04	0.0160	0.4840	0.59	0.2224	0.2776	1.14	0.3729	0.1271	1.69	0.4545	0.0455	2.26	0.4881	0.0119	2.83	0.4977	0.0023
0.05	0.0199	0.4801	0.60	0.2257	0.2743	1.15	0.3749	0.1251	1.70	0.4554	0.0446	2.27	0.4884	0.0116	2.84	0.4977	0.0023
0.06	0.0239	0.4761	0.61	0.2291	0.2709	1.16	0.3770	0.1230	1.71	0.4564	0.0436	2.28	0.4887	0.0113	2.85	0.4978	0.0022
0.07	0.0279	0.4721	0.62	0.2324	0.2676	1.17	0.3790	0.1210	1.72	0.4573	0.0427	2.29	0.4890	0.0110	2.86	0.4979	0.0021
0.08	0.0319	0.4681	0.63	0.2357	0.2643	1.18	0.3810	0.1190	1.73	0.4582	0.0418	2.30	0.4893	0.0107	2.87	0.4979	0.0021
0.09	0.0359	0.4641	0.64	0.2389	0.2611	1.19	0.3830	0.1170	1.74	0.4591	0.0409	2.31	0.4896	0.0104	2.88	0.4980	0.0020
0.10	0.0398	0.4602	0.65	0.2422	0.2578	1.20	0.3849	0.1151	1.75	0.4599	0.0401	2.32	0.4898	0.0102	2.89	0.4981	0.0019
0.11	0.0438	0.4562	0.66	0.2454	0.2546	1.21	0.3869	0.1131	1.76	0.4608	0.0392	2.33	0.4901	0.0099	2.90	0.4981	0.0019
0.12	0.0478	0.4522	0.67	0.2486	0.2514	1.22	0.3888	0.1112	1.77	0.4616	0.0384	2.34	0.4904	0.0096	2.91	0.4982	0.0018
0.13	0.0517	0.4483	0.68	0.2517	0.2483	1.23	0.3907	0.1093	1.78	0.4625	0.0375	2.35	0.4906	0.0094	2.92	0.4982	0.0018
0.14	0.0557	0.4443	0.69	0.2549	0.2451	1.24	0.3925	0.1075	1.79	0.4633	0.0367	2.36	0.4909	0.0091	2.93	0.4983	0.0017
0.15	0.0596	0.4404	0.70	0.2580	0.2420	1.25	0.3944	0.1056	1.80	0.4641	0.0359	2.37	0.4911	0.0089	2.94	0.4984	0.0016
0.16	0.0636	0.4364	0.71	0.2611	0.2389	1.26	0.3962	0.1038	1.81	0.4649	0.0351	2.38	0.4913	0.0087	2.95	0.4984	0.0016
0.17	0.0675	0.4325	0.72	0.2642	0.2358	1.27	0.3980	0.1020	1.82	0.4656	0.0344	2.39	0.4916	0.0084	2.96	0.4985	0.0015
0.18	0.0714	0.4286	0.73	0.2673	0.2327	1.28	0.3997	0.1003	1.83	0.4664	0.0336	2.40	0.4918	0.0082	2.97	0.4985	0.0015
0.19	0.0753	0.4247	0.74	0.2704	0.2296	1.29	0.4015	0.0985	1.84	0.4671	0.0329	2.41	0.4920	0.0080	2.98	0.4986	0.0014
0.20	0.0793	0.4207	0.75	0.2734	0.2266	1.30	0.4032	0.0968	1.85	0.4678	0.0322	2.42	0.4922	0.0078	2.99	0.4986	0.0014
0.21	0.0832	0.4168	0.76	0.2764	0.2236	1.31	0.4049	0.0951	1.86	0.4686	0.0314	2.43	0.4925	0.0075	3.00	0.4987	0.0013
0.22	0.0871	0.4129	0.77	0.2794	0.2206	1.32	0.4066	0.0934	1.87	0.4693	0.0307	2.44	0.4927	0.0073	3.01	0.4987	0.0013
0.23	0.0910	0.4090	0.78	0.2823	0.2177	1.33	0.4082	0.0918	1.88	0.4699	0.0301	2.45	0.4929	0.0071	3.02	0.4987	0.0013
0.24	0.0948	0.4052	0.79	0.2852	0.2148	1.34	0.4099	0.0901	1.89	0.4706	0.0294	2.46	0.4931	0.0069	3.03	0.4988	0.0012
0.25	0.0987	0.4013	0.80	0.2881	0.2119	1.35	0.4115	0.0885	1.90	0.4713	0.0287	2.47	0.4932	0.0068	3.04	0.4988	0.0012
0.26	0.1026	0.3974	0.81	0.2910	0.2090	1.36	0.4131	0.0869	1.91	0.4719	0.0281	2.48	0.4934	0.0066	3.05	0.4989	0.0011
0.27	0.1064	0.3936	0.82	0.2939	0.2061	1.37	0.4147	0.0853	1.92	0.4726	0.0274	2.49	0.4936	0.0064	3.06	0.4989	0.0011
0.28	0.1103	0.3897	0.83	0.2967	0.2033	1.38	0.4162	0.0838	1.93	0.4732	0.0268	2.50	0.4938	0.0062	3.07	0.4989	0.0011
0.29	0.1141	0.3859	0.84	0.2995	0.2005	1.39	0.4177	0.0823	1.94	0.4738	0.0262	2.51	0.4940	0.0060	3.08	0.4990	0.0010
0.30	0.1179	0.3821	0.85	0.3023	0.1977	1.40	0.4192	0.0808	1.95	0.4744	0.0256	2.52	0.4941	0.0059	3.09	0.4990	0.0010
0.31	0.1217	0.3783	0.86	0.3051	0.1949	1.41	0.4207	0.0793	1.96	0.4750	0.0250	2.53	0.4943	0.0057	3.10	0.4990	0.0010
0.32	0.1255	0.3745	0.87	0.3078	0.1922	1.42	0.4222	0.0778	1.97	0.4756	0.0244	2.54	0.4945	0.0055	3.11	0.4991	0.0009
0.33	0.1293	0.3707	0.88	0.3106	0.1894	1.43	0.4236	0.0764	1.98	0.4761	0.0239	2.55	0.4946	0.0054	3.12	0.4991	0.0009
0.34	0.1331	0.3669	0.89	0.3133	0.1867	1.44	0.4251	0.0749	1.99	0.4767	0.0233	2.56	0.4948	0.0052	3.13	0.4991	0.0009
0.35	0.1368	0.3632	0.90	0.3159	0.1841	1.45	0.4265	0.0735	2.00	0.4772	0.0228	2.57	0.4949	0.0051	3.14	0.4992	0.0008
0.36	0.1406	0.3594	0.91	0.3186	0.1814	1.46	0.4279	0.0721	2.01	0.4778	0.0222	2.58	0.4951	0.0049	3.15	0.4992	0.0008
0.37	0.1443	0.3557	0.92	0.3212	0.1788	1.47	0.4292	0.0708	2.02	0.4783	0.0217	2.59	0.4952	0.0048	3.16	0.4992	0.0008
0.38	0.1480	0.3520	0.93	0.3238	0.1762	1.48	0.4306	0.0694	2.03	0.4788	0.0212	2.60	0.4953	0.0047	3.17	0.4992	0.0008
0.39	0.1517	0.3483	0.94	0.3264	0.1736	1.49	0.4319	0.0681	2.04	0.4793	0.0207	2.61	0.4955	0.0045	3.18	0.4993	0.0007

z	area between mean and z	area beyond z
0.40	0.1554	0.3446
0.41	0.1591	0.3409
0.42	0.1628	0.3372
0.43	0.1664	0.3336
0.44	0.1700	0.3300
0.45	0.1736	0.3264
0.46	0.1772	0.3228
0.47	0.1808	0.3192
0.48	0.1844	0.3156
0.49	0.1879	0.3121
0.50	0.1915	0.3085
0.51	0.1950	0.3050
0.52	0.1985	0.3015
0.53	0.2019	0.2981
0.54	0.2054	0.2946

z	area between mean and z	area beyond z
0.95	0.3289	0.1711
0.96	0.3315	0.1685
0.97	0.3340	0.1660
0.98	0.3365	0.1635
0.99	0.3389	0.1611
1.00	0.3413	0.1587
1.01	0.3438	0.1562
1.02	0.3461	0.1539
1.03	0.3485	0.1515
1.04	0.3508	0.1492
1.05	0.3531	0.1469
1.06	0.3554	0.1446
1.07	0.3577	0.1423
1.08	0.3599	0.1401
1.09	0.3621	0.1379

z	area between mean and z	area beyond z
1.50	0.4332	0.0668
1.51	0.4345	0.0655
1.52	0.4357	0.0643
1.53	0.4370	0.0630
1.54	0.4382	0.0618
1.55	0.4394	0.0606
1.56	0.4406	0.0594
1.57	0.4418	0.0582
1.58	0.4429	0.0571
1.59	0.4441	0.0559
1.60	0.4452	0.0548
1.61	0.4463	0.0537
1.62	0.4474	0.0526
1.63	0.4484	0.0516
1.64	0.4495	0.0505

z	area between mean and z	area beyond z
2.05	0.4798	0.0202
2.06	0.4803	0.0197
2.07	0.4808	0.0192
2.08	0.4812	0.0188
2.09	0.4817	0.0183
2.10	0.4821	0.0179
2.11	0.4826	0.0174
2.12	0.4830	0.0170
2.13	0.4834	0.0166
2.14	0.4838	0.0162
2.15	0.4842	0.0158
2.16	0.4846	0.0154
2.17	0.4850	0.0150
2.18	0.4854	0.0146
2.19	0.4857	0.0143
2.20	0.4861	0.0139
2.21	0.4864	0.0136

z	area between mean and z	area beyond z
2.62	0.4956	0.0044
2.63	0.4957	0.0043
2.64	0.4959	0.0041
2.65	0.4960	0.0040
2.66	0.4961	0.0039
2.67	0.4962	0.0038
2.68	0.4963	0.0037
2.69	0.4964	0.0036
2.70	0.4965	0.0035
2.71	0.4966	0.0034
2.72	0.4967	0.0033
2.73	0.4968	0.0032
2.74	0.4969	0.0031
2.75	0.4970	0.0030
2.76	0.4971	0.0029
2.77	0.4972	0.0028
2.78	0.4973	0.0027

z	area between mean and z	area beyond z
3.19	0.4993	0.0007
3.20	0.4993	0.0007
3.21	0.4993	0.0007
3.22	0.4994	0.0006
3.23	0.4994	0.0006
3.24	0.4994	0.0006
3.25	0.4994	0.0006
3.30	0.4995	0.0005
3.35	0.4996	0.0004
3.40	0.4997	0.0003
3.45	0.4997	0.0003
3.50	0.4998	0.0002
3.60	0.4998	0.0002
3.70	0.4999	0.0001
3.80	0.4999	0.0001
3.90	0.49995	0.00005
4.00	0.49997	0.00003

Appendix B
t distribution

Directional p Non-directional p	0.4 0.8	0.25 0.5	0.1 0.2	0.05 0.1	0.025 0.05	0.01 0.02	0.005 0.01	0.001 0.002
Degrees of freedom								
1	0.325	1.000	3.078	6.314	12.706	31.821	63.657	318.31
2	0.289	0.816	1.886	2.920	4.303	6.965	9.925	22.326
3	0.277	0.765	1.638	2.353	3.182	4.541	5.841	10.213
4	0.271	0.741	1.533	2.132	2.776	3.747	4.604	7.173
5	0.267	0.727	1.476	2.015	2.571	3.365	4.032	5.893
6	0.265	0.718	1.440	1.943	2.447	3.143	3.707	5.208
7	0.263	0.711	1.415	1.895	2.365	2.998	3.499	4.785
8	0.262	0.706	1.397	1.860	2.306	2.896	3.355	4.501
9	0.261	0.703	1.383	1.833	2.262	2.821	3.250	4.297
10	0.260	0.700	1.372	1.812	2.228	2.764	3.169	4.144
11	0.260	0.697	1.363	1.796	2.201	2.718	3.106	4.025
12	0.259	0.695	1.356	1.782	2.179	2.681	3.055	3.930
13	0.259	0.694	1.350	1.771	2.160	2.650	3.012	3.852
14	0.258	0.692	1.345	1.761	2.145	2.624	2.977	3.787
15	0.258	0.691	1.341	1.753	2.131	2.602	2.947	3.733
16	0.258	0.690	1.337	1.746	2.120	2.583	2.921	3.686
17	0.257	0.689	1.333	1.740	2.110	2.567	2.898	3.646
18	0.257	0.688	1.330	1.734	2.101	2.552	2.878	3.610
19	0.257	0.688	1.328	1.729	2.093	2.539	2.861	3.579
20	0.257	0.687	1.325	1.725	2.086	2.528	2.845	3.552
21	0.257	0.686	1.323	1.721	2.080	2.518	2.831	3.527
22	0.256	0.686	1.321	1.717	2.074	2.508	2.819	3.505
23	0.256	0.685	1.319	1.714	2.069	2.500	2.807	3.485
24	0.256	0.685	1.318	1.711	2.064	2.492	2.797	3.467
25	0.256	0.684	1.316	1.708	2.060	2.485	2.787	3.450
26	0.256	0.684	1.315	1.706	2.056	2.479	2.779	3.435
27	0.256	0.684	1.314	1.703	2.052	2.473	2.771	3.421
28	0.256	0.683	1.313	1.701	2.048	2.467	2.763	3.408
29	0.256	0.683	1.311	1.699	2.045	2.462	2.756	3.396
30	0.256	0.683	1.310	1.697	2.042	2.457	2.750	3.385
40	0.255	0.681	1.303	1.684	2.021	2.423	2.704	3.307
60	0.254	0.679	1.296	1.671	2.000	2.390	2.660	3.232
120	0.254	0.677	1.289	1.658	1.980	2.358	2.617	3.160
∞	0.253	0.674	1.282	1.645	1.960	2.326	2.576	3.090

Appendix C
χ^2-square

df	0.99	0.98	0.95	0.90	0.80	0.70	0.50	0.30	0.20	0.10	0.05	0.02	0.01	0.001
1	0.00016	0.00063	0.0039	0.016	0.064	0.15	0.46	1.07	1.64	2.71	3.84	5.41	6.64	10.83
2	0.02	0.04	0.10	0.21	0.45	0.71	1.39	2.41	3.22	4.60	5.99	7.82	9.21	13.82
3	0.12	0.18	0.35	0.58	1.00	1.42	2.37	3.66	4.64	6.25	7.82	9.84	11.34	16.27
4	0.30	0.43	0.71	1.06	1.65	2.20	3.36	4.88	5.99	7.78	9.49	11.67	13.28	18.46
5	0.55	0.75	1.14	1.61	2.34	3.00	4.35	6.06	7.29	9.24	11.07	13.39	15.09	20.52
6	0.87	1.13	1.64	2.20	3.07	3.83	5.35	7.23	8.56	10.64	12.59	15.03	16.81	22.46
7	1.24	1.56	2.17	2.83	3.82	4.67	6.35	8.38	9.80	12.02	14.07	16.62	18.48	24.32
8	1.65	2.03	2.73	3.49	4.59	5.53	7.34	9.52	11.03	13.36	15.51	18.17	20.09	26.12
9	2.09	2.53	3.32	4.17	5.38	6.39	8.34	10.66	12.24	14.68	16.92	19.68	21.67	27.88
10	2.56	3.06	3.94	4.86	6.18	7.27	9.34	11.78	13.44	15.99	18.31	21.16	23.21	29.59
11	3.05	3.61	4.58	5.58	6.99	8.15	10.34	12.90	14.63	17.28	19.68	22.62	24.72	31.26
12	3.57	4.18	5.23	6.30	7.81	9.03	11.34	14.01	15.81	18.55	21.03	24.05	26.22	32.91
13	4.11	4.76	5.89	7.04	8.63	9.93	12.34	15.12	16.98	19.81	22.36	25.47	27.69	34.53
14	4.66	5.37	6.57	7.79	9.47	10.82	13.34	16.22	18.15	21.06	23.68	26.87	29.14	36.12
15	5.23	5.98	7.26	8.55	10.31	11.72	14.34	17.32	19.31	22.31	25.00	28.26	30.58	37.70
16	5.81	6.61	7.96	9.31	11.15	12.62	15.34	18.42	20.46	23.54	26.30	29.63	32.00	39.29
17	6.41	7.26	8.67	10.08	12.00	13.53	16.34	19.51	21.62	24.77	27.59	31.00	33.41	40.75
18	7.02	7.91	9.39	10.86	12.86	14.44	17.34	20.60	22.76	25.99	28.87	32.35	34.80	42.31
19	7.63	8.57	10.12	11.65	13.72	15.35	18.34	21.69	23.90	27.20	30.14	33.69	36.19	43.82
20	8.26	9.24	10.85	12.44	14.58	16.27	19.34	22.78	25.04	28.41	31.41	35.02	37.57	45.32
21	8.90	9.92	11.59	13.24	15.44	17.18	20.34	23.86	26.17	29.62	32.67	36.34	38.93	46.80
22	9.54	10.60	12.34	14.04	16.31	18.10	21.34	24.94	27.30	30.81	33.92	37.66	40.29	48.27
23	10.20	11.29	13.09	14.85	17.19	19.02	22.34	26.02	28.43	32.01	35.17	38.97	41.64	49.73
24	10.86	11.99	13.85	15.66	18.06	19.94	23.34	27.10	29.55	33.20	36.42	40.27	42.98	51.18
25	11.52	12.70	14.61	16.47	18.94	20.87	24.34	28.17	30.68	34.38	37.65	41.57	44.31	52.62
26	12.20	13.41	15.38	17.29	19.82	21.79	25.34	29.25	31.80	35.56	38.88	42.86	45.64	54.05
27	12.88	14.12	16.15	18.11	20.70	22.72	26.34	30.32	32.91	36.74	40.11	44.14	46.96	55.48
28	13.56	14.85	16.93	18.94	21.59	23.65	27.34	31.39	34.03	37.92	41.34	45.42	48.28	56.89
29	14.26	15.57	17.71	19.77	22.48	24.58	28.34	32.46	35.14	39.09	42.56	46.69	49.59	58.30
30	14.95	16.31	18.49	20.60	23.36	25.51	29.34	33.53	36.25	40.26	43.77	47.96	50.89	59.70

Index